VETERINARY
ANESTHESIA
and ANALGESIA

Third Edition

VETERINARY ANESTHESIA and ANALGESIA

Diane McKelvey, BSc, DVM
Kamloops Veterinary Clinic
Kamloops, British Columbia, Canada

K. Wayne Hollingshead, MSc, DVM
Assistant Professor, Small Animal Medicine and Surgery
Animal Health Technology
The University College of the Cariboo
Kamloops, British Columbia, Canada

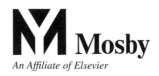

Mosby
An Affiliate of Elsevier

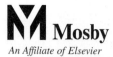
Mosby
An Affiliate of Elsevier

11830 Westline Industrial Drive
St. Louis, Missouri 63146

NOTICE

Pharmacology is an ever-changing field. Standard safety precautions must be followed, but as new research and clinical experience broaden our knowledge, changes in treatment and drug therapy may become necessary or appropriate. Readers are advised to check the most current product information provided by the manufacturer of each drug to be administered to verify the recommended dose, the method and duration of administration, and contraindications. It is the responsibility of the treating veterinarian, relying on experience and knowledge of the patient, to determine dosages and the best treatment for each individual patient. Neither the Publisher nor the editor assume any liability for any injury and/or damage to persons or property arising from this publication.

Previous editions copyrighted 1994, 2000

ISBN-13: 978-0-323-01988-0
ISBN-10: 0-323-01988-9

Publishing Director: Linda L. Duncan
Managing Editor: Teri Merchant
Project Manager: Joy Moore
Design Coordinator: Teresa Breckwoldt
Cover Art: Studio Montage
Internal Design: Top Graphics

Printed in the United States of America

Last digit is the print number: 9   8   7   6   5   4

CONTRIBUTORS

Paul Flecknell, MA, VetMB, PhD, DLAS, DiplECVA, DipECLAM, MRCVS
Comparative Biology Centre Medical School
University of Newcastle-upon-Tyne
Framlington Place
Newcastle-upon-Tyne, United Kingdom

Meghan Richey
Orlando, Oklahoma

Chuck McGrath
Orlando, Oklahoma

PREFACE

Since the publication of the second edition of *Small Animal Anesthesia and Analgesia,* the field of veterinary anesthesia has continued to evolve. New drugs and techniques have been introduced, and specialized equipment such as capnometers and blood pressure monitoring devices are increasingly available in practice.

The role of the veterinary technician in veterinary anesthesia also continues to expand, particularly in the fields of laboratory animal anesthesia, large animal anesthesia, and pain recognition and control. In an attempt to respond to this need, we have added two new chapters, Anesthesia of Rodents and Rabbits and Large Animal Anesthesia. These additions required a new title for the book, *Veterinary Anesthesia and Analgesia.* We have also expanded the chapters on anesthetic monitoring and pain control to reflect advances in these areas.

Our goal in writing this book is to support quality care, anesthetic management, and analgesia of veterinary patients. We hope that our readers find this edition helpful in achieving that goal.

Diane McKelvey
K. Wayne Hollingshead

ACKNOWLEDGMENTS

We wish to thank the many people who assisted us in preparing the third edition of this book. In particular, we thank Dr. John Ludders, who reviewed the manuscript and made many valuable suggestions. We also acknowledge with thanks the contributions of Dr. Paul Flecknell and Dr. Chuck McGrath.

We also wish to thank our editor, Teri Merchant, and the staff at Elsevier Health Science, who made the preparation of this edition a relatively smooth and painless task.

Finally, we wish to recognize the patient support that we received from our families during the long process of writing and revising this edition.

CONTENTS

VETERINARY
ANESTHESIA
and ANALGESIA

CHAPTER 1

The Preanesthetic Period

PERFORMANCE OBJECTIVES

After completion of this chapter, the reader will be able to:
- Define the term *preanesthetic period*.
- Understand the reasons for preoperative patient evaluation.
- Understand the need for obtaining a proper history, know how to take a complete history, and know what pitfalls may be encountered when taking a history.
- List the information that makes up the minimum database for a patient.
- Understand the rationale for obtaining the owner's consent for anesthesia.
- Describe the components of a proper physical examination.
- Understand the importance of species, breed, weight, and body condition as they relate to the use and choice of anesthetic drugs.
- List the five physical classifications for patients as specified by the American Society of Anesthesiologists.
- Describe the components of preanesthetic preparation, including diagnostic tests, choice of protocol, withholding food, and correction of preexisting problems.
- List the reasons why an intravenous (IV) catheter is advisable for anesthetized patients.
- Describe the types of IV fluids that can be used and why they might be chosen.
- List the preanesthetic agents in common use, the reasons for their use, their mode of action and effects on the body, and their potential adverse effects.

P*reanesthesia* is a term that describes the period immediately preceding the induction of anesthesia. Throughout the preanesthetic period and the anesthetic period that follows, the goal of the technician is to work with the veterinarian to achieve efficient, safe, and effective anesthesia with minimal stress to the patient. This chapter describes the responsibilities of the technician during the preanesthetic period.

One of the most important duties of the technician in the preanesthetic period is to help obtain patient information through history, physical examination, and diagnostic tests. This information is useful not only to the technician/anesthetist but also to the veterinarian, who must determine the patient's physical condition, identify high-risk patients before anesthesia, and select the anesthetic protocol. The technician may also be responsible for preanesthetic care of the patient, including fasting, intravenous (IV) catheterization, and other procedures ordered by the veterinarian. To prepare for anesthesia, the technician must also ensure that the necessary equipment and supplies are available and in good working order (further described in Chapter 4). Finally, the technician is usually responsible for administering preanesthetic drugs to the patient, as requested by the veterinarian, and must have a thorough knowledge of the actions and adverse effects associated with these drugs.

PATIENT EVALUATION

Technicians working as anesthetists in small animal practice soon become accustomed to the wide variety of patients they see. Animals vary in age, in temperament, and in physical appearance. Some are healthy, and some are critically ill or injured. Some are brought in for minor procedures; others will undergo complicated and lengthy operations. Given this diversity, it is unrealistic to assume that the same anesthetic techniques should be used for all patients. Furthermore, it would be dangerous to expect all patients to react to a given anesthetic agent in the same way. Before initiating anesthesia, the veterinarian and technician must gather as much information as possible on each patient to discover any factor that might lead to anesthetic complications. Accordingly, it is recommended that a minimum patient database be obtained for each patient. If the information obtained on a given animal reveals a potential problem, the veterinarian may choose to alter the planned anesthetic procedure or postpone (or even cancel) the anesthesia.

The minimum patient database should include the following (at the discretion of the veterinarian):
1. Patient history
2. The nature of the procedure to be performed with the patient under anesthesia
3. A complete physical examination
4. Diagnostic tests requested by the supervising veterinarian, which may include radiography, electrocardiography, urinalysis, hematology, clinical chemistry, and routine screening tests (for example, heartworm testing)
5. In consultation with the veterinarian, determination of the patient's physical status and anesthetic risk

Some veterinary clinics routinely recommend that animals scheduled for elective operations be brought into the clinic for an appointment before the day of surgery so that information can be gathered for the minimum patient database outlined previously. During the visit, the veterinarian may also administer necessary vaccinations, give information on preanesthetic fasting of the animal, obtain signed consent forms, and give the owner an estimate of surgery and anesthesia fees. If such an appointment is scheduled several days before the planned operation, unforeseen problems can be discovered and addressed well in advance of surgery.

Patient History

No examination of an animal is complete without an adequate history. Obtaining a thorough history requires skill and care. Like all arts, it must be continually practiced and refined. If the technician asks questions that require only a "yes" or "no" answer, the history may be incomplete or misleading. Thus asking, "Does your dog drink much water?" would not encourage the client to provide specific information. Asking, "How much water does your dog drink?" is the preferred option because it requires the owner to describe the amount of water consumed but not judge whether he or she believes the amount to be abnormal. If, for example, the client replied, "About 2 liters," the questioner would then be able to evaluate the information, perhaps deciding that 2 liters (8 cups) of water per day is excessive for a 4-kg Chihuahua, despite the owner's belief that this is normal.

Another common error is to ask leading questions of the owner. In this example, asking the question, "Your dog doesn't drink much water, does she?" would suggest to the owner that the appropriate response should be "No, I guess not." A technician asking such a question would fail to obtain an accurate patient history.

To obtain a complete history for any patient requiring anesthesia, the following questions should be asked:

1. What is the procedure to be performed on the animal?
2. How old is the animal?
3. Has the animal had any previous illnesses, and if so, what was the medical or surgical treatment? Obviously the patient's record may supplement the owner's information. A history that includes abnormalities of the heart and circulatory system, respiratory system, kidneys, liver, blood, nervous system, endocrine organs, or gastrointestinal tract may be of significance to the anesthetist and surgeon and should be brought to the attention of the veterinarian.
4. Has the animal exhibited any signs of illness in the past 24 hours, including lack of appetite, coughing, sneezing, vomiting, diarrhea, or any other condition that is of concern to the owner? When was the animal last sick or ill, and has the animal recovered from this disease as far as the owner knows? A report of recent illness should alert the veterinarian or technician to focus particular attention on the physical examination of that organ system. Animals with disease may be at increased risk of anesthetic complications because of dehydration, fever, or electrolyte abnormalities. Sick animals may also introduce pathogens into the hospital, posing a risk to other patients unless they are placed in isolation.
5. How well does the animal tolerate exercise? The owner may be able to describe the type and amount of daily exercise or play that is normal for the animal. Dyspnea or fatigue after mild exercise (such as walking up a flight of stairs) may indicate the presence of a cardiovascular or respiratory disease, which should be of concern to the anesthetist.
6. Has the animal undergone recent treatment with drugs or insecticides? Many medications, including anticonvulsants, antidepressants, antibiotics, drugs used for chemotherapy, and flea control products, may alter the effect of anesthetics. For example, tricyclic antidepressants such as amitriptyline may predispose patients to cardiac arrhythmias, especially if certain drugs (ketamine, pancuronium) are given during the anesthetic period.
7. Is there any history of allergies or drug reactions? The owner may be able to recall the animal's reaction to anesthetic agents used in the past. This information is particularly important if the animal has experienced difficulties such as prolonged recovery or personality changes after a previous anesthesia. In addition, if the animal has exhibited signs of an anaphylactic or other allergic reaction to any medication, this should be noted on the record and the information conveyed to the veterinarian.
8. When was the animal last vaccinated and against what diseases? Many veterinary clinics require current vaccinations for all healthy patients that are to be hospitalized to prevent the spread of contagious diseases among patients.

9. What is the reproductive status of the animal? Has the animal been spayed or castrated? In the case of an intact female, has the owner observed any recent estrous cycle activity? Is it possible that the animal is pregnant? These questions are of particular importance if the animal is scheduled for an ovariohysterectomy because the animal's reproductive status may affect the length and difficulty of the operation. Animals in heat also may have increased blood-clotting times because of the effect of estrogen on the clotting cascade. This may result in excessive bleeding during surgery.

10. Has the owner observed any of the following in the animal: abnormal bleeding or bruising, fainting, seizures, unexplained weakness, excessive thirst, or difficulty in passing stool or urine? If the owner answers yes to any of these questions, the veterinarian should be consulted because a serious illness may be present.

At the same time the patient history is obtained, it is advisable to give the owner a written estimate of the expected charges. It is also customary to obtain a signed release authorizing anesthesia and surgery. It is illegal in most jurisdictions to undertake surgery or anesthesia on an animal without the owner's written or oral consent. Such consent must be informed, meaning that the owner is warned beforehand of any unusual risks associated with the anesthesia or surgery. Standard consent forms (available from practice management consultants and from state and provincial veterinary associations) often state that anesthesia and surgery are never without risk. Many consent forms also include a statement giving the veterinarian permission to perform cardiopulmonary resuscitation (CPR) if the patient's condition requires it. Owners should be asked to provide a telephone number at which they may be reached during the day, in case an emergency or unforeseen complication should arise.

Consent forms may also state that some of the drugs used in anesthesia have not received approval from the Food and Drug Administration for this purpose. This is termed *extra-label* use and is common in veterinary anesthesia, particularly in dogs, cats, and exotic patients such as reptiles or birds.

Obviously a great deal of information must be exchanged before anesthesia is initiated. Ideally, the history is obtained in person by the veterinarian or technician. A trained receptionist may be able to assist, particularly when a young, healthy animal is scheduled for an elective operation such as castration or ovariohysterectomy. The hospital employee who admits a patient and speaks to the owner must not only obtain a history but also relay that information to the anesthetist by means of a written record or oral report.

In some cases it may be difficult to obtain the history in person. Some clinics prefer to have the owner fill out a prepared history form, particularly if the clinic has a high volume of patients. In any practice, difficulties may arise when an animal's owner is in a hurry and reluctant to stop and answer questions. However, it is usually possible to obtain a telephone number and call for more information at a prearranged time. Occasionally the person bringing the animal into the clinic is not the owner and is unfamiliar with the pet. In this case, every effort should be made to contact the owner by telephone to obtain a more complete history.

In a busy practice it may seem difficult to set aside adequate time to obtain a good history, and the technician may be tempted to take shortcuts or omit one or more questions. **The importance of obtaining a complete history on each animal cannot be overemphasized.** The experienced anesthetist knows that a thorough history will help avoid unpleasant surprises during anesthesia and surgery. A dog that has been coughing regularly and that tires easily when chasing a ball may have a cardiac problem unknown to the owner. If an adequate history is not taken, the heart disease may not be suspected and the technician may only become aware of the problem when the anesthetized animal suddenly shows signs of circulatory failure during the procedure.

Physical Examination

A complete physical examination should be conducted on every animal scheduled for anesthesia. Although the examination is usually carried out by a veterinarian, the technician should be familiar with the procedure. In some jurisdictions, veterinary technicians are authorized to perform basic physical examinations provided they are acting under the supervision of a licensed veterinarian.

The physical examination is important because it may reveal the following:

- *The presence of respiratory or cardiovascular disease.* These can increase the risk of anesthetic complications and even lead to death during anesthesia.
- *The presence of a disorder such as an enlarged liver or abnormally small kidneys.* Either of these may indicate a reduced ability to metabolize or excrete anesthetic agents.
- *Dehydration.* A dehydrated patient has an increased risk of problems during anesthesia.
- *Conditions requiring veterinary attention.* Some of the more common disorders that are easily detected by physical examination include ear mite infestation, otitis externa due to bacteria or yeast, dental disease, overgrown nails, the presence of fleas, and anal sac impaction. The owner is often unaware that these disorders are present and once informed of them will authorize the veterinarian to treat the animal while it is hospitalized.
- *Physical factors that may affect the procedure to be performed.* One surprisingly common example is the discovery that a cat brought in for an ovariohysterectomy is actually a male. It is far better to discover this mistake before undertaking anesthesia than to become aware of the problem during surgery. Another common example is the presentation of a cryptorchid animal for castration. The owner should be informed that the animal is a cryptorchid and that an increased fee may be charged for the operation.

It is often helpful to have the owner present during the physical examination to give pertinent history about any physical abnormalities that are found. If the technician examines the animal, any unusual findings should be brought to the attention of the veterinarian for confirmation. It is the veterinarian's responsibility to formulate an appropriate treatment plan and advise the owner and hospital staff accordingly.

The complete physical examination should include the signalment, disposition, and activity level of the animal and an examination of the organ systems.

Signalment

The signalment includes the patient's species, breed, weight, age, sex, and reproductive status. Some of this information can be obtained as part of the animal's history, but as previously mentioned, it is wise to double-check the owner's information on issues such as the animal's sex.

Species and breed. Each species has a characteristic response to specific drugs. The metabolism of many drugs differs significantly even between cats and dogs, and the recommended dose of many drugs reflects this fact (for example, the dose of morphine recommended for cats is less than that recommended for dogs). The technician, or veterinarian, may occasionally encounter an unfamiliar species, such as an iguana or parrot, and should consult specialty references and the veterinarian before administering anesthesia.

Differences in anatomy and physiology among the various breeds also may affect the animal's response to anesthetic drugs and procedures. For example, endotracheal intubation may be difficult in a brachycephalic dog such as a bulldog because of excess soft tissue in the oropharyngeal area. For the same reason, brachycephalic dogs are more likely to have breathing difficulties during anesthetic recovery. Sighthounds such as the greyhound or saluki may experience a prolonged recovery from thiobarbiturate anesthesia because of their relative absence of body fat and slow metabolism of barbiturates compared with other breeds of dogs.

Weight. Anesthetic dosages and IV fluid drip rates are calculated according to body weight. Estimating an animal's weight may lead to incorrect dosages, particularly in smaller patients. All animals should therefore be accurately weighed each time they visit the clinic. Animals lighter than 15 kg should be weighed on a pediatric scale. The patient's weight should be compared with previous weights (found in the patient's medical record) to determine whether weight gain or loss has occurred. Changes in weight may reflect changes in the patient's food intake, activity level, or overall state of health.

Age. The age of the patient can be an important consideration when deciding the anesthetic protocol or types of drugs used. The neonate (up to 2 weeks of age) or pediatric animal (2 to 8 weeks of age) is much less capable of metabolizing injectable drugs than is the adult animal because the necessary liver metabolic pathways are not fully developed. At the other end of the scale, a geriatric animal may be unable to tolerate normal doses of some drugs because of poor hepatic or renal function. The net result in either case may be a slow recovery from anesthesia, particularly when excessive doses of injectable agents are used.

Disposition and activity level

Before initiating anesthesia, the veterinary technician should observe the animal's temperament and activity level, both of which will affect the selection of anesthetic agent and the route of administration. For example, an animal that is anxious or aggressive may not become adequately sedated if a phenothiazine tranquilizer is used. In this case, combining a phenothiazine tranquilizer with an opioid or giving a more potent agent such as medetomidine may be preferable. On the other hand, geriatric or high-risk patients may be excessively sedated with a standard dose of acepromazine, and the veterinarian may choose to reduce the dose of acepromazine, give a milder agent such as diazepam, or omit sedation entirely.

Aggressive or fearful animals are occasionally scheduled for anesthesia and surgery. Special handling techniques such as anesthetic chamber inductions, oral administration of ketamine, or the use of intramuscular (IM) medetomidine or tiletamine-zolazepam may be necessary to restrain such patients without endangering hospital staff. Orally administered anesthetics are slower to take effect than injectable agents (a range of 30 to 90 minutes has been reported), and larger doses may be necessary. Oral administration of anesthetics generally constitutes extra-label use and requires the owner's informed consent.

Examination of organ systems

There are probably as many ways to perform a thorough physical examination as there are veterinarians and technicians. The examination should be done in a systematic manner (for example, from head to tail) and ideally should include all of the following:

1. *Observation of overall body condition (for example, dehydrated, emaciated, obese, weak, or pregnant).* All patients should be routinely evaluated for hydration status, which indicates if the amount of body water is normal. Table 1-1 outlines the parameters used to determine whether a patient is dehydrated, including the appearance of the skin, eyes, and oral cavity. Clinical chemistry and hematology tests may also give clues about the hydration status of an animal. If the animal appears significantly dehydrated, this should be corrected if possible before

TABLE 1-1

Evaluation of State of Hydration Using Clinical Signs

PHYSICAL FEATURE	MILD (5%) DEHYDRATION	MODERATE (6%-9%) DEHYDRATION	PROFOUND (10%-12%) DEHYDRATION
Eyelid pinch	Mild tenting; pinch slowly relaxes	Severe tenting; pinch persists	Severe tenting; pinch persists
Cornea	Cornea moist; tearing still possible	Cornea drier and tearing is infrequent	Dry cornea and no tearing
Position of eyeball in orbit	Minimal (1-2 mm) space between medial canthus and globe	Pronounced space (2-4 mm) between medial canthus	A space of more than 4 mm between medial canthus and globe
Skin of neck	Decreased pliability	Tented skin persists 3-5 seconds	Tented skin persists more than 5 seconds
Oral mucous membranes	Moist, warm, and pink	Warm, sticky, and pale	Dry mucous membranes; cold, cyanotic or very pale; poor capillary perfusion
General condition	Standing; extremities are warm	Often recumbent	Often mentally depressed; extremities are cold; weak rapid pulse
Lab findings	Normal	Increased PCV and total protein, decreased urine volume	Increased PCV and total protein, decreased urine volume

Modified from *Veterinary teaching hospital manual*, Guelph, Ontario, Canada, 1992, Ontario Veterinary College.

anesthesia, because dehydration may impair blood circulation within the tissues, leading to increased anesthetic risk. Fluid therapy is further discussed on p. 21.

Obesity is commonly observed in companion animals scheduled for anesthesia, and this condition poses some difficulties for the anesthetist. Obese animals may have reduced exercise tolerance and may show signs of dyspnea at rest, indicating inadequate cardiovascular and respiratory function. Venipuncture, auscultation, and assessment of hydration may be difficult in these animals. When obese animals are anesthetized, injectable drug dosages should be calculated according to the animal's ideal weight (however difficult this is to imagine) rather than the actual weight. Although the animal's size is increased by the deposition of fat stores, the size of the target organ of anesthesia (that is, the brain) is unaffected.

Excessive thinness is also of concern to the anesthetist because it may indicate the presence of an underlying disorder such as hyperthyroidism or chronic parasitism. Animals with little body fat may be unusually sensitive to the effects of some anesthetics and also are prone to hypothermia.

2. *Measurement of body temperature.* The normal temperature range in the cat is 37.8° to 39.2° C (100.0° to 102.5° F). The normal range in the dog is 37.5° to 39.2° C (99.5° to 102.5° F). The veterinarian should be informed if the patient's temperature is outside the normal range.

3. *Examination of the head, including eyes, oral cavity, pharynx, ears, and nose.* The technician should observe the animal for wheezing or noisy respirations, which may indicate that the airway is partially obstructed. Any disorder that could impede endotracheal intubation, such as the presence of redundant tissue in the oropharynx or difficulty in opening the mouth, should be noted. If the mouth cannot be opened (for example, if severe myositis is present), normal endotracheal procedures are difficult, and it may be necessary to use an alternate means of intubation (such as the use of a stylet or intubation through a tracheotomy incision). The gingivae should be observed for mucous membrane color and capillary refill time (CRT, see p. 77). If the gingivae are pigmented, mucous membrane color and CRT may be observed at other sites, such as the conjunctiva of the lower eyelid, the entrance to the vulva, or the tip of the prepuce.

4. *Observation of the pupillary light reflex and consensual light reflex* (Fig. 1-1). The pupillary light reflex is elicited by shining a beam of light (usually from a penlight or other portable light source) into one eye and noting whether the pupil of that eye constricts in response (direct reflex). Pupil constriction (miosis) is the normal response; failure to constrict or dilation of the pupil (mydriasis) in the presence of light is abnormal. At the same time, change in pupil size should be observed in the other eye (consensual reflex). Again, miosis is the expected response. In healthy animals the pupils are initially the same size and demonstrate both a direct and a consensual light reflex in each eye, although this reflex may be altered in excited animals or after the administration of some preanesthetic and anesthetic drugs.

5. *Auscultation of the heart and lungs.* Auscultation of the chest is performed to determine the heart rate and rhythm and to check for the presence of abnormal heart or lung sounds. Auscultation of the lungs is best performed by listening to at least four different areas of the chest (called *quadrants*), including the right

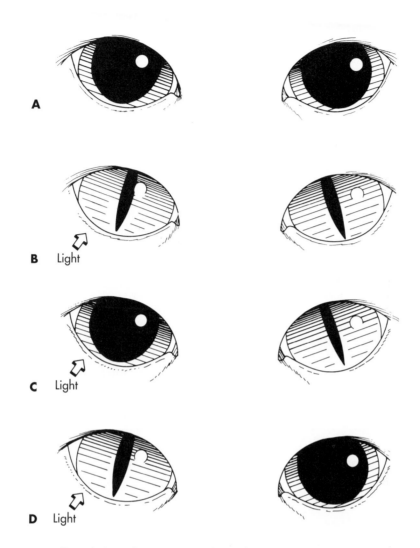

FIG. 1-1 Pupillary light reflex. A, Normal pupils. B, Direct and consensual light reflex (normal). C, Consensual but no direct light reflex (abnormal). D, Direct but no consensual light reflex (abnormal).

and left anteroventral lung fields and the right and left dorsal lung fields. Auscultation of the heart should also be performed on both the left and right sides of the chest. Evaluate each of the four valves of the heart: the pulmonic, aortic, and mitral valves on the left side of the chest and the tricuspid valve on the right side of the chest. Heart murmurs in cats are sometimes most easily heard next to the sternum.

The normal range of heart rates for dogs is 60 to 180 beats per minute (bpm), with pediatric patients and smaller breeds tending to have rates more rapid than those of larger breeds. The heart rate in giant breeds should be less than 100 bpm. The normal range of heart rates for cats is 110 to 220 bpm. The rhythm in both dogs and cats should be reasonably regular (called *sinus rhythm*), although it is common for the heart rate to increase slightly during inspiration (called *sinus arrhythmia*). Sinus arrhythmia is more commonly found in the dog than in the cat.

Exercise or the stress of handling may cause the heart rate to increase. The heart rate should be measured on a calm animal and, if possible, not immediately after inserting a rectal thermometer or collecting a blood sample. The heart rate should be checked repeatedly, particularly after premedication, and before and immediately after induction.

6. *Palpation of the pulse and comparison of pulse rate and heart rate.* For the dog and cat, the pulse is most easily palpated at the femoral artery, on the medial side of the rear leg. Other sites that may be palpated include the metatarsal and metacarpal arteries (Fig. 1-2). Palpation of the pulse gives some indication of blood pressure: a weak or absent pulse may indicate hypotension (low blood pressure), whereas a bounding pulse may indicate hypertension (high blood pressure). The heart rate should be compared with the pulse rate. If the heart rate exceeds the pulse rate, a pulse deficit exists, which may indicate the presence of cardiovascular disease.

7. *Determination of respiratory rate and observation for dyspnea.* The normal respiratory rate for dogs is 10 to 30 breaths per minute, and for cats it is 25 to 40 breaths per minute. Animals experiencing dyspnea (that is, difficult or labored breathing) may exhibit signs such as mouth breathing, flared nostrils, excessive panting, exaggerated chest or abdominal movements on inspiration, wheezing, and reluctance to lie down. In extreme cases, an animal with breathing difficulty may exhibit cyanosis (that is, mucous membranes that appear purple or

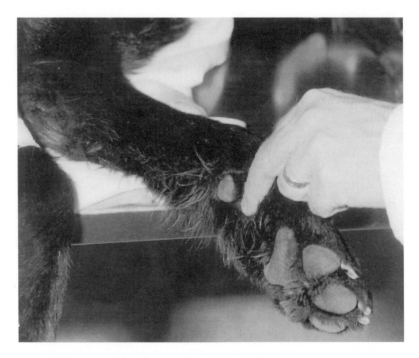

FIG. 1-2   Palpation of the metatarsal/metacarpal artery.

blue). Any animal showing signs of dyspnea should be brought to the veterinarian's attention immediately. Dyspnea must be differentiated from normal rapid breathing (tachypnea) or panting.

8. *Examination of the thorax, abdomen, and limbs* to note the condition of hair coat and presence of parasites or any cutaneous lesions. Although examination of the skin is seldom relevant to the anesthesia itself, it may indicate the presence of a disorder requiring treatment.

9. *Observation for lameness or localized pain in the extremities.*

10. *Palpation of superficial lymph nodes.* Enlarged lymph nodes may indicate the presence of inflammation or neoplasia, both of which would be of concern to the anesthetist and surgeon.

11. *Abdominal palpation* for pain, organ size, and location and the presence of fluid, gas, fetuses, or feces.

12. *Observation of mammary glands* for signs of lactation or lumps, particularly if the animal is an unspayed female. The vulva should also be observed for indications of estrus or the presence of a discharge.

Diagnostic Tests

After the history and physical examination are completed, the veterinarian decides which diagnostic tests (if any) are recommended for a given patient. The technician's responsibilities include obtaining blood and urine samples and either performing the tests or forwarding the samples to a diagnostic laboratory. All test results should be reviewed by the veterinarian.

There are no universal guidelines for preanesthetic diagnostic tests. Depending on the clinic policy, certain tests may be routinely performed on every animal scheduled for anesthesia. The veterinarian may request additional tests on the basis of the patient's age, history, and the results of the physical examination. Economic considerations may limit the number and type of tests approved by the client.

Preoperative diagnostic tests and procedures that provide information of particular interest to the anesthetist and supervising veterinarian include the complete blood count, urinalysis, blood chemistries, blood clotting tests, electrocardiogram, and radiographs.

Complete blood cell count

One commonly requested preanesthetic test is a complete blood cell count (CBC). The CBC includes the determination of packed cell volume (PCV), hemoglobin (Hb), and total plasma protein (TPP) and the evaluation of a blood smear for white blood cell, red blood cell, and platelet abnormalities. Normal values for these parameters in the dog and cat are given in Table 1-2. Some variation may be expected depending on age, breed, and geographic location.

The information obtained from the PCV and Hb indicates the ability of the blood to deliver oxygen to the tissues. A PCV above normal limits suggests that the relative amount of red blood cells has increased. This is most often a result of fluid loss leading to dehydration. An elevated PCV is of concern to the anesthetist because hemoconcentration and increased blood viscosity will be present. These in turn lead to poor tissue perfusion and a reduction in cardiac output. On the other hand, a PCV below the normal range may indicate anemia caused by blood loss,

TABLE 1-2

Normal Values for Selected Parameters in Dogs and Cats

PARAMETER	CANINE	FELINE
Heart rate (bpm)	60-180	110-220
Temperature	99.5°-102.5° F	100.0°-102.5° F
	37.5°-39.2° C	37.8°-39.2° C
Respiratory rate (bpm)	10-30	25-40
Hb (g/dl)	14-18	9-16
TPP (g/dl)	5.7-7.8	6.3-8.3
PCV (%)	35-54	29-45
Total leucocyte ($\times$ 10^9/L)	6.0-18	6.0-20
Pao$_2$ (mm Hg)	91-97	91-115
Paco$_2$ (mm Hg)	30-43	28-43
Arterial pH	7.36-7.46	7.34-7.43

Modified from Muir WW III, Hubbell JAE: *Handbook of veterinary anesthesia*, St Louis, 1989, Mosby.

hemolysis, or failure to produce adequate numbers of red blood cells. The net result in each case is a decreased capacity to supply oxygen to the tissues. A PCV less than 25% in the dog or cat indicates that tissue oxygenation may be inadequate, especially for the heart, and the veterinarian may recommend that anesthesia should be postponed until the anemia is corrected.

The TPP value is also of interest to the anesthetist. An increase in TPP, similar to an increase in PCV, may indicate dehydration. A decreased TPP usually indicates hypoproteinemia, which may be a result of renal, hepatic, or gastrointestinal disease. Alterations in TPP are particularly significant to the anesthetist because they indicate that the patient's response to anesthetic drugs may be altered. Many anesthetic agents are distributed in the blood such that a portion circulates freely and another portion is bound to plasma proteins. Only the portion of the drug that is free and unbound to plasma proteins can affect the drug receptors. In the patient with hypoproteinemia, a decreased proportion of drug is bound to plasma proteins. This results in an increased proportion of unbound drug and, consequently, increased drug potency for that particular patient.

The CBC should also include a differential white blood cell count and an examination of white blood cells, which may indicate that the animal is undergoing severe infection or stress. Such conditions may be exacerbated by anesthesia and surgery and also increase anesthetic risk.

Urinalysis

The results of a urinalysis (particularly the urine specific gravity) provide information about kidney and hormonal function. If a urine sample has a low specific gravity (less than 1.025 in a canine sample or less than 1.035 in a feline sample), the veterinarian should be notified because further tests may be needed. Urine dipstick results are also useful, allowing rapid screening for conditions such as diabetes mellitus and urinary tract infection. The interpretation of urinalysis results may be aided by microscopic examination of urine and by blood chemistry results such as blood urea nitrogen (BUN).

Blood chemistry

Some patients scheduled for anesthesia may be known or suspected to have renal, hepatic, endocrine, or other disease. In many cases the degree of organ dysfunction can be determined through appropriate biochemical tests. The most common of these include tests for alanine aminotransferase (ALT), alkaline phosphatase (AP), BUN, creatinine, blood glucose, and serum electrolytes such as sodium, chloride, and potassium. Interpretation of test results requires specialized knowledge of disease and is therefore the responsibility of the veterinarian.

Blood clotting tests

Blood clotting tests usually are performed only on animals with suspected coagulation disorders or animals of breeds known to be commonly affected by von Willebrand's disease (such as the Doberman pinscher and Scottish terrier). A toenail cuticle or buccal bleeding time gives a rough estimate of blood clotting ability and can be easily performed on any anesthetized animal. For a toenail cuticle bleeding time to be performed, the nail is cut slightly short with a pair of nail trimmers so that the quick is entered and a small amount of bleeding results. The nail is allowed to bleed without any effort to wipe away accumulated blood. In a healthy animal, bleeding should stop within 4 minutes. The buccal bleeding time is performed by nicking the tissue on the inside of the cheek with a small lancet. As with the toenail bleeding time, bleeding should stop within 4 minutes. One can also put whole blood in a plain "red top" tube and observe for clotting, which normally occurs within a few minutes. More precise evaluation of hemostasis can be obtained through the use of more sophisticated tests such as partial prothrombin time (PPT) and platelet counts. A patient with reduced ability to clot blood will require special handling by the anesthetist and the surgeon because hemorrhage during surgery may result in prolonged recovery, shock, or death.

Electrocardiogram

The electrocardiogram (ECG) monitors the electrical activity of the heart muscle, allowing the veterinarian to assess the pattern and rhythm of the myocardial contractions. Abnormalities in the size, duration, shape, and rhythm of the ECG tracing provide useful information about cardiac function. An ECG is not routinely done on every patient before anesthesia but is usually recommended for those patients with known or suspected heart disease, chest trauma, or electrolyte disturbances such as hyperkalemia (abnormally high potassium concentration in the blood). The ECG also can be used to screen for cardiac disease before anesthetics are given to higher-risk animals, such as geriatric patients. The ECG assists the veterinarian in determining the presence of cardiac dysfunction and evaluating the risk of anesthesia for a particular patient. Electrocardiograms are further discussed in Chapter 2.

Radiography

Because of economic considerations, chest radiographs are not routinely obtained for every patient scheduled to receive a general anesthetic. Radiography may be warranted in animals that show signs of dyspnea or those in which abnormal heart or lung sounds are detected during the physical examination. It is also advisable that animals that have had major trauma (such as being hit by a car) undergo chest radiographs before any surgery, including fracture repair. This will alert the veterinarian to the presence of pneumothorax, pleural effusion, pulmonary trauma, or diaphragmatic hernia before making the decision to anesthetize the patient.

Patients must not be stressed during radiography procedures, particularly if dyspnea is present. In some cases the patient may be less uncomfortable or anxious if radiographed in the standing position, instead of being placed in lateral or dorsal recumbency. Oxygen delivery by mask or nasal cannula will often reduce dyspnea and increase patient safety during radiography and other procedures.

Miscellaneous tests

Depending on the geographic location of the practice, other diagnostic tests may be routinely performed before anesthesia. For example, veterinary practices in some areas require a heartworm test for all canine patients before anesthesia.

Classification of Patient Status

The veterinarian should evaluate the patient's minimum database (that is, physical examination, history, and results of diagnostic tests) and assign a status to the patient before the anesthetic protocol is chosen and the anesthesia is initiated. The most widely accepted classification system is the one proposed by the American Society of Anesthesiologists (ASA). It is summarized in Table 1-3. In general, class I and class II patients can be safely anesthetized with standard protocols and techniques. Patients with class III or higher physical status should be stabilized before surgery, if possible, and special techniques and anesthetic protocols may be advisable.

Classification of risk is subject to personal interpretation. Two anesthetists might disagree, for example, on whether a particular animal should be assigned to class II (slight risk) or class III (moderate risk). Whatever the preoperative status assigned to an animal, it should be recorded in the animal's hospital record and in the anesthetic logbook. The anesthetist should also recognize that a patient's ASA status may change. For example, patients that receive appropriate therapy such as IV fluids before surgery may have their ASA classification changed to a lower-risk category. On the other hand, a patient whose condition is deteriorating may be changed to a higher-risk category.

The technician acting as anesthetist should not hesitate to discuss abnormal findings from the minimum database with the veterinarian because such information may lead to changes in the planned anesthetic protocol. The presence of organ dysfunction in an animal does not necessarily require that anesthesia be postponed or canceled, although this may be the wisest course in some situations. Often anesthesia may be successfully achieved by selecting the agents that are least likely to have adverse effects on the animal. For example, if the physical examination and diagnostic tests suggest that heart disease is present in a 13-year-old dog scheduled for a dental procedure, the veterinarian may choose to use isoflurane instead of halothane because isoflurane is less likely to induce potentially dangerous cardiac arrhythmias.

If the patient is very ill, the veterinarian may decide that the animal's condition must be stabilized before an anesthetic is administered. Patients that are severely

TABLE 1-3

Classification of Patient Physical Status

CATEGORY	PHYSICAL CONDITION	EXAMPLES OF CLINICAL SITUATIONS
CLASS I Minimal risk	Normal healthy animal No underlying disease	Ovariohysterectomy, castration, declawing operation, hip dysplasia radiograph
CLASS II Slight risk, minor disease is present	Animals with slight to mild systemic disturbances Animal able to compensate	Neonate or geriatric animals, obesity, skin tumor, uncomplicated hernia, local infection
CLASS III Moderate risk, obvious disease is present	Animals with moderate systemic disease or disturbances Mild clinical signs	Anemia, moderate dehydration, fever, low-grade heart murmur or cardiac disease
CLASS IV High risk, significantly compromised by disease	Animals with preexisting systemic disease or disturbances of a severe nature	Severe dehydration, shock, uremia, or toxemia, high fever, uncompensated heart disease, diabetes, pulmonary disease, emaciation
CLASS V Extreme risk, moribund	Surgery often performed in desperation on animals with life-threatening systemic disease or disturbances not often correctable by an operation; includes all moribund animals not expected to survive 24 hours	Advanced cases of heart, kidney, liver, lung, or endocrine disease; profound shock; major head injury; severe trauma; pulmonary embolus; terminal malignancy

dehydrated, are profoundly anemic, or have a serious systemic disease or electrolyte imbalance are poor anesthetic risks, and every attempt should be made to correct the condition before anesthesia, if time allows. If the planned procedure is not immediately necessary to save the patient's life and the patient's condition may be improved by nursing care, it is likely that anesthesia can be safely postponed.

SELECTION OF THE ANESTHETIC PROTOCOL
Factors That Influence Selection

In all jurisdictions in the United States and Canada, it is the veterinarian, rather than the veterinary technician, who chooses (that is, prescribes) the anesthetic drugs for a given patient. The veterinarian also chooses the dose and the route of administration of each agent. In most hospitals the veterinarian establishes one or two standard anesthetic protocols to be used for routine operations on healthy patients. However, the standard protocol must be evaluated for its suitability for each individual patient, and changes should be made to the protocol when necessary for the safety of the patient. The technician who has a good understanding of anesthetic principles and who demonstrates sincere interest in patient care and monitoring can communicate valuable observations and suggestions to the veterinarian. Nevertheless, the supervising veterinarian has the ultimate responsibility for the patient's safety and must make the final decision regarding the anesthetic protocol.

The patient's physical status is not the only factor that determines the anesthetic protocol to be used. Other factors that affect the veterinarian's decision include the following.

Availability of facilities and equipment

Some anesthetic techniques require the use of specialized equipment. For example, halothane and isoflurane anesthesia require the use of a vaporizer designed for use with a volatile liquid anesthetic and an oxygen supply. This is somewhat impractical for equine field anesthesia, so injectable drugs are used.

Familiarity with the agent

For most patients, any one of several anesthetic procedures is likely to result in successful and safe anesthesia, and it is reasonable to use the method with which the anesthetist is most familiar, provided patient safety is ensured. It is seldom beneficial to anesthetize a critically ill patient with a new combination of drugs that the anesthetist may have heard or read about but never tried before.

Nature of the procedure requiring anesthesia

Procedures vary in their anticipated duration and in the amount of analgesia (pain relief) and restraint required. For example, local anesthesia may be suitable for short procedures in which the patient requires only minimal restraint. On the other hand, patients that are to undergo thoracic or abdominal surgery require general anesthesia and provision of adequate pain control.

Special patient circumstances

Anesthetics that may be appropriate for animals undergoing a routine operation (such as ovariohysterectomy or castration) may not be the first choice for every surgical procedure. For example, the choice of anesthetic for a cesarean section is partially determined by the need to avoid agents that may cause respiratory depression in the newborn puppy or kitten. Anesthetic protocols may also be altered depending on the temperament of the patient (for example, docile, fearful, excited, or aggressive).

Cost

Anesthetic agents vary in cost. In a situation in which two agents are of equal value from the standpoint of patient safety, it is reasonable to choose the less expensive option.

Speed

Critically injured animals may require rapid induction of anesthesia to initiate emergency therapy. For example, a patient that is in danger of shock because of ongoing, uncontrolled hemorrhage cannot wait for a premedication given subcutaneously (SC) or IM that needs 15 to 20 minutes to take effect. A combination of minimal sedation and a rapid induction agent is desirable in this case.

PREANESTHETIC PATIENT CARE

During the preanesthetic period the technician should ensure that the patient receives appropriate nursing care, including fasting, IV catheterization, and any other procedures requested by the veterinarian. The technician must also ensure that each patient is clearly identified, usually by means of a card attached to its cage or an identification band placed around the animal's neck. All diagnostic procedures and treatments should be recorded in the medical record. A checklist of procedures may be helpful, particularly if more than one person is responsible for preanesthetic care.

Withholding Food Before Anesthesia

Animals that are anesthetized without prior fasting may vomit or regurgitate stomach contents during anesthesia or during the recovery period. This may cause esophageal irritation. Even more seriously, vomitus in the airway may be aspirated into the trachea, bronchi, and lung alveoli. If the vomitus blocks the airways, immediate respiratory arrest may result. An animal that survives the initial episode may develop aspiration pneumonia several days after the incident.

To prevent vomiting during the anesthetic period, food should be withheld from adult dogs and cats for 8 hours before anesthesia. Some veterinarians also suggest that water should be withheld for 2 hours before anesthesia. Birds, pocket pets such as hamsters and guinea pigs, and dogs and cats younger than 3 months should be fasted for a shorter period or not at all because of their tendency to develop hypoglycemia. The technician must ensure that dehydrated animals receive adequate IV fluids to prevent further dehydration when water is withheld.

If a patient is known to have eaten within 12 hours of the proposed surgery and the surgery cannot be postponed, the veterinarian may choose to administer a preanesthetic that is likely to cause vomiting in the unfasted patient (for example, xylazine in cats or morphine in dogs).

Despite every precaution, vomiting may occur during the anesthetic or recovery period. Possible explanations for vomiting in an animal that was supposedly fasted include individual patient variation and owner noncompliance. If vomiting occurs in the anesthetized patient, there is some protection against aspiration and airway blockage if a cuffed endotracheal tube is in place. This is the reason why the endotracheal tube is usually left in place until the animal regains the swallowing reflex during recovery. Vomiting during anesthesia is discussed further in Chapter 6.

Animals undergoing gastrointestinal procedures may require special feeding and care to minimize the amount of digestive material within the gastrointestinal tract at the time of surgery. If a surgical procedure involving the stomach or intestine is planned, food is generally withheld for 24 hours, and water is withheld for 8 to 12 hours before anesthesia. If endoscopy or surgery of the colon is planned, it may be advisable to administer enemas or cathartic agents before the procedure.

The anesthetist should be aware that although preanesthetic fasting is recommended, prolonged fasting might be detrimental to the animal. Many seriously ill animals are anorexic and may refuse to eat for several days before and after anesthesia. For example, a dog that has been hit by a car may arrive at the veterinary clinic with a fractured femur and pneumothorax. The veterinarian may elect to postpone fracture repair for several days to allow the pneumothorax to resolve. The animal may be too uncomfortable, too frightened, or too weak to eat throughout this period. By the time the operation is performed, the animal may have gone without eating for more than 4 days. This may be harmful to the animal because lack of nutrition impedes the healing process and prolongs recovery. Efforts should be made to reestablish caloric intake in the anorexic animal by hand-feeding palatable foods, syringe bolus feeding, the use of feeding tubes, or total parenteral nutrition.

Correction of Preexisting Problems

Animals scheduled for anesthesia sometimes have systemic disorders such as dehydration, anemia, respiratory distress, shock, and hypothermia. As already mentioned, these patients are at increased anesthetic risk, and in the interest of patient safety, it may be best to postpone anesthesia to allow time for appropriate nursing care. In some cases (for example, a patient with a gastric torsion or uncontrolled internal bleeding) the veterinarian may decide that the risk of delaying surgery outweighs the increased anesthetic risk and will elect to proceed with anesthesia. These patients may pose the greatest challenge to the technician's skills as an anesthetist and as an intensive care nurse.

Intravenous Catheterization
Reasons for catheterization

Not all animals are catheterized before anesthesia; however, the presence of an IV catheter is of potential benefit to both the patient and the anesthetist. Reasons for catheterization include the following:

1. IV catheterization allows the administration of balanced electrolyte solutions or saline during surgery. Fluid administration helps to maintain blood volume and support blood pressure in the anesthetized patient. It is not mandatory for routine operations in healthy animals but is highly recommended. Fluid administration is particularly important for the following:
   - Animals undergoing any operation that may result in significant blood loss, including cesarean sections
   - Animals that are debilitated or dehydrated because of renal, gastrointestinal, metabolic, or other systemic disease
   - Animals with electrolyte abnormalities (for example, hyperkalemia)
   - Animals undergoing prolonged anesthesia (more than 1 hour)
   - Animals that are at risk of hypotension (low blood pressure) or shock. Even mild hypotension is a potential problem in anesthetized animals because it leads to decreased blood flow to the kidneys and other vital organs.
2. IV or butterfly catheters allow the rapid and easy administration of emergency drugs such as epinephrine. They are useful not only during the anesthetic period itself, but also during the recovery period, when treatment of complications such as respiratory obstruction or seizures may require intravenous access.

3. Some animals require a constant infusion of anesthetics, analgesics, electrolytes, or drugs such as insulin during anesthesia. These animals are usually catheterized, and the drug is administered through a syringe pump or mixed with IV fluids. One example of constant infusion of anesthetic is the use of propofol to maintain anesthesia in a patient undergoing bronchoscopy. The drug is given intravenously by repeated injection or constant infusion, in amounts adequate to maintain unconsciousness. In these animals, use of an IV catheter is preferable to needle and syringe because the accidental manipulation of a needle and syringe can lead to perivascular drug injection or inadvertent administration of excessive amounts of drug.

4. IV catheters are a convenient way to administer anesthetic agents that can be irritating if injected perivascularly, such as thiopental. IV catheters also allow concurrent injection of incompatible drugs (such as diazepam and oxymorphone) through the use of separate syringes and a catheter adapter.

Types of intravenous catheters

Two types of IV catheters are used in veterinary medicine: through the needle (used for long-term fluid administration, especially through the jugular vein) and over the needle. In the latter type, a plastic catheter is inserted into a vein with a long thin needle called a *stylet*. Once the vein is entered, the catheter is advanced and the inner stylet is withdrawn and discarded (Fig. 1-3). Typically, 18- to 22-gauge, 1- to 2-inch catheters are used in small animal anesthesia, and 12- to 16-gauge, 5¼-inch catheters are used in cattle and horses.

Risks of catheterization

There are several potential complications associated with the administration of fluids and drugs through an IV catheter. These include the following:

- *The introduction of air.* This should be avoided, although significant air embolism is unlikely if a peripheral vein is used.
- *Broken catheter tip.* Do not repeatedly advance and withdraw the catheter over the stylet. This can break off the catheter tip, creating a catheter embolus.
- *Accidental overhydration.* If fluid administration is too rapid, the volume of fluid entering the animal may overwhelm the circulation and cause problems such as pulmonary edema or cerebral edema. Animals weighing less than 5 kg and those with cardiac or renal disease are at greatest risk. Fluid bags should be labeled with the patient's name and the starting fluid level indicated by tape or a marker to avoid overhydration. The use of a burette (Fig. 1-4) or microdrip/pediatric drip set is advisable in small patients because it allows accurate measurement and administration of small volumes of fluids rather than direct administration from a bag or bottle.

   When monitoring any anesthetized patient that is receiving IV fluids, especially those with cardiac or renal insufficiency, the anesthetist should be alert for signs of overhydration. These include ocular and nasal discharge, chemosis (edema and swelling of the conjunctiva), SC edema, increased lung sounds, increased respiratory rate, and dyspnea. In the awake animal, coughing and restlessness may be seen. Measurement of central venous pressure (see p. 88) allows early detection of overhydration.

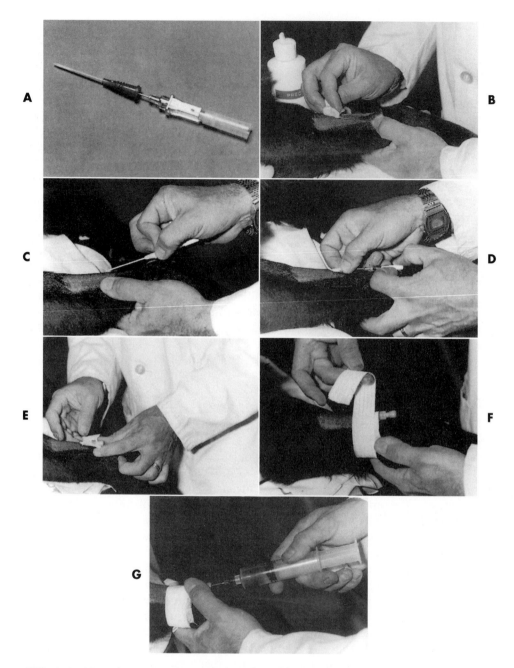

FIG. 1-3 Use of an intravenous (IV) catheter for injection of a barbiturate. A, IV catheter showing metal stylet used for placement of catheter in vein. B, Surgical preparation of cephalic vein. C, Insertion of catheter into vein. D, Catheter is advanced over stylet. E and F, Taping of catheter in place. G, Injection of drug into catheter cap.

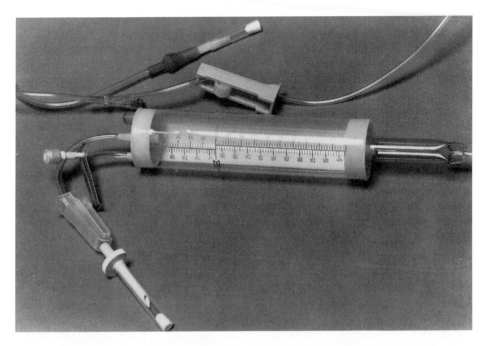

FIG. 1-4   Burette.

- *Catheter-induced sepsis.* Careful antiseptic technique helps reduce the risk of bacteria colonizing the catheter site. This includes wiping the injection port with 70% isopropyl alcohol before giving an injection through the catheter and using an antibiotic ointment at the catheter placement site.
- *Overrapid administration of drugs.* Most drugs are best given by slow IV injection, over a period of 15 to 60 seconds. It is helpful to pause between each bolus and allow several milliliters of fluid to run through the line.

Fluid administration rates

The rate of fluid administration varies depending on the patient and the procedure. The following guidelines may be useful.

Maintenance fluids. Daily maintenance fluids are commonly given to hospitalized patients at a rate of 2 ml/kg/hr (large dogs) to 4 ml/kg/hr (small dogs/cats).

Fluids given during anesthesia. During anesthesia, fluids can be administered from an IV bag, with an administration set that delivers 10 or 15 drips per milliliter if the patient weighs more than 10 kg and an administration set that delivers 60 drips per milliliter if the patient weighs less than 10 kg. If prolonged or accurate administration is required, it is helpful to use an automated constant rate infusion device (Fig. 1-5). Anesthetic drugs, analgesics, and emergency drugs can also be continuously infused with these devices.

A fluid infusion rate of 5 to 10 ml/kg/hr is the standard fluid administration rate during routine anesthesia and surgery and is safe for almost all patients. This rate is significantly higher than the maintenance requirement and is intended to compensate for the vasodilation and increase in insensible fluid loss that can occur during anesthesia.

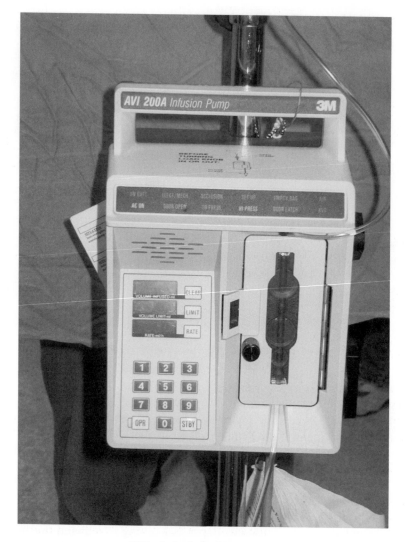

FIG. 1-5   Infusion pump.

Animals with cardiovascular or respiratory disease are at increased risk of overhydration, and a slower infusion rate during surgery (for example, 5 ml/kg/hr) is advisable.

Some patients benefit from more rapid administration rates, particularly if bleeding or decreased blood pressure is encountered during surgery. Healthy young dogs tolerate an infusion rate of 40 ml/kg for 1 hour, with half of this given over the first 15 minutes if hypotension is present. Cats are more susceptible to overhydration than dogs, and for this reason the fluid infusion rate should not exceed 20 ml/kg/hr unless the cat is in shock. If excessive blood loss occurs, the anesthetist should ensure that 3 ml of fluids are given for every 1 ml of blood lost. If a blood transfusion is given, the amount of blood given should approximately equal the amount of blood lost.

Fluid therapy for animals in shock. Fluids are given at rapid flow rates when treating shock (for example, up to 90 ml/kg for the first hour in dogs and 50 ml/kg

TABLE 1-4								
Composition of Intravenous Fluids and Plasma								
			mEq/LITER					
SOLUTION	pH	CARBOHYDRATE	Na$^+$	K$^+$	Ca$^+$	Mg^{+2}	Cl$^-$	HCO$_3^-$
Plasma	7.5	100 mg/dl	144	5	5	1.5	107	27
0.9% NaCl	5.4	None	154	0	0	0	154	0
5% Dextrose	5.0	5 gm/dl	0	0	0	0	0	0
Lactated ringer's	6.5	None	130	4	3	0	109	28

Data from Short CE: *Principles and practice of veterinary anesthesia*, Baltimore, 1987, Williams & Wilkins; and Broadstone R: Fluid therapy and newer drug products, *Vet Clin North Am Small Anim Pract* 29(3):618, 1999.

for the first hour in cats). Often, a 10- to 20-ml/kg bolus is given, and the patient is reevaluated, with further boluses given as necessary. When in doubt, the technician should consult with the veterinarian about the optimum fluid administration rate and should carefully monitor the total amount of fluids being given to the patient during surgery.

Types of IV fluids

Crystalloid solutions. The choice of IV fluids is governed by the animal's condition and the veterinarian's preference. Crystalloid solutions are the most commonly administered type of fluid. Depending on the fluid used, crystalloid solutions may provide water, electrolytes, alkalinizing agents such as lactate, and dextrose (Table 1-4). Other constituents may be added, including 50% dextrose, potassium, and B-complex vitamins. Crystalloid solutions are appropriate for most patients, provided the PCV is 20% or greater and the total protein is no less than 3.5 g/dl. There are three types of crystalloid solutions:

- *Balanced electrolyte solutions.* As the term implies, these solutions contain several electrolytes (most often sodium, potassium, chloride, magnesium, and calcium) in concentrations that reflect the electrolyte composition of blood. Lactated Ringer's solution is one of the most commonly used balanced electrolyte solutions. The lactate is broken down in the liver to produce bicarbonate, which is helpful in correcting metabolic acidosis.
- *Saline solutions.* Physiologic saline (0.9% saline) and other saline solutions contain only sodium and chloride ions in water. These solutions may be preferable to lactated Ringer's solution in some animals (for example, patients with liver disease). Very concentrated (up to 7.5%) hypertonic saline solutions may be administered to patients in shock along with one of the other crystalloids previously mentioned. Hypertonic saline solution should never be administered alone and must be given slowly (for example, 3 to 5 ml/kg IV over a 5-minute period) to avoid hypotension, bradycardia, and bronchoconstriction.
- *Dextrose solutions.* Solutions of 2.5% or 5% dextrose in water or saline are commonly used in animals with hypoglycemia or hyperkalemia and in animals receiving insulin. Dextrose solutions are also useful in neonatal animals and in debilitated animals, both of which benefit from a ready source of dextrose during anesthesia.

The dextrose provides very few calories but helps maintain a normal blood glucose level. Dextrose in water should not be used as the sole maintenance fluid because it lacks necessary electrolytes (sodium, potassium, chloride) and could result in the dilution of these electrolytes in serum, leading to serious consequences. It is also unsuitable for patients in shock because most of the fluid leaves the vessels and enters the intracellular space.

The anesthetist must exercise caution when administering drugs and crystalloid fluids concurrently because undesirable interactions may occur. Diazepam, for example, precipitates in IV fluids. Thiopental is incompatible with lactated Ringer's solution. Sodium bicarbonate and whole blood products should not be mixed with fluids containing calcium.

Colloid solutions. Some patients require the administration of colloid solutions, which contain large molecules that do not freely diffuse across membranes and therefore stay in the blood. Colloid solutions are sometimes able to maintain circulating blood volume and blood pressure more effectively than crystalloid solutions. Examples of colloid solutions include the following:

- *Plasma or blood.* Transfusions of plasma or blood are particularly useful in treating animals that have acute blood loss or severe anemia. Patients with extensive burns may also have severe plasma loss, and a plasma transfusion may be required. Plasma or blood is also useful in animals with hypoproteinemia and in patients with coagulation disorders.
- *Synthetic colloids.* Patients in shock or with hypoproteinemia are sometimes given synthetic colloids such as dextran, pentastarch, and hetastarch. Hetastarch can be combined with regular fluid therapy, is given at a rate of 5 ml/kg over 5 minutes, and can be repeated up to 4 times over a 24-hour period. More rapid administration is preferred if the patient is in shock.
- *Blood substitute.* Oxyglobin is an oxygen-carrying fluid derived from bovine hemoglobin. It absorbs and releases oxygen in a manner similar to red blood cells, but no crossmatching or blood typing is required. It may cause transient discoloration of mucous membranes and urine, and may alter some clinical chemistry results. Oxyglobin is most commonly used to treat animals with acute hemorrhage or chronic anemia.

Other Preanesthetic Patient Care

On occasion the veterinarian may direct the technician or another staff member to provide specific preoperative care. Some patients require the administration of medication such as insulin or anticonvulsant medication. Antibiotics may be required for animals that have infections or that are scheduled for surgery involving a contaminated area (such as the gastrointestinal tract). The technician should obtain specific instructions from the veterinarian on the route, dose, and type of medication to be administered to each patient.

PREANESTHETIC AGENTS

Preanesthetic agents are drugs that are administered to an animal before general anesthesia. The most commonly used preanesthetic agents are atropine, acepromazine, xylazine, medetomidine, diazepam, and opioids (formerly called narcotics). Either a single drug or a combination of drugs may be administered to an animal.

Suggested dosages of the common preanesthetic agents for use in healthy dogs and cats are given in Table 1-5. Dosages should be adjusted according to the patient's health status.

Reasons for Use

The potential benefits associated with the use of preanesthetic agents are summarized in Table 1-6. The most important reasons for the administration of preanesthetic agents are the following:

1. *To calm or sedate an excited, frightened, or vicious animal.* Sedation not only enhances patient comfort but also simplifies the task of the anesthetist. However, not every patient requires the same degree of sedation: geriatric, debilitated, injured, or sick animals may need only very light sedation or none at all, so as not to cause excessive central nervous system (CNS) depression. Conversely, some healthy animals may be unaffected by even high doses of tranquilizing medications.

TABLE 1-5

Suggested Dosage Ranges of Common Preanesthetic Medications for Use in Healthy Dogs and Cats*

DRUG	ROUTE	CANINE DOSAGE (mg/kg)	FELINE DOSAGE (mg/kg)
Acepromazine	SC, IM, IV	0.02-0.1 SC or IM 0.01-0.05 IV Maximum 3 mg (1 mg geriatrics) Use with caution in boxers	Same
	Oral	1-3	Same
Atropine	SC, IM, IV	0.02-0.04	Same
Butorphanol	SC, IM	0.1-0.5	Same
	IV	0.05	Same
Diazepam	IM	0.2-0.4 (not always effective)	Same
	IV	0.1-0.5 (max 10 mg)	Same
Glycopyrrolate	SC, IM	0.01-0.02	Same
Medetomidine	IM	10-20 µg/kg	10-40 µg/kg
	IV	5-10 µg/kg	10-20 µg/kg
Meperidine	SC, IM	3-5	5
Midazolam	IM, IV	0.1-0.2 (max 10 mg)	Not recommended as sole agent
Morphine	SC, IM	0.25-1.0	0.1-0.3 (may produce excitement)
Oxymorphone	IM	0.1-0.3	Same
	IV	0.05-0.10 Maximum 3 mg	0.02 Maximum 1 mg
Xylazine	IM	0.25-2	Same
	IV	0.2-0.5	Same

Data from Morgan RV: *AAHA formulary*, Denver, 1988, American Animal Hospital Association; Muir WW III, Hubbell JAE: *Handbook of veterinary anesthesia*, St Louis, 1989, Mosby; Warren RG: *Small animal anesthesia*, St Louis, 1983, Mosby; Ko JCH: Anesthetic potency: how to use medetomidine and atipamezole, *Vet Tech* 18(10):695-702, 1997.
*For analgesic dosages, see Tables 8-3 and 8-4.

TABLE 1-6

Benefits Associated with the Use of Selected Preanesthetic Agents

WHAT THE PREANESTHETIC CAN DO	WHICH PREANESTHETIC?
Tranquilize or sedate the animal to facilitate catheterization, masking, or injection of an induction agent; reduce patient apprehension; allow calm recovery and reduce postanesthetic excitement	• Phenothiazines (acepromazine) • Thiazines (xylazine, medetomidine) • Opioids (meperidine, butorphanol, oxymorphone) • Benzodiazepines (diazepam, midazolam: debilitated animals only)
Decrease amount of general anesthetic required	All of the above
Muscle relaxation	• Xylazine, medetomidine • Diazepam, midazolam
Induce vomiting in unfasted animal	• Xylazine (cats) • Morphine (dogs)
Minimize bradycardia that occurs during intubation, handling of viscera, or as side effect of many anesthetics	• Atropine • Glycopyrrolate
Minimize salivation	• Atropine • Glycopyrrolate
Decrease gastrointestinal tract (GIT) motility, thereby preventing vomiting, diarrhea, and flatulence that may occur with some opioids	• Atropine • Glycopyrrolate
Provide intraoperative or postoperative analgesia	• Opioids • Nonsteroidal antiinflammatory drugs (NSAIDs)
Prevent intraoperative or postoperative seizures	• Diazepam

2. *To reduce or eliminate possible adverse effects resulting from the use of general anesthetics.* Injectable anesthetics such as barbiturates or ketamine and the inhalation anesthetics such as halothane or isoflurane may cause undesirable side effects in addition to their anesthetic action. For example, ketamine causes excessive salivation in some patients. Some opioid drugs may induce bradycardia, vomiting, diarrhea, and flatulence. Preanesthetic agents, particularly the anticholinergics (atropine and glycopyrrolate), are sometimes given to prevent these effects.

3. *To reduce the amount of general anesthetic required to induce anesthesia.* The administration of preanesthetic tranquilizers and opioids causes significant sedation in most veterinary patients. Although this level of sedation is insufficient to allow surgery, the animal will likely require smaller doses of general anesthetics to produce surgical anesthesia. Reduction of the amount of general anesthetic given to the patient minimizes the adverse effects of the general anesthetic on the respiratory and cardiovascular systems. This approach to anesthesia, in which low doses of several preanesthetic and general anesthetic agents are used in combination to achieve a satisfactory anesthetic state, is termed *balanced anesthesia.*

4. *To decrease pain and discomfort during surgery and in the postoperative period and allow a smoother anesthetic recovery.* If the period of anesthesia is brief, drugs given during the preanesthetic period may exert some analgesic effect even during the recovery period.

Preanesthetic drugs have many other uses, even in animals that are not undergoing anesthesia. For example, tranquilizers are used to calm patients for transport, physical examination, and minor procedures. They are helpful in preventing animals from chewing wounds and bandages. Phenothiazines are useful antiemetics for animals with gastrointestinal disease. Most opioids are effective cough suppressants.

Preanesthetic agents are chosen from one or more of several classes of drugs, including tranquilizers and sedatives, opioids (narcotics), and anticholinergics. The type of drug or combination of drugs is chosen by the veterinarian on the basis of the nature of the procedure; the veterinarian's personal preference; the facilities and equipment available; and the patient's species, breed, physical status, and temperament.

The timing of the administration of the drug will also vary among patients. The veterinarian will usually choose to administer a preanesthetic well before the general anesthetic is given, allowing at least 15 to 20 minutes for the preanesthetic to gradually exert its effects. Drugs with a sedative effect, such as acepromazine and opioids, work best if the animal is left undisturbed until the full effect of the drug is evident.

Preanesthetics are usually given by IM or SC injection. Some agents can be given intravenously, but caution should be used when giving any preanesthetic or general anesthetic by this route because drug potency and the potential for adverse effects are increased. IV dosages are typically less than those used for IM or SC injection. Some agents can also be given orally, but response to oral administration is slow and less predictable than that seen after injection.

No preanesthetic agent is entirely free of side effects, and no single agent is safe for every animal. Table 1-7 gives a summary of the precautions and contraindications associated with the commonly used preanesthetic agents. The anesthetist should be aware that all preanesthetics except glycopyrrolate cross the placental barrier, and adverse effects may be observed in the newborn animal if the agents are administered shortly before birth.

Anticholinergics (Parasympatholytics)

Anticholinergic drugs are sometimes given to patients before anesthesia. The two anticholinergic agents commonly used in veterinary medicine are atropine and glycopyrrolate (Robinul-V). Atropine is derived from the deadly nightshade plant, and glycopyrrolate is a synthetic quaternary ammonium derivative of atropine. Both drugs may be given by the IV, IM, or SC routes. The IV route is generally recommended only for emergency situations (treatment of very slow heart rates, cardiac resuscitation), when a rapid effect is required. The SC or IM route is used for preanesthesia for most patients. As is common for anesthetic agents, the SC and IM dosages are considerably greater than the IV dosage.

Atropine is available in several concentrations, including 0.4 mg/ml, 0.54 mg/ml (1/120 grain/ml), 2.2 mg/ml, and 15 mg/ml. It is important to ensure that the atropine drawn into the syringe is the same concentration as that used to calculate the dose, or an incorrect amount will be administered. For example, an anesthetist

TABLE 1-7	
Precautions for the Use of Selected Preanesthetic Agents	
ANESTHETIC OR PREANESTHETIC	USE WITH CAUTION IN WHICH SITUATIONS?
Atropine	Tachycardia (heart rate over 140 in a dog, 180 in a cat)
	Constipation or obstruction
Acepromazine	Hypotension (shock)
	Seizure disorders, head trauma
	Hypothermia
Diazepam	Cesarean section
	Neonatal patients
Xylazine and medetomidine	Cardiovascular disease or respiratory disease
	Debilitated animals
	Neonates or geriatrics
	Pregnant animals
	Large dogs prone to bloat
Opioids	Respiratory disease
	Head trauma or spinal cord injury
	Chest injury
	Shock

who calculates a dose of 0.5 ml of atropine using a concentration of 0.4 mg/ml will cause atropine toxicity in a patient if the 0.5 ml is drawn from a bottle containing the drug at a concentration of 15 mg/ml.

Mode of action

Anticholinergic drugs such as atropine exert their effect by blocking certain receptors for the neurotransmitter acetylcholine. Acetylcholine is produced by the parasympathetic part of the autonomic nervous system and is the transmitter at both the nicotinic and muscarinic receptors (Fig. 1-6). Atropine blocks the action of acetylcholine at the muscarinic receptors, which are the terminal ends of the parasympathetic nervous system. It therefore acts to reverse parasympathetic effects and is therefore called a *parasympatholytic drug*. Atropine has no effect on the nicotinic receptors.

The muscarinic receptors are found in the heart, gastrointestinal tract, bronchi, several secretory glands, and the iris of the eye, and in these locations the effect of atropine is readily observed by the anesthetist (Fig. 1-7). When the parasympathetic system is activated (as often occurs during anesthesia), the muscarinic receptors are stimulated by acetylcholine. This is sometimes undesirable because it may result in bradycardia, gastrointestinal stimulation, salivation, and pupil constriction. By blocking the muscarinic receptors, atropine helps to prevent these parasympathetic effects.

Effects of atropine

Atropine has many effects that make it a useful drug in veterinary anesthesia, although its use is not without hazard.

1. *Atropine blocks stimulation of the vagus nerve.* Several anesthetic procedures and agents may stimulate the vagus nerve, which is an important part of the parasym-

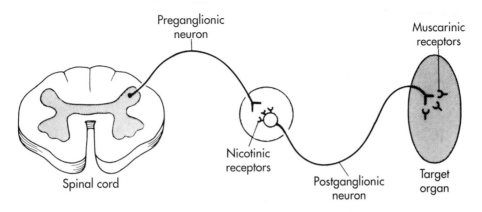

FIG. 1-6 Schematic view of the parasympathetic nervous system. Preganglionic neuron releases acetylcholine at the nicotinic receptors. Postganglionic neuron releases acetylcholine at the muscarinic receptors of the target organ. Atropine affects only the muscarinic receptors.

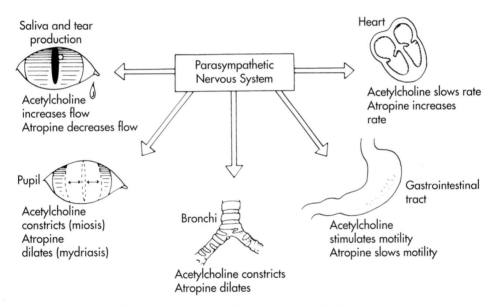

FIG. 1-7 Effect of atropine on the parasympathetic nervous system.

pathetic nervous system. Procedures that stimulate the vagus nerve include endotracheal intubation, handling of the viscera during surgery, and the administration of several commonly used anesthetic agents (including inhalation agents, xylazine, and some opioids). Stimulation of the vagus nerve may be undesirable during anesthesia because it causes increased parasympathetic activity, resulting in bradycardia and reduced cardiac output. By blocking the stimulation of the vagus nerve, atropine prevents bradycardia and in some cases will cause the heart rate to increase. For this reason, atropine is said to "protect the heart" during anesthesia. However, atropine may also cause very fast heart rates and should be avoided in animals with heart problems such as congestive heart failure or hyperthyroidism. Atropine should not be given to animals with preexisting rapid heart rates (more 140 bpm in dogs and 180 bpm in cats).

2. *Atropine reduces salivation (antisialagogic activity).* Several anesthetic agents, particularly ketamine, stimulate the parasympathetic nerves that promote salivation. This may predispose the animal to aspiration of saliva and possible upper airway blockage. Atropine markedly reduces the production of saliva in these patients.

3. *Atropine reduces gastrointestinal activity.* Some anesthetic agents (particularly the opioids) increase the peristaltic movement of the gastrointestinal tract, leading to flatulence, vomiting, and diarrhea. Atropine counters these effects by inhibiting intestinal peristalsis. This action also accounts for the inclusion of atropine in several popular antidiarrheal preparations. Atropine should be avoided in animals with constipation or ileus because these drugs will further reduce peristaltic action of the intestines. Atropine can cause gut stasis in healthy horses and ruminants even at clinical doses.

4. *Atropine causes pupil dilation (mydriasis).* This effect is not commonly seen when dogs are given the usual preanesthetic doses of atropine. In cats, however, mydriasis may occur even at the preanesthetic dosage rates. Mydriasis has been associated with temporary blurred vision and may also predispose the animal to retinal damage if the eyes are exposed to bright light for a considerable time. The anesthetist should also be aware that animals given atropine may show reduced pupillary light reflex because of the mydriatic effect. This reflex is commonly used to assess depth of anesthesia but may be unreliable in patients that have received atropine.

5. *Atropine reduces tear secretions.* In the awake animal, the cornea is lubricated by the secretion of tears. Atropine causes a marked reduction in tear production, and the corneas of animals receiving atropine should be protected from drying by instilling an ophthalmic ointment. This effect is particularly important when an anesthetic agent such as ketamine is used in addition to atropine. (Animals anesthetized with ketamine do not close their eyelids, resulting in an even greater tendency toward corneal drying.) Atropine should be avoided in animals with glaucoma.

6. *Atropine promotes bronchodilation.* Atropine dilates bronchioles in the lungs, increasing the diameter of these airways. This results in increased anatomic dead space. This term refers to the parts of the respiratory system that contain air but where oxygen and carbon dioxide exchange do not occur. A certain amount of anatomic dead space is present in every patient, but if the amount of dead space is excessive the patient is at risk of hypoxemia (low blood oxygen).

7. *The use of atropine may be associated with the production of thick mucous secretions within the airways, particularly in cats.* This may predispose the animal to airway blockage, and for this reason, some veterinarians avoid the use of atropine in cats.

Use of atropine

Atropine and glycopyrrolate are still commonly used by veterinary anesthetists, however, less so now than in the past. Most modern anesthetic agents do not stimulate salivation or gastrointestinal secretions, and bradycardia is well tolerated by most patients. Because of the potential for significant adverse effects, particularly tachycardia, thick mucous secretions, decreased tear production, and mydriasis, many authorities question the routine use of anticholinergics. However, anticholinergics are beneficial for some patients (for example, those with preexisting bradycardia and patients receiving ketamine or opioids at high dosages). Some authorities continue to advocate the routine use of atropine or glycopyrrolate as part of preanesthetic mixtures for healthy patients. Atropine is also given during surgery to treat some patients with bradycardia or excessive salivation, and it is also used for treatment of cardiac arrest. It is also commonly given before reversal of neuromuscular blocking agents.

The onset of atropine action occurs approximately 20 minutes after SC injection, and therefore it should be administered at least 20 to 30 minutes before anesthetic induction. Atropine may be mixed in a syringe with most other preanesthetic and anesthetic agents, including acepromazine and ketamine (but not diazepam) and given SC, IM, or IV. Because the onset of action is rapid after IV administration of atropine (30 seconds to 2 minutes), it offers almost immediate protection when given in this way, but there is a greater risk of adverse effects, particularly on the heart. Some anesthetists prefer to reserve the use of intravenous atropine for treatment of severe bradycardia or cardiac arrest.

The duration of effect of atropine is 60 to 90 minutes (less if strong parasympathetic tone is present). It is common to see a reduction in heart rate at the end of a long anesthesia, due in part to the loss of atropine activity.

Atropine toxicity

An overdose of atropine may cause drowsiness in some animals and excitement in others. It may also cause dry mucous membranes and thirst, ataxia, muscle tremors, dilated pupils, hyperthermia, and tachycardia. Dogs are more susceptible to atropine toxicity than are cats. Atropine overdose can be treated with physostigmine at a dose of 0.02 mg/kg to a maximum of 0.5 mg per animal IV over several minutes. The dosage can be repeated every 5 to 10 minutes if required to a total maximum dose of 2 mg per animal.

Glycopyrrolate

The effects of glycopyrrolate are similar to those of atropine, but the duration of effect is much longer (atropine is effective for approximately 60 minutes after SC injection, whereas glycopyrrolate is effective for 2 to 3 hours). Glycopyrrolate may have less tendency to cause tachycardia and cardiac arrhythmias than atropine and is therefore safer to use in some animals with preexisting heart problems. Glycopyrrolate also suppresses salivation more effectively than atropine. Glycopyrrolate does not cross the placental barrier in pregnant animals. For these reasons glycopyrrolate may be preferable to atropine for some procedures in both the cat and the dog, despite its greater expense. Although many anesthetists prefer to use glycopyrrolate as a preanesthetic, atropine is still considered to be the better drug for rapid treatment of slow heart rates, because of its faster onset of effect.

Tranquilizers and Sedatives

A *sedative* and a *tranquilizer* are not exactly the same thing. A tranquilizer is a drug that reduces anxiety but does not necessarily decrease awareness and wakefulness.

A sedative is a drug that causes reduced mental activity and sleepiness. Diazepam (Valium) is a good example of a true tranquilizer, whereas medetomidine is a sedative. Most veterinarians, however, use the terms *sedative* and *tranquilizer* interchangeably, and this will also be the case in this book.

The main reason for giving tranquilizers/sedatives before anesthesia is to calm the patient and allow easy handling. A quiet induction period is safer for the patient (because there is less epinephrine release and fewer cardiac arrhythmias are seen) and may lead to a less stressful recovery.

Because sedation is seen with most preanesthetic drugs, patients that have received these drugs should not be left unattended on a table because they could easily fall and be injured. The technician must also be aware that animals that appear sedated may suddenly become aroused and even aggressive, particularly if stimulated suddenly (for example by pain).

Three classes of tranquilizers/sedatives are used in veterinary medicine: phenothiazines, benzodiazepines, and alpha-2 agonists (α-2 agonists). Agents from each of these classes act on the central nervous system, resulting in a more tranquil or calmer animal. These drugs may also cause ataxia and prolapse of the nictitating membrane (also called the *third eyelid*, Fig. 1-8). Only the alpha-2 agonists have analgesic (pain-relieving) effects; phenothiazines and benzodiazepines have none.

Phenothiazines

The phenothiazine group of drugs includes such agents as acepromazine maleate (also known as acetylpromazine), chlorpromazine, and triflupromazine. Phenothiazines are among the most commonly used sedatives in veterinary medicine. Unlike opioids (narcotics), they are not subject to detailed record-keeping requirements. They do not cause significant respiratory or cardiac depression and have a wide margin of safety in healthy patients. They are effective in many species and may be given in combination with other agents, such as atropine, opioids, and ketamine. Phenothiazines may be administered orally, subcutaneously, intramuscularly, or (with caution) intravenously.

Effects of phenothiazines

Phenothiazines have the following clinical effects:
1. *Sedation.* Phenothiazines affect the reticular activating center of the brain, causing sedation. This effect may last up to 24 hours, especially when used at higher doses. Sedation is less pronounced in cats than in dogs and in both species is less than that seen with alpha-2 agonist sedatives such as medetomidine. The sedative effect not only is useful for preanesthesia of animals, but also helps calm patients that are fearful during thunderstorms, anxious when traveling in a car, or showing signs of excitement after administration of an opioid such as morphine.
2. *Antiemetic effect.* Phenothiazines, even at very low doses, help prevent vomiting during the anesthetic period. They are also used to prevent vomiting caused by gastrointestinal disease or motion sickness.
3. *Antiarrhythmic effect.* Some anesthetics, such as halothane, have a potential to cause cardiac arrhythmias, which may result in decreased cardiac output. Phenothiazines may partially antagonize this effect.

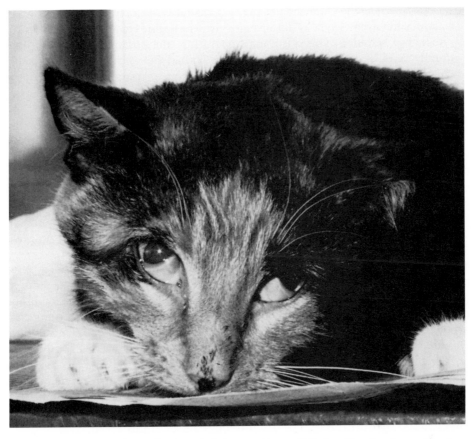

FIG. 1-8 Prolapse of the third eyelid. (*From Warren RG:* Small animal anesthesia, *St Louis, 1983, Mosby.*)

4. *Antihistamine effect.* Histamine is a chemical released by the body as part of the allergic response. Phenothiazines prevent the release of histamine and therefore help reduce allergic reactions. For this reason, phenothiazines should not be used to sedate animals that are to undergo allergy testing.

5. *Peripheral vasodilation.* Phenothiazine agents dilate blood vessels, particularly when given by the IV route. The heart rate may increase as a reflex response to vasodilation. Vasodilation may result in increased heat loss, leading to hypothermia. Even more seriously, vasodilation may lead to a fall in blood pressure (hypotension). Consequently, phenothiazines are not the preanesthetic agents of choice for animals with low blood pressure, including animals in circulatory shock. Animals that experience significant hypotension from phenothiazine administration should be given IV fluids to raise blood pressure. The veterinarian may also prescribe drugs that increase blood pressure by constricting the arteries, including alpha sympathomimetics such as phenylephrine.

6. *Effects on personality.* Occasionally, the administration of a phenothiazine or other tranquilizing agent (such as diazepam or medetomidine) may induce excitement rather than sedation. This effect may persist into the postanesthetic period but usually resolves within 48 hours. Owners should be warned that personality changes sometimes occur after the administration of tranquilizing agents, and care should be used when handling patients returning home within 48 hours of anesthesia.

7. *Penile prolapse.* Acepromazine and other sedatives have been reported to cause prolapse of the penis in horses. The risk of permanent prolapse is low; however, some veterinarians choose not to use acepromazine in breeding stallions.

8. *Lack of analgesia.* Acepromazine has no analgesic (pain-relieving) effect. Patients that are restless or excited because they are in pain are better managed with an opioid or nonsteroidal antiinflammatory drug.

As is evident from the previous discussion, the use of phenothiazines is not without risk. There is currently no reversing agent available for phenothiazines, and adverse effects are therefore somewhat difficult to treat.

It has been suggested that the manufacturer's recommended dose for acepromazine is higher than that actually required for preanesthesia and should be reduced by 50% or more to minimize the danger of side effects. High doses of phenothiazine drugs do not result in increased levels of sedation and may induce significant hypotension. The anesthetist should be particularly aware that phenothiazines have increased potency in geriatric animals, neonates, and animals with liver dysfunction, and the dose should be reduced by at least one half in these patients to avoid excessive sedation and prolonged recovery. Hypotensive, anemic, or dehydrated patients are at increased risk of having severe hypotension with phenothiazine use. Some anesthesiologists believe that boxers may be abnormally sensitive to phenothiazines and that the dosage may need to be reduced in this breed.

Benzodiazepines

The benzodiazepine group includes diazepam (Valium), as well as zolazepam (a component of Telazol), midazolam (Versed), and lorazepam (Ativan). Diazepam, although commonly used in veterinary anesthesia as a preanesthetic or combination induction agent, is not licensed in the United States or Canada for use in animals.

Effects of benzodiazepines

Benzodiazepines probably exert their effects through the release of endogenous gamma-aminobutyric acid (GABA), an inhibitory neurotransmitter in the brain. The following properties of diazepam are also seen in other drugs in this class:

1. *Antianxiety and calming effect.* Benzodiazepines, unlike phenothiazines, do not cause significant CNS sedation in healthy young animals unless used in combination with other drugs such as ketamine or opioids. A healthy young animal that is given diazepam without other drugs does not usually appear drowsy; instead, the animal appears less anxious but still alert. With its normal inhibitions and anxieties removed by the drug, the animal may actually become more difficult to control. Although its use as the sole sedative in healthy young animals is often disappointing, diazepam is much more effective in geriatric or debilitated animals. Diazepam also enhances the sedation and analgesia of other

agents, and its relative safety makes it a popular drug for protocols with drug combinations. The anesthetist should be aware that benzodiazepines, like phenothiazines, have no analgesic effect and when used alone will not be effective in calming animals that are experiencing pain.

2. *Skeletal muscle relaxation.* Benzodiazepines are excellent skeletal muscle relaxants and often are used to counteract the muscle rigidity seen with agents such as ketamine and etomidate.

3. *Anticonvulsant activity.* Diazepam is an excellent anticonvulsant drug. To take advantage of this effect, many anesthetists use diazepam in combination with agents that have a potential to cause seizures, including ketamine and local anesthetics. It is also the preanesthetic of choice for some animals with seizure disorders. Diazepam can be given intravenously or rectally as a treatment for many types of seizures, including those that occur in the postanesthetic period.

4. *Minimal adverse effects.* At therapeutic dosages, benzodiazepines have minimal adverse effects on the cardiovascular and respiratory systems and therefore have a high margin of safety. This property makes them particularly useful for anesthesia of high-risk and geriatric animals. If adverse effects are seen after the use of a benzodiazepine, flumazenil can be administered to reverse these agents (dose: 1 mg of flumazenil for each 13 mg of benzodiazepine).

   Benzodiazepines should be used with caution in neonates and in animals with known liver dysfunction because these agents are poorly metabolized in these patients. Some veterinarians avoid its use in cesarean sections.

5. *Other properties.* Benzodiazepine agents are used for a variety of purposes in veterinary medicine other than anesthesia. Diazepam and midazolam are effective appetite stimulants in cats, and oral diazepam is sometimes used to modify undesirable behavior such as inappropriate urination in cats. Both of these effects may arise from the action of benzodiazepine agents on neurotransmitters within the brain.

Methods of use

Diazepam. The most effective and least painful way to administer diazepam is by the IV route, rather than the IM or SC routes.* When given intravenously, diazepam should be injected slowly because rapid administration may cause cardiac arrhythmias.

Unfortunately, diazepam is not water soluble and is therefore not physically compatible with most other preanesthetic agents. It should not be mixed in a single syringe with atropine, acepromazine, barbiturates, or opioids because a precipitate may result. The only anesthetic agent that is physically compatible with diazepam is ketamine. Ketamine and diazepam can be mixed together in equal volumes in the same syringe, but prolonged storage is not recommended. Diazepam is very soluble in plastic and over time is absorbed by syringes and IV bags.

Diazepam is most commonly used in combination with drugs that induce anesthesia. Although it is not possible to induce anesthesia in a healthy animal through

---

*Diazepam can also be administered through a syringe or feeding tube passed into the rectum, at twice the IV dose. This provides rapid sedation for dogs and cats with seizures, in which IV access may be difficult.

the use of diazepam alone, it is an effective supplement to other agents. In particular, the combination of ketamine and diazepam has gained wide acceptance as a safe and effective IV induction agent in small animals and horses. Diazepam may also be administered concurrently with opioids, propofol, or thiopental (provided separate syringes are used) to achieve safe, smooth induction of high-risk patients. If diazepam is given in combination with opioids, thiopental, or propofol, an IV catheter should be used and a saline flush given after each injection of anesthetic agent.

Diazepam is light sensitive and for this reason is often provided in brown glass vials. If stored in a clear glass container, diazepam should be kept in a safe or other location away from light.

Diazepam is classified as a controlled drug in Canada and the United States. Some potential for human abuse and theft exists, so this drug should be stored in a secure location, and appropriate records must be kept.

Midazolam. Another benzodiazepine agent, midazolam, appears to have some advantages over diazepam. It is water soluble and therefore can be mixed with other preanesthetic and anesthetic agents. It is less irritating to tissues than diazepam and is also more reliably absorbed after IM or SC injection. Effects are usually apparent within 3 minutes of IM injection.

Like diazepam, midazolam produces minimal sedation when used on its own and may in fact cause excitement in healthy cats and dogs. If midazolam is used as the sole preanesthetic agent, the patient often becomes more difficult to restrain. In dogs, midazolam is usually combined with ketamine, thiopental, or an opioid for induction of anesthesia. In feline patients, it is most commonly given in combination with ketamine (0.2 mg/kg midazolam and 10 mg/kg ketamine IM).

Midazolam has minimal cardiovascular effects. Like diazepam, midazolam crosses the placenta and may cause CNS depression in neonates delivered by cesarean section.

Alpha-2 Agonists

Alpha-2 agonists are potent sedatives widely used in both large and small animal patients. Xylazine (Rompun, Anased), medetomidine (Domitor), detomidine (Dormosedan), and romifidine (Sedivet) are members of this class of drugs, which are also called the *thiazine derivatives*. These drugs have several useful properties, including fast onset, reliable and potent effect, reversibility, and analgesia (pain relief). Because they are not controlled by legislation, no special record keeping is required.

The intended site of action is receptors found on sympathetic nerves within the brain and spinal cord, called *alpha-2 adrenoreceptors*. Xylazine and other alpha-2 adrenoreceptor agonists stimulate these receptors, causing a decrease in the level of the neurotransmitter norepinephrine. The result is sedation, analgesia, and muscle relaxation. When these drugs are combined with other tranquilizers or analgesic agents, the result tends to be additive (even synergistic) in nature.

Alpha-2 agonists also affect receptors in the heart and blood vessels, which leads to a significant potential for cardiovascular side effects. Compared with xylazine, medetomidine has greater potency and fewer adverse effects. However, all members of this class should be used with caution, and standard doses of these drugs should be given only to young, healthy patients. These drugs are generally avoided in geriatric, diabetic, pregnant, pediatric, or sick patients. Careful monitoring of patient status is always essential after receiving these drugs. Fortunately, reversing agents are available and can be used if adverse effects are seen.

Effects of alpha-2 agonists

Alpha-2 agonists are potent sedatives and muscle relaxants. Unlike phenothiazines and diazepam, alpha-2 agonists also provide analgesia. When combined with other tranquilizers, ketamine, opioid agents, local anesthetics, or nitrous oxide, they may provide sufficient analgesia and sedation to allow minor surgical procedures. The sedative effect of alpha-2 agonists may last for several hours in some patients, however the analgesia may be short-lived (approximately 20 minutes for xylazine) and should be supplemented with another agent if a prolonged effect is required.

Xylazine and medetomidine can be absorbed through skin abrasions and mucous membranes, and as little as 0.1 ml medetomidine can cause hypotension and sedation in humans. Hospital employees handling these agents should ensure that any of the drugs spilled on human or animal skin is immediately washed off.

Methods of use

Xylazine. Xylazine is supplied as a 2% solution (20 mg/ml) for small animal use and as a 10% solution (100 mg/ml) for equine use. The 10% solution can be diluted with sterile water for use in small animals.

Xylazine can be used alone or in combination with ketamine, opioids, and many other agents. The required doses of other agents are substantially reduced when they are given in combination with xylazine, particularly barbiturates (up to 80% reduction) and inhalation agents (up to 50% reduction). Whether given alone or in combination with other agents, xylazine can be administered IM or IV. Subcutaneous injections have much less effect and are generally avoided.

Medetomidine Medetomidine (Domitor) is supplied as a 1-mg/ml solution for small animal use. In the United States and Canada, medetomidine is approved for dogs only although it has been used extensively in many other species, including cats, horses, and exotic animals. Like xylazine, medetomidine is commonly used in combination with other agents. One combination in widespread use is medetomidine (10 µg/kg) and butorphanol (0.2 mg/kg). The two drugs can be mixed in the same syringe and given IV or (preferably) IM. Medetomidine can also be mixed with opioids or with ketamine. Animals should be left in a quiet environment for 20 to 30 minutes after injection to allow the drug to take maximum effect. If a short, minimally invasive procedure is planned (such as an ear flush, bandage change, or x-ray procedure), the sedation provided by medetomidine/butorphanol and other combinations may be adequate without a general anesthetic. The sedation can be supplemented with a local block if minor surgery such as suturing a laceration or removal of a superficial skin tumor is planned. Although these patients are too awake for intubation, some veterinarians choose to provide supplemental oxygen by face mask. Caution should be used when using medetomidine combinations for minor operations, because sudden arousal has been reported even in heavily sedated patients. Severe bites to hospital personnel have resulted in some cases.

If the sedated animal is to undergo more extensive surgery, an injectable or inhalant general anesthetic (for example, thiopental, propofol, or isoflurane) can be given.

The dose of general anesthetic required will be significantly less than that required for a nonsedated animal, and caution must be exercised to avoid overdosage.

Adverse effects

Alpha-2 agonists have considerable potential for adverse effects. These are reported most commonly when the drugs are given by the IV route and include the following:

1. Bradycardia, reduced cardiac output, and second-degree heart block (faulty conduction of the electrical impulse between the right atrium and the ventricles, see p. 95) are commonly seen after administration of alpha-2 agonists. These drugs also sensitize the heart to the arrhythmogenic effect of epinephrine, making cardiac arrhythmias more common, especially in excited animals. Blood pressure rises initially after alpha-2 agonists are given but soon falls to normal or hypotensive levels (especially with xylazine). Because of these serious effects on the cardiovascular system, the use of alpha-2 agonists should be avoided in animals that are debilitated or that have cardiovascular disease.

   To reduce the incidence of adverse cardiac effects, some veterinarians give atropine or glycopyrrolate as a premedication. However, atropine is not always effective in preventing or treating the cardiovascular side effects of medetomidine and may in fact increase the workload of the heart and exacerbate hypertension. (Hypertension is often present, due to medetomidine-induced vasoconstriction.) If bradycardia occurs with either medetomidine or xylazine, the best treatment is reversal of the alpha-2 agonist effects with atipamezole or other reversing agent (see p. 39).

2. Respiratory effects of alpha-2 agonists vary from animal to animal and among species and are more severe when other drugs are given in combination with the alpha-2 agonist. Some animals show respiratory depression, whereas others show no ill effects. Cyanosis may occasionally result from the use of these agents, particularly in brachycephalic dogs. In some cases cyanosis is due to reduced local blood flow to the tissues, rather than hypoxia, and blood gas values usually remain within acceptable limits. As a general rule, however, alpha-2 agonists should not be administered to animals showing signs of respiratory disease.

3. Xylazine causes vomiting in up to 50% of dogs and 90% of cats. The emetic action of xylazine appears to be unpleasant for the animal but may be somewhat reduced if the animal is premedicated with atropine. Medetomidine is less likely to cause vomiting than xylazine, especially at low doses.

4. Xylazine depresses gastrointestinal activity and has been reported to cause bloat in ruminants and gastrointestinal stasis in dogs. For this reason it should not be used as a preanesthetic in breeds of dogs prone to gastric dilation and torsion, such as German shepherds, Great Danes, Saint Bernards, Irish setters, basset hounds, and other large, deep-chested dogs.

5. Alpha-2 agonists have been associated with temporary behavior and personality changes in both dogs and cats. This effect also has been reported for other preanesthetic agents, including acepromazine, opioids, and diazepam.

6. Alpha-2 agonists reduce the secretion of insulin by the pancreas. Transient hyperglycemia may be seen, which is not harmful to the animal but may confuse the interpretation of blood samples collected during this period. Urination is commonly observed 90 to 120 minutes after administration of medetomidine and is due to an osmotic diuresis from the hyperglycemia.

7. Xylazine causes increased intrauterine pressure in cattle and has the potential to cause abortion in the last trimester.

Alpha-2 agonists are metabolized in the liver, and the metabolites are excreted in the urine. Adequate hepatic and renal function are therefore important requirements for any animal receiving this drug.

Use of reversing agents

Because of the adverse cardiovascular effects and long duration of sedation that can occur after xylazine or medetomidine administration, use of a reversing agent is often advisable. Yohimbine (Yobine), given IV at a dose of 0.1 mg/kg, is an effective reversing agent for xylazine. Reversal of sedation and the cardiovascular effects of xylazine occurs within a few minutes of IV administration of yohimbine. Tolazoline, given IV at a dose rate of 1 to 2 mg/kg, is more effective than yohimbine in cattle and is also used to reverse detomidine in horses. Yohimbine and tolazoline should be given slowly because they are occasionally associated with unwanted side effects, including rapid arousal, excitement, rage, and tremors. Tolazoline may also cause vasodilation and hypotension.

Medetomidine has a specific antagonist, atipamezole (Antisedan). Atipamezole may be given IM or IV, although it is currently only approved for IM administration in the United States. The dosage for atipamezole is 5 times that of medetomidine; however, because the formulation of atipamezole is 5 times more concentrated than medetomidine (atipamezole 5 mg/ml, medetomidine 1 mg/ml), equal volumes of the two drugs should be administered to dogs. Cats appear to be more sensitive to the effects of atipamezole, and only half this dose should be used. In both cats and dogs, total reversal of effects typically occurs within 20 minutes of IM atipamezole administration. It is suggested that if the initial dose of IM atipamezole is not effective, administration of an amount equivalent to one half of the IM dose should be given by the IV route.

Atipamezole will reverse all of the clinical effects of medetomidine, both detrimental (bradycardia) and beneficial (analgesia). To maintain analgesia it may be appropriate to administer another analgesic agent just before the reversal of medetomidine. Atipamezole does not reverse the effects of other drugs given concurrently with medetomidine (ketamine, opioids, general anesthetics). High doses of atipamezole are associated with panting, excitement, muscle tremors, hypotension, and tachycardia, especially if given intravenously.

Opioids (Narcotics)

The term *narcotic* has traditionally been applied to the class of drugs derived from morphine. This term has been replaced with *opiate* or *opioid* depending on whether the drug is a natural chemical (opiate) or synthetically derived (opioid). The term *narcotic* is properly reserved for those agents that induce physical dependence and addiction and are therefore subject to stringent regulations regarding storage, use, and record keeping. Several opioids, such as buprenorphine, have little tendency to induce physical dependence and therefore are not considered to be narcotics. For the purposes of this text, the term *opioid* will be used for all members of this class, both narcotic and nonnarcotic.

Opioids are a versatile class of drugs that may be used as preanesthetics, induction agents, and analgesics. As a group they have excellent pain-relieving properties and also have a sedative effect, especially when used in combination with other agents. They have a wide safety margin and can be used on both healthy and debilitated patients. This chapter discusses the general characteristics of this class of drugs, with emphasis on their use as preanesthetics and as neuroleptanalgesics. Information on the use of opioids as induction agents is found in Chapter 3, and detailed information on specific opioid agents and their use for postoperative analgesia is presented in Chapter 8.

Mode of action

The site of action of opioids has been the subject of a great deal of research. Although opioid receptors are found on neurons throughout the body, the analgesic and sedative effects are chiefly the result of their action on receptors located in the brain and spinal cord. The natural stimulants of these receptors are chemicals produced by the body, such as endorphins and enkephalins. At least four types of opioid receptors have been identified: mu (μ), kappa (κ), sigma (σ), and delta (δ). Opioid agents differ in their action at each of these sites and therefore in their overall effects on the body (Table 1-8).

An opioid agent may act as an agonist (stimulating agent) or antagonist (blocking agent) at each type of receptor. Some agents (including morphine, oxymorphone, and fentanyl) are pure agonists in that they stimulate all four types of receptors. Other agents (for example, butorphanol) are considered mixed agonists/antagonists in that they block one type of receptor and stimulate another type. Still other opioids

TABLE 1-8

Effect of Opioid Drugs on Receptors

RECEPTOR	EFFECTS	AGONISTS	ANTAGONISTS OR MINIMAL EFFECT
Mu (μ)	Respiratory depression Euphoria Addiction Analgesia Sedation Miosis	Morphine Meperidine Fentanyl Oxymorphone Buprenorphine (partial)	Naloxone Butorphanol
Kappa (κ)	Analgesia Sedation Respiratory depression Miosis	Morphine Meperidine Fentanyl Oxymorphone Butorphanol	Naloxone
Sigma (σ)	Hallucinations Euphoria/dysphoria	Morphine Meperidine Fentanyl Oxymorphone Butorphanol	Naloxone
Delta (δ)	Analgesia Motor dysfunction	Morphine Fentanyl Meperidine	

Modified from Orsini J: Butorphanol tartrate: pharmacology and clinical indications, *Compendium* 10:849, 1988.

(for example, naloxone) block all types of receptors and are therefore considered to be pure antagonists. These antagonists have no clinical effect on their own but are used to reverse the effects of the pure agonists and the mixed agonists/antagonists.

Beneficial effects

Opioid agents have the following two effects on the nervous system that account for their use in veterinary anesthesia:

1. *CNS effects.* Depending on the dose, the particular opioid agent, and the species in which the agent is used, an opioid agent may cause CNS depression or excitement. In dogs the predominant effect is sedation. Most dogs exhibit a combination of CNS depression and analgesia within 60 seconds of IV administration and 15 minutes after IM administration. If high doses are given (particularly to a sick animal), a hypnotic state called *narcosis* may be produced in which the patient appears profoundly sedated yet can be aroused by sufficient stimulation. Narcosis is typically more profound than the sedation seen with acepromazine, xylazine, or diazepam. Although swallowing may persist, endotracheal intubation is often possible. Recovery is often slow (up to 6 hours in some animals) unless a reversing agent is given.

    Cats may react to some opioids by exhibiting bizarre behavior patterns, including anxiety or excitement, particularly if the drug is given intravenously. For this reason, some opioids (for example, morphine) must be used at low doses in cats, and IV injection is avoided. Dogs that are not in pain may also show excitement (for example, whining and barking) after opioid administration, particularly if a tranquilizing agent is not used concurrently.

2. *Analgesia.* Opioids have long been considered to be the most effective agents known to medicine for the treatment of pain. The degree of analgesia varies between members of the class: pure agonists such as morphine and oxymorphone are more effective for treatment of severe pain than the mixed agonist/antagonists such as butorphanol. Opioids are particularly useful as premedications for patients undergoing surgery for painful conditions (for example, repair of fractures).

    With the routine use of general anesthetics that have limited analgesic properties (for example, isoflurane, sevoflurane, halothane, propofol, and barbiturates) and the current emphasis on prevention of postoperative pain, the analgesic effect of opioids remains one of the chief reasons for their use in veterinary medicine. (See Chapter 8 for more information on the use of opioids for pain control.)

Method of use

Opioid agents are used in many ways in veterinary anesthesia. For detailed discussion of individual agents, see Chapter 8.

1. They are a common component of preanesthetic protocols. For high-risk patients, some anesthetists prefer to use an opioid such as morphine or oxymorphone as the sole preanesthetic agent. More commonly, however, the opioids are mixed with a tranquilizer (such as acepromazine, diazepam, or medetomidine) and/or an anticholinergic (atropine or glycopyrrolate) and given during the preanesthetic period. Many combinations are used: one example is butorphanol 0.2 mg/kg, midazolam 0.2 mg/kg, and glycopyrrolate 0.01 mg/kg (useful for sick animals

BOX 1-1 Formulas for Preanesthetic Mixtures

PREMIX
Contains per ml:

1 mg acepromazine
0.2 mg atropine
20 mg meperidine

To Make up a 20-ml Solution, Mix Together the Following:

Acepromazine	2 ml of 10 mg/ml solution = 20 mg
Atropine	8 ml of 0.5 mg/ml solution = 4 mg
Meperidine	4 ml of 100 mg/ml of solution = 400 mg

Make the mixture up to 20 ml by adding 6 ml of sterile saline.
For dosage rates for cats and dogs, see the chart below.

BAA (BUTORPHANOL-ACE-ATROPINE)
Contains per ml:

1 mg acepromazine
0.2 mg atropine
2 mg butorphanol

To Make up a 20-ml Solution, Mix Together the Following:

Acepromazine	2 ml of 10 mg/ml solution = 20 mg
Atropine	8 ml of 0.5 mg/ml solution = 4 mg
Butorphanol	4 ml of 10 mg/ml solution = 40 mg

Make the mixture up to 20 ml by adding 6 ml of sterile saline.
NOTE: Sedation is usually greater than for Premix. Alternatively, the acepromazine
can be reduced to half this dose (1 ml of 10 mg/ml solution = 10 mg, in 20 ml of
total solution) for sedation comparable to Premix. For minimal sedation or for use
in geriatric animals, reduce acepromazine to one fourth of this dose (0.5 ml of
10 mg/ml solution = 5 mg).

DOSAGE RATE FOR CATS (FOR BAA OR PREMIX)

Wt (kg)	1	2	3	4	5	6	7	8	9	10
Dose (ml)	0.2	0.35	0.45	0.55	0.65	0.75	0.85	0.95	1	1.1
Wt (kg)	1	2	3	4	5	6	7	8	9	10
Dose (ml)	0.1	0.15	0.2	0.25	0.3	0.35	0.4	0.45	0.5	0.55
Wt (kg)	11	12	13	14	15	16	17	18	19	20
Dose (ml)	0.6	0.65	0.65	0.7	0.75	0.8	0.8	0.85	0.9	0.95
Wt (kg)	21	22	23	24	25	26	27	28	29	30
Dose (ml)	0.95	1	1	1.1	1.1	1.2	1.2	1.2	1.2	1.3

BOX 1-1 Formulas for Preanesthetic Mixtures—cont'd

DOSAGE RATES FOR DOGS (FOR BAA OR PREMIX)

Wt (kg)	31	32	33	34	35	36	37	38	39	40
Dose (ml)	1.3	1.3	1.4	1.4	1.4	1.5	1.5	1.5	1.6	1.6
Wt (kg)	41	42	43	44	45	46	47	48	49	50
Dose (ml)	1.6	1.7	1.7	1.7	1.7	1.7	1.8	1.8	1.9	1.9
Wt (kg)	51	52	53	54	55	56	57	58	59	60
Dose (ml)	1.9	1.9	2	2	2	2	2.1	2.1	2.1	2.2
Wt (kg)	61	62	63	64	65	66	67	68	69	70
Dose (ml)	2.2	2.2	2.2	2.3	2.3	2.3	2.3	2.4	2.4	2.4
Wt (kg)	71	72	73	74	75	76	77	78	79	80
Dose (ml)	2.4	2.5	2.5	2.5	2.5	2.6	2.6	2.6	2.7	2.7

Data courtesy of Doris Dyson, Ontario Veterinary College, Guelph, Ontario; and Donald Sawyer, Education Services, Okemos, Mich.

but not adequate sedation for healthy patients) or butorphanol 0.2 mg/kg, atropine 0.02 mg/kg, midazolam 0.2 mg/kg, and xylazine 0.2 mg/kg.

Ideally, these drugs should be chosen on the basis of individual patient need and drawn up into a syringe immediately before use. Some practices prepare these mixtures in advance and administer a set dose by IM or SQ injection according to patient weight. (Sample formulas are given in Box 1-1.) This is more convenient than individual dosing, but there is some risk of inappropriate treatment, particularly if the patient is geriatric, debilitated, or has significant organ dysfunction (for example, liver disease).

2. Opioids are used to prevent and treat postoperative pain (see Chapter 8).
3. Opioid agents are sometimes used at higher dosages and in combination with a tranquilizer to achieve a state of profound sedation and analgesia termed *neuroleptanalgesia*. Neuroleptanalgesic combinations may be used in both the cat and dog and can be prepared within the clinic with tranquilizing agents (such as acepromazine, medetomidine, or diazepam) and opioids (such as morphine, meperidine, oxymorphone, or butorphanol). The drugs are mixed in the same syringe in some cases, or they may be injected separately by the IM or IV

route after pretreatment with atropine (separate syringes are necessary if diazepam is used). Safe use of neuroleptanalgesic agents by the IV route requires slow injection.

Combinations of drugs used to induce neuroleptanalgesia are also available commercially in some countries, for example, Hypnorm (fentanyl/fluanisone), Innovar-Vet (fentanyl/droperidol), and Immobilon (etorphine/methotrimeprazine).

Animals that are given these agents lie quietly in lateral recumbency but can be aroused by sufficient noise or surgical stimulation. Neuroleptanalgesia with an opioid/tranquilizer combination is commonly used for procedures that require significant CNS depression and analgesia but not general anesthesia. Examples include minor surgery such as porcupine quill removal and diagnostic procedures such as endoscopy or radiography. Neuroleptanalgesic combinations can also be used to induce anesthesia, especially in very sick patients (see Chapter 3). One example is oxymorphone (0.1 mg/kg) given slowly IV at the same time as 0.1 mg/kg diazepam. Two syringes are used, because these two drugs cannot be mixed together. The drugs are injected alternately, with small doses given until the animal is adequately anesthetized. Although this type of induction is slow and may cause some respiratory depression and bradycardia, it is safe for most patients, especially if the patient is subsequently intubated and ventilation is assisted. This protocol does not induce anesthesia in healthy animals, unless supplemented with an inhalation agent given by mask.

For all neuroleptanalgesic combinations, the opioid component can be reversed with naloxone or another narcotic antagonist (see p. 45). However, the tranquilizer component cannot be reversed unless a specific antagonist such as atipamezole or flumazenil is available. The ability to partially reverse neuroleptanalgesia is particularly useful in geriatric and other higher-risk patients.

Adverse effects

Because of associated side effects, opioids must be administered with caution.

1. *Effect on respiration.* One serious potential side effect of opioids is their tendency to depress respiration, particularly when used with a tranquilizing agent. Although this effect is not seen at low dose rates (such as those used for pain control), opioids given at high dose rates may cause a decrease in both respiratory rate and tidal volume, resulting in decreased blood oxygen levels (Pao_2) and increased carbon dioxide levels ($Paco_2$). This effect is particularly noticeable if the opioid is given in combination with another drug that is a respiratory depressant, such as medetomidine or inhalation agents. Respiratory depression is dose dependent for many opioid agents, meaning the effect is more pronounced at high doses. Other opioids (for example, butorphanol) show a "ceiling effect" in that high doses show no greater depression of respiration than do low doses.

   Interestingly, despite the tendency of opioids to depress respiration, some animals pant after opioid administration. This is due to a direct effect of opioids on the temperature-regulating center of the brain, which mistakenly interprets normal body temperature as being elevated.

2. *Effect on gastrointestinal function.* The effect of opioids on the gastrointestinal tract is twofold. The initial effect of many agents is an increase in peristaltic movement, resulting in diarrhea, vomiting, and flatulence. Pretreatment with atropine

or acepromazine usually moderates this effect. After the initial stimulation of peristalsis, a prolonged period of gastrointestinal stasis may occur, resulting in constipation. Because of the emetic effect of some opioid agents (particularly morphine), these drugs should be avoided in animals in which vomiting would be detrimental (for example, animals with gastrointestinal obstruction).

3. *Physical dependence (addiction).* Prolonged use of some opioid agents can lead to physical dependence. Human patients given morphine develop tolerance for its effects in approximately 2 to 3 weeks. Not all opioids are addictive: those with minimal or antagonistic activity at mu receptors (for example, butorphanol) have less potential for causing physical dependence.

4. *Drug interactions.* Some opioids, particularly meperidine, may cause fatal reactions when given to animals receiving monamine oxidase inhibitors such as selegiline (Anipryl) and should be avoided in these patients. Animals receiving tricyclic antidepressants may also undergo severe reactions when given opioids, particularly within the first 3 weeks of starting the antidepressant medication.

Other reported effects of opioid agents include the following:

- Bradycardia due to increased vagal tone (a dose-related effect that is less pronounced in animals pretreated with atropine)
- Morphine and meperidine may cause facial swelling and hypotension after rapid intravenous administration because of histamine release
- Miosis in dogs and mydriasis in cats
- Increased responsiveness to noise
- Excessive salivation
- Increased intraocular and intracranial pressure

Reversibility

One advantage of the opioid class as a whole is the reversibility of these agents. Several narcotic antagonists (reversing agents) are available, including naloxone hydrochloride, levallorphan tartrate, nalorphine hydrochloride, nalmefene, and nalbuphine. Technically, levallorphan and nalorphine are classified as mixed agonist/antagonists, whereas naloxone and nalmefene are pure antagonists. Butorphanol (a mixed agonist/antagonist) has also been used to reverse pure opioid agonists such as morphine. Of these drugs, naloxone is the preferred reversing agent because it is the most effective and causes the least respiratory depression. Opioid antagonists are effective in reversing opioid agents only and cannot be used to reverse the effects of phenothiazines, thiazine derivatives, and other nonopioid agents.

Opioid antagonists exert their effect by binding to opioid receptors and thus acting as blocking agents. By displacing other opioid agents from receptors, they reverse the agonist effect of those agents. Reversal of sedation, dysphoria, panting, respiratory depression, hypotension, bradycardia, and gastrointestinal effects occurs within minutes of IV injection of the antagonist. Unfortunately, reversal of analgesia also occurs. Reversal of analgesia can be avoided by titrating the dose of reversing agent such that respiratory depression is only partially relieved, allowing an acceptable level of analgesia to be maintained, or by using a reversing agent such as butorphanol that has, in itself, some analgesic effect.

Reversal of opioid effects through the use of an antagonist is expensive and is usually unnecessary for routine anesthesia. However, the technique is extremely useful in emergency overdose situations and rapid reversal of anesthesia in the compromised patient. They are also helpful in reviving neonates delivered by a cesarean section when the operation is performed with the patient under opioid agents. One drop of naloxone, placed under the tongue of each puppy or kitten, is usually sufficient to reverse the respiratory depression caused by fentanyl, morphine, or other opioids given to the mother.

When used as a reversal agent, naloxone is given at a dose rate of 0.04 mg/kg IV, SC, or IM, every 2 hours as needed. The calculated dose should be diluted in 10 ml of saline and slowly given IV until the desired level of reversal is achieved. The remainder of the calculated dose can then be given SC. The effects of opioid antagonists are usually observed within 30 seconds of IV injection.

Reversing agents may not remove all sedative effects in some animals, and additional doses are usually ineffective in such cases. In fact, repeated doses of some reversing agents may cause CNS and respiratory depression through overload and stimulation of opioid receptors. Occasionally, animals treated with opioid antagonists may show symptoms of sympathetic system activity, including tachycardia and cardiac arrhythmias, which can precipitate acute heart failure.

Regulatory considerations

Most opioid agents are subject to government regulation regarding purchase, handling, and dispensing. The need for detailed record keeping and the potential for abuse or theft of opioid agents are significant disadvantages of this class of drugs. In the United States, the Controlled Substances Act assigns each opioid to one of five drug schedules according to each drug's potential for abuse. In a similar way, Canadian legislation has classified each opiate as a narcotic, controlled, or prescription drug. Agents classified as narcotics in Canada or as Schedule II substances in the United States cannot be dispensed or drawn into a syringe except under the direct supervision of a licensed veterinarian. Regulated substances should be kept in a locked cabinet, safe, or other secure storage place and should not be left on countertops or in other public areas. After a dose from a bottle of controlled substance is withdrawn, the bottle should be immediately returned to locked storage. Usage must be accurately recorded in a drug logbook, and inventory must be periodically checked to ensure that no drug is unaccounted for.

KEY POINTS

1. The technician's duties during the preanesthetic period may include obtaining an adequate patient history, performing a physical examination, and performing diagnostic tests, as requested by the veterinarian.
2. Preanesthetic care of the patient may include fasting and intravenous (IV) catheterization. Preparation of equipment and administration of drugs are also the responsibility of the anesthetist.
3. No single anesthetic protocol is ideal for all patients. Rather, the anesthetic techniques and agents used are tailored to the needs of the individual patient. Factors such as previous or concurrent illness; patient age, temperament, and species; nature of the procedure; and preference of the veterinarian are all considered in determining the choice of anesthetic protocol.

4. Diagnostic tests such as the complete blood cell count (CBC) and urinalysis may provide valuable information regarding the patient's ability to tolerate anesthesia. Procedures such as radiography and electrocardiography also may be useful in selected patients but are not done on a routine basis.

5. The risk of anesthesia to the patient should be assessed before initiating the procedure. The patient should be assigned to a class on the basis of physical condition, as outlined by the American Society of Anesthesiologists.

6. The patient should be in stable condition, when possible, before being anesthetized; preexisting problems such as dehydration or shock should be corrected.

7. Although IV catheterization offers enhanced patient safety and convenience for the anesthetist, this procedure is associated with the risk of accidental overhydration. A fluid infusion rate of 10 ml/kg/hr is considered safe for most patients.

8. Preanesthetic agents increase the safety and convenience of anesthesia by reducing the dose of general anesthetic needed, by preventing bradycardia and other parasympathetic effects, and by reducing patient stress and discomfort. All preanesthetic agents, however, have side effects that may be harmful in some patients.

9. Anticholinergics (such as atropine and glycopyrrolate) help prevent bradycardia, bronchoconstriction, excessive salivation, and gastrointestinal activity. Anticholinergic agents may be harmful when used in animals with preexisting tachycardia, constipation, or ileus.

10. Tranquilizing agents include phenothiazines, benzodiazepines, and alpha-2 agonists. Phenothiazines have a wide margin of safety but may cause hypotension in some patients. Benzodiazepines have a calming effect on geriatric and debilitated animals and are excellent for prevention and treatment of seizures. Alpha-2 agonists are potent sedatives and produce excellent muscle relaxation but may cause serious cardiovascular and respiratory complications in some patients.

11. Opioids may be used as preanesthetic agents, as induction agents, as postoperative analgesics, and (in combination with tranquilizers) as neuroleptanalgesics. Their greatest advantage is the profound analgesia they produce in most patients. They have the potential to cause adverse effects on the cardiovascular, respiratory, and gastrointestinal systems, and prolonged administration may be associated with addiction. Their use is subject to government regulation regarding purchase, handling, and dispensing.

12. The action of some preanesthetic agents may be reversed through the use of specific agents such as yohimbine, atipamezole, and naloxone.

REVIEW QUESTIONS

1. Given the busy nature of a veterinary practice, it is probably best to assume that the same anesthetic protocol should be used on all patients.
   True   False
2. The following question would be a good example of how to ask a question: "Your dog does not exercise much, does he, Mrs. Jones?"
   True   False
3. Dogs and cats may differ in how they react to or metabolize a drug.
   True   False
4. An obese dog will require more anesthetic than a normal-weight dog of the same breed.
   True   False
5. Blood tests such as ALT have minimal value for an anesthetist.
   True   False
6. It is always best to withhold food and water from any patient scheduled to receive a general anesthetic for at least 12 hours before the scheduled procedure.
   True   False
7. Which of the following is not a crystalloid solution?
   a. Lactated Ringer's solution
   b. Normal saline solution
   c. Dextran
   d. 5% dextrose
8. Which of the following is not a valid reason for administering a preanesthetic medication?
   a. It reduces the amount of general anesthetic required for induction.
   b. It may calm an excited animal.
   c. It may reduce possible adverse side effects from the general anesthetic.
   d. It increases patient safety by allowing the animal to stay under the general anesthetic for a longer time.
9. Most preanesthetics will not cross the placental barrier.
   True   False
10. It is recommended that atropine not be given to an animal that has tachycardia.
    True   False
11. Anticholinergic drugs such as atropine block the release of acetylcholine at the:
    a. Muscarinic receptors of the parasympathetic system
    b. Nicotinic receptors of the parasympathetic system
    c. Muscarinic receptors of the sympathetic system
    d. Nicotinic receptors of the sympathetic system
12. Phenothiazine tranquilizers such as acepromazine sedate the animal and give some analgesia.
    True   False

13. High doses of opioids can cause bradycardia and respiratory depression.
　　True　　　　　　　False

14. A patient that is anemic or moderately dehydrated would be classified as a

　　_____ anesthetic risk.
　　a. Class I
　　b. Class II
　　c. Class III
　　d. Class IV
　　e. Class V

15. Severe bradycardia after the use of medetomidine should be treated with the following drug:
　　a. Atropine
　　b. Naloxone
　　c. Epinephrine
　　d. Atipamezole

For the following questions, more than one answer may be correct.

16. The suggested minimum database for any patient may include:
　　a. History
　　b. Physical examination
　　c. Diagnostic tests
　　d. Name of the required procedure

17. Which of the following are alpha-2 agonists?
　　a. Atipamezole
　　b. Xylazine
　　c. Acepromazine
　　d. Medetomidine

18. Effects that atropine may have on the body include:
　　a. Decreased salivation
　　b. Increased vagal tone
　　c. Decreased gastrointestinal motility
　　d. Mydriasis

19. Effects that are commonly seen after premedication with the phenothiazine tranquilizers include:
　　a. Sedation
　　b. Antiarrhythmic effect
　　c. Peripheral vasodilation
　　d. Reduced salivation

20. Characteristic effects of the benzodiazepines include:
　　a. Pronounced sedation in healthy young animals
　　b. Muscle relaxation
　　c. Significant decrease in respiratory function
　　d. Minimal effect on cardiovascular system

21. Physical effects that may be seen after administration of xylazine include:
    a. Bradycardia
    b. Mydriasis
    c. Bloat
    d. Hypoventilation
    e. Vomiting
22. Effects of opioid administration include the following:
    a. Analgesia
    b. Increased sensitivity to noise
    c. Panting
    d. Decreased tear production
23. Opioids may be reversed with:
    a. Atipamezole
    b. Naloxone
    c. Atropine
    d. Yohimbine
24. Which of the following drugs will precipitate out when mixed with other drugs or solutions?
    a. Atropine
    b. Acepromazine
    c. Diazepam
    d. Butorphanol
25. A neuroleptanalgesic is a combination of:
    a. An opioid and an anticholinergic
    b. An anticholinergic and a tranquilizer
    c. An opioid and a tranquilizer
    d. An anticholinergic and a benzodiazepine

ANSWERS FOR CHAPTER 1

1. False	**2.** False	**3.** True	**4.** False	**5.** False
6. False	**7.** c	**8.** d	**9.** False	**10.** True
11. a	**12.** False	**13.** True	**14.** c	**15.** d
16. a, b, c, d	**17.** b, d	**18.** a, c, d	**19.** a, b, c	**20.** b, d
21. a, c, d, e	**22.** a, b, c	**23.** b	**24.** c	**25.** c

Selected Readings

Haskins SC: Opinions in small animal anesthesia, *Vet Clin North Am Small Anim Pract* 22:326-469, 1992.

Ko JCH: Anesthetic potency: how to use medetomidine and atipamezole, *Vet Tech* 18:695-702, 1997.

Mama K: New drugs in feline anesthesia, *Compendium* 20(2):125-137, 1998.

Muir WW III, Hubbell JAE, Skarda RT, et al: *Handbook of veterinary anesthesia,* ed 3, St Louis, 2000, Mosby.

Paddleford RR: *Manual of small animal anesthesia,* Philadelphia, 1999, WB Saunders.

Paddleford RR, Harvey RC: Alpha-2 agonists and antagonists, *Vet Clin North Am Small Anim Pract* 29:737-746, 1999.

Short CE: *Principles and practice of veterinary anesthesia,* Baltimore, 1987, Williams & Wilkins.

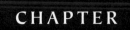

CHAPTER *2*

General Anesthesia

PERFORMANCE OBJECTIVES

After completion of this chapter, the reader will be able to:
- Define or explain the following terms: *general anesthesia, balanced anesthesia, titration, induction, endotracheal intubation, hypoventilation, hyperventilation, tachypnea, apneustic breathing, hypostatic congestion, atelectasis, cyanosis, bagging, anatomic dead space, mechanical dead space, laryngospasm, hypertension, hypotension, vital sign,* and *reflex.*
- Identify and describe the components of general anesthesia, including the various stages and planes.
- Understand the techniques, advantages, and disadvantages of intravenous (IV), intramuscular (IM), and inhalation anesthesia.
- Describe the technique of endotracheal intubation and understand the benefits and hazards of this procedure.
- Understand the importance of monitoring an anesthetized patient and be able to effectively and safely monitor an anesthetized patient.
- Describe appropriate ways to position an animal during anesthesia.
- Describe the various tasks that need to be performed during the recovery period.
- Understand the concept of patient safety as it relates to general anesthetics.

Through the use of the preanesthetic drugs described in Chapter 1, the anesthetist is able to profoundly sedate and provide analgesia for the small animal patient. This level of central nervous system (CNS) depression is adequate for minor procedures; however, a state of general anesthesia is usually required to provide sufficient analgesia and muscle relaxation for major operations. This chapter describes the components of general anesthesia, including induction, maintenance, and recovery. The classical stages and planes of general anesthesia and the anesthetic procedures and monitoring associated with each stage are also described.

DEFINITION OF GENERAL ANESTHESIA

General anesthesia is a state of controlled and reversible unconsciousness achieved through the use of injectable and/or inhaled drugs and characterized by the absence of pain perception, memory, motor response to stimuli, or reflex responses. Ideally, this state is achieved without significantly affecting the patient's vital systems, particularly respiration and circulation. Safe anesthesia is achieved through appropriate selection of drugs, careful administration, and constant monitoring.

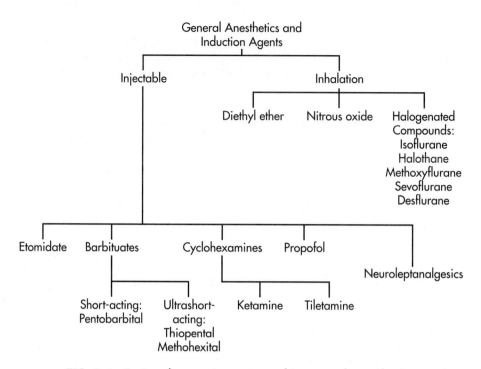

FIG. 2-1   Past and present agents used in general anesthesia.

In any given patient, general anesthesia may be accomplished through the use of injectable anesthetics, inhalation anesthetics, or both (Fig. 2-1). *Injectable anesthetics* include barbiturates (for example, thiopental, methohexital, and pentobarbital); cyclo-hexamines (for example, ketamine, tiletamine); propofol; and etomidate. Neuroleptanalgesic agents may also be used to induce anesthesia. *Inhalation anesthetics* used in veterinary medicine include halothane, isoflurane, sevoflurane, desflurane, and nitrous oxide. Patients may be anesthetized with one drug or with several agents used in combination in a technique called *balanced anesthesia*. This chapter describes the characteristics of general anesthesia, and the properties, advantages, and disadvantages of specific agents are discussed in detail in Chapter 3.

COMPONENTS OF GENERAL ANESTHESIA

General anesthesia is achieved through the use of techniques and agents chosen by the veterinarian that is called the *anesthetic protocol*. As discussed in Chapter 1, the choice of anesthetic protocol for any animal varies according to such variables as temperament and physical status of the patient, nature of the procedure to be done, cost and availability of various drugs, and preference of the veterinarian. Regardless of the anesthetic protocol chosen, any anesthetic procedure may be divided into the following components: preanesthesia, induction, maintenance, and recovery.

Preanesthesia

The preanesthetic period is the time immediately preceding anesthesia in which patient data are collected, the patient is fasted and adequate hydration ensured, and preanesthetic drugs are administered. This period is discussed in Chapter 1.

Induction

The process by which an animal leaves the normal conscious state and enters an unconscious state is known as *induction*. Usually the induction process is initiated only after the animal has received premedication drugs as ordered by the veterinarian and enough time has lapsed for these drugs to take effect. The minimum time is 10 minutes if the drugs are given through the intramuscular (IM) route and 20 minutes if the subcutaneous (SC) route is used. Occasionally, premedications and induction agents may be administered simultaneously (for example, when acepromazine, atropine, and ketamine are mixed in a syringe and given intravenously to a cat).

The induction agent may be administered to the patient either by injection or inhalation. When injection is used, it is often followed by intubation with an endotracheal tube to allow the administration of an inhalation (gas) anesthetic by means of an anesthetic machine. Alternatively, the animal may be directly induced by means of a gas anesthetic delivered by a mask or anesthetic chamber, in which case no injectable anesthetic is necessary.

Initially the animal may show signs of incoordination or excitement, followed by progressive relaxation and unconsciousness. Ideally, excitement and struggling should be avoided during induction, because this is unpleasant for the patient and predisposes the animal to cardiac arrhythmias and perivascular drug injection. The onset of general anesthesia is also characterized by the loss of some protective reflexes, including the ability to swallow and cough.

Maintenance

After the induction period, the animal enters the maintenance period, during which sufficient anesthetic is supplied to keep the patient at an appropriate depth of anesthesia. Surgery and other procedures are commonly performed during this period. As with induction, a predictable sequence of events occurs during the maintenance period, including the onset of analgesia, skeletal muscle relaxation and cessation of movement, further loss of protective reflexes including the palpebral (eye blink) reflex, and the occurrence of mild respiratory and cardiovascular depression. If anesthetic depth increases, the patient may show more severe respiratory and cardiovascular depression, and in the unusual event of an anesthetic overdose, respiratory and cardiac arrest can occur. Close monitoring is essential throughout this period.

Recovery

The maintenance period ends and recovery begins when the concentration of anesthetic in the brain begins to decrease. The method by which the anesthetic is eliminated from the brain and circulatory system varies according to the anesthetic agent:
- Most injectable drugs are removed from the blood by the liver and undergo metabolism by liver enzymes. The metabolites are excreted by the urinary system. Some drugs do not undergo metabolism and are excreted unchanged by the kidneys (for example, ketamine in the cat).

- In the case of short-acting thiobarbiturates, the level of anesthetic in the brain falls as the drug is rapidly redistributed to other tissues, especially muscle and fat. This redistribution results in lower levels of the drug in the brain and thus the arousal of the patient. In this case, the patient awakens from the anesthetic even though the drug is still present in the body.
- Inhalation agents are eliminated mainly through the respiratory tract. Anesthetic molecules leave the brain, entering first the blood and then the alveoli of the lung, and are exhaled.
- Recovery from either injectable or inhalation anesthesia may be hastened by the action of analeptic agents such as doxapram. Some injectable agents (for example, opioids, medetomidine, and xylazine) have specific reversing agents, as discussed in Chapter 1.

However it is achieved, recovery from anesthesia is in many respects the reverse of the induction process. Reflex activity, muscle tone, and sensitivity to pain are regained as consciousness returns.

SAFETY OF GENERAL ANESTHESIA

General anesthesia is not without risk. The administration of any anesthetic may affect the patient's vital centers, which are the areas of the brain that control cardio-vascular and respiratory function and thermoregulation. Death may occur if the activity of these centers is not maintained throughout anesthesia. Every anesthetized patient is at risk of serious complications such as hypotension (decreased blood pressure), hypoventilation (decreased respiratory rate and/or volume), hypoxia (decreased availability of oxygen to the tissues), and hypothermia (low body temperature). It is therefore vitally important that the animal be closely monitored during induction, maintenance, and recovery from any general anesthetic to detect complications of anesthesia at the earliest possible point. Monitoring by a trained individual is the single most important factor in preventing serious anesthetic problems. Particular attention should be focused on heart rate, pulse quality, ventilation, mucous membrane color, and perfusion (capillary refill).

The anesthetist may use several strategies to increase the safety of anesthesia and minimize the adverse effects of general anesthetic agents:

- The patient's history, physical examination findings, and laboratory data should be evaluated before selecting the anesthetic protocol. The routine use of a single, standard protocol for all patients should be discouraged.
- If possible, significant physiologic abnormalities such as dehydration, hypotension, and anemia should be corrected before anesthesia.
- Preanesthetic drugs such as atropine or acepromazine may be given to prevent cardiac abnormalities such as bradycardia and cardiac arrhythmias during general anesthesia.
- Preanesthetic sedatives such as acepromazine, alpha-2 agonists, and opioids help reduce the dose of general anesthetic required to induce and maintain anesthesia, thus minimizing the adverse effects of the general anesthetic agent. In some patients, multiple general anesthetic and preanesthetic agents (such as a combination of nitrous oxide, an opioid, and a muscle relaxant) may be used in a balanced anesthesia technique to further minimize the required dose of each agent used.
- All injectable drug dosages should be double-checked before administration to the animal, and the anesthetist should ensure that the concentration of an agent

drawn into a syringe is the same as that used for the drug calculations. It is a good idea to label all syringes containing injectable anesthetic agents with the name of the patient, the name of the drug, and the drug concentration.

- When inducing an animal or maintaining an animal already under anesthesia, the anesthetist should administer only the minimum dose of drug needed to achieve the desired level of anesthesia. Many injectable agents are given "to effect," which means that only the amount of injectable anesthetic necessary to produce unconsciousness is given, rather than administering the entire dose calculated on a milligram per kilogram basis. This technique is necessary because the amount of drug needed to induce or maintain anesthesia cannot be accurately predicted for a given patient. In fact, the dose needed is affected by many patient factors, including age, breed, physical condition, and liver and kidney function. For example, the amount of thiobarbiturate required to induce a quiet, older dog may be one half or less of the dose required for an active 2-year-old dog, even though the dogs weigh the same. Similarly, a cat with a urinary obstruction may be deeply anesthetized after receiving less than 10 mg of intravenous (IV) ketamine, whereas a healthy cat may require 30 mg of IV ketamine to reach the same depth of anesthesia.

  The drugs used for premedication also affect the dose of general anesthetic required. For example, a patient that has not received any premedications may require 15 mg/kg of body weight of thiopental to induce it to a moderate plane of anesthesia, whereas a patient that has been premedicated with a tranquilizer and an opioid analgesic (for example, acepromazine and hydromorphone) may be induced to a comparable plane of anesthesia with only 5 mg/kg of thiopental.

  Because the anesthetist can seldom predict the exact dose that a given patient will require, it is safer to give the drug as a series of bolus injections, observing the animal for signs of anesthesia and discontinuing the administration of anesthetic when the desired depth is reached. This process is known as *titration*.

  Just as the amount of drug required to induce anesthesia varies among patients, so the amount of inhalation or injectable agent required to maintain anesthesia also varies. At a given concentration of halothane gas, for example, one patient may show brisk reflexes and appear to be only lightly anesthetized, whereas another may show the absence of all reflexes and a relatively slow heart rate, indicating deep anesthesia. The knowledgeable anesthetist monitors the patient closely and alters the amount of anesthetic given to suit the patient's requirements, rather than relying solely on a calculated dose recommended by a textbook.

- Endotracheal intubation is recommended for patients undergoing general anesthesia because it allows the anesthetist to efficiently administer oxygen (even if the patient is breathing poorly or not at all) and protects the airway from aspiration or obstruction.

- Close observation of a patient during the recovery period is also critical. Various untoward events, such as vomiting, laryngospasm, and seizures, may occur during this time. Problems that may be encountered during the recovery period are described in Chapter 6.

CLASSICAL STAGES AND PLANES OF ANESTHESIA

During the course of general anesthesia, the animal passes through a series of anesthetic stages and planes roughly correlated with changes in anesthetic depth.

With the induction of anesthesia, the patient enters stage I. As anesthetic depth increases, the animal passes through stage II and stage III (the anesthetic depth most appropriate for surgical procedures) and in some cases may enter stage IV. As the animal passes through each stage, there is a progressive loss of pain perception, motor coordination, consciousness, reflex responses, muscle tone, and (eventually) cardiopulmonary function. These stages and planes are summarized in Table 2-1. Although they were first developed on the basis of work done with the anesthetic agent diethyl ether, the stages may be adapted to describe the effect of other agents, including inhalation and some injectable anesthetics. The signs listed in the table vary somewhat, depending on the agent used and the individual patient's response.

Stage I

Immediately after the administration of an inhalation or injectable agent, the animal enters the initial stage of anesthesia, stage I. Animals in this stage are conscious but disoriented and show reduced sensitivity to pain. Respiration and heart rate are normal or increased, and all reflexes are present. The patient is still awake and may show struggling, urination, defecation, and other signs of fear or anxiety.

Stage II

Stage II begins with the loss of consciousness. All reflexes are still present and in fact may appear exaggerated. The animal is able to chew and swallow, and yawning is common. The pupils are dilated but will constrict in response to intense light.

As the higher centers of the brain release voluntary control of body functions, the animal may exhibit involuntary excitement in the form of rapid movement of the limbs, vocalization, and struggling. Breathing may be irregular, or the animal may appear to be holding its breath. Although animals in stage II may appear to be "fighting" the anesthesia, the actions are not under conscious control. Rather, they are thought to occur because the anesthetic selectively depresses neurons in the brain that normally inhibit and control the function of motor neurons.

Stage II is unpleasant for the animal and potentially hazardous to hospital personnel. There is a risk of epinephrine release and the possibility of cardiac arrhythmias or arrest. The struggling patient may injure itself, the restrainer, or the anesthetist. Therefore it is desirable that the induction be planned to avoid this stage or quickly pass through it, by continuing the administration of anesthetic until stage III is reached. In fact, premedicated animals that are rapidly induced with an injectable anesthetic usually seem to pass directly from stage I to stage III. Although these patients pass through stage II, it is not clinically evident. Stage II ends when the animal shows signs of muscle relaxation, slower respiration rate, and decreased reflex activity.

Stage III

The third stage is subdivided into four planes, representing increasing anesthetic depth from plane 1 through plane 4. In plane 1 the respiratory pattern becomes regular, and involuntary limb movements cease. The eyeballs start to rotate ventrally, the pupils may become partially constricted, and the pupillary response to bright light is diminished. The gagging and swallowing reflexes are depressed such that an endotracheal tube may be successfully passed, allowing the patient to

TABLE 2-1

Depth Indicators of Anesthetic Stages and Planes

STAGE OF ANESTHESIA	BEHAVIOR	RESPIRATION	CARDIOVASCULAR FUNCTION	RESPONSE TO SURGERY	DEPTH	EYE POSITION	PUPIL SIZE	PUPIL RESPONSE TO LIGHT	MUSCLE TONE	REFLEX RESPONSE
I	Disoriented	Normal, may be panting; respiration rate 20-30 breaths/min	Heart rate unchanged	Struggle	Not anesthetized	Central	Normal	Yes	Good	All present
II "Excitement stage"	Excitement: struggling, vocalization, paddling, chewing, yawning	Irregular, may hold breath or hyperventilate	Heart rate may increase	Struggle	Not anesthetized	Central, may be nystagmus	May be dilated	Yes	Good	All present, may be exaggerated
III— PLANE 1 Light anesthesia	Anesthetized	Regular; rate 12-20 breaths/min	Pulse strong; Heart rate >90 bpm	May respond with movement	Light	Central or rotated, may be nystagmus	Normal	Yes	Good	Swallowing poor or absent, others present but diminished
III— PLANE 2 Medium (surgical anesthesia)		Regular (may be shallow); rate 12-16 breaths/min	Heart rate >90 bpm	Heart and respiration rates may increase	Moderate	Often rotated ventrally	Slightly dilated	Sluggish	Relaxed	Patellar, ear flick, palpebral, and corneal may be present; others absent
III— PLANE 3 Deep anesthesia		Shallow; rate <12 breaths/min	Heart rate 60-90 bpm; CRT increased; pulse less strong	None	Deep	Usually central, may rotate ventrally	Moderately dilated	Very sluggish or absent	Greatly reduced	All reflexes diminished or absent
III— PLANE 4		Jerky	Heart rate <60 bpm; prolonged CRT; pale mucous membranes	None	Overdose	Central	Widely dilated	Unresponsive	Flaccid	No reflex activity
IV	Moribund	Apnea	Cardiovascular collapse	None	Dying	Central	Widely dilated	Unresponsive	Flaccid	No reflex activity

be connected to a gas anesthetic machine. Other reflexes (such as the palpebral reflex) are present; however, responses are less brisk than in stage II. Although appearing to be unconscious, the patient will not tolerate surgical procedures at this light plane of anesthesia and will move, exhibit increased heart and respiratory rates, or otherwise react to a painful stimulus.

Animals in plane 2 of stage III are generally considered to be at medium depth of anesthesia, suitable for most surgical procedures. Surgical stimulation may evoke a mild response such as increased heart rate or respiration rate, but the patient usually remains unconscious and immobile. The pupillary light response is sluggish, the eyeballs may be central or rotated, and the pupils are slightly dilated. The respirations are regular but shallow, with a respiratory rate between 12 and 16 breaths per minute in the dog and slightly higher in the cat. Heart rate and blood pressure are mildly decreased. The skeletal muscle tone becomes more relaxed, and many of the normal protective reflexes (for example, pedal, laryngeal, and palpebral) are diminished or lost.

In plane 3 of stage III, the patient appears to be deeply anesthetized. Significant depression of circulation and respiration is often present, and for this reason plane 3 is considered to be excessively deep for most surgical procedures. In the dog or cat, the respiratory rate is less than 12 breaths per minute, and respirations are shallow. Ventilation assistance in the form of "bagging" with the reservoir bag or assistance from a mechanical ventilator may be desirable in some patients. Heart rate is also notably reduced in patients at this plane, even in the presence of surgical stimulation. Pulse strength may be reduced because of a fall in blood pressure. The capillary refill time (CRT) may be increased to 1.5 to 2 seconds. The pupillary light reflex is poor throughout this plane and may be absent. The eyeballs become central, and the pupils are moderately dilated. Reflex activity is often totally absent. Skeletal muscle relaxation is marked to the degree that no resistance occurs when the mouth is opened (that is, jaw tone is slack).

Plane 4 of stage III can be recognized by a "rocking" ventilatory pattern in which the abdominal muscles are increasingly responsible for ventilation while the thoracic muscles become less active. The overall effect is a decrease in effective ventilation. Plane 4 is also characterized by fully dilated pupils and the absence of a pupillary light reflex. The eyes may be dry because of the absence of lacrimal secretions. Muscle tone is flaccid. More important, there is obvious depression of the cardiovascular system as marked by a dramatic drop in heart rate and blood pressure, accompanied by pale mucous membranes and a prolonged CRT. The patient in this plane is too deeply anesthetized for safety and is in danger of respiratory and cardiac arrest.

Stage IV

If anesthetic depth is increased past stage III, plane 4, the animal enters stage IV of anesthesia. At this stage there is a cessation of respiration, which may be followed by circulatory collapse and death. Immediate resuscitation is necessary to save the patient's life.

Overview of Anesthetic Stages and Planes

Although these stages and planes appear easy to differentiate on paper, they are not well defined in every animal. A given patient may show some signs that indicate stage III, plane 2, anesthesia and other signs that indicate stage III, plane 3. The anesthetist must assess as many variables as possible to come to a conclusion about the patient's depth of anesthesia (see p. 104 for examples of depth assessment). The anesthetist must also be aware that some agents (notably, ketamine and tiletamine) do not affect the CNS in the same manner as inhalants and injectables such as barbiturates do, and therefore the anesthetic stages and planes are difficult to recognize with these drugs. The appearance of the anesthetic stages and planes also varies among inhalation anesthetic agents. For example, halothane may cause bradycardia at a surgical plane, but isoflurane has minimal effect on heart rate.

What, then, is the ideal depth of anesthesia? This question has no easy answer. The anesthetist must ensure that the patient does not perceive a surgical stimulus. At the same time, the anesthetist must avoid excessive anesthetic depth, which may result in depression of the cardiovascular and respiratory systems. When in doubt about the depth of anesthesia, it is usually safer for the patient if the anesthetist decreases or stops the administration of anesthetic by turning down the vaporizer or stopping the injection of anesthetic. The patient should then be closely monitored to ensure that an appropriate depth has been achieved.

INDUCTION TECHNIQUES AND AGENTS
Injectable Agents

Anesthesia may be induced by IV or IM injection of general anesthetic agents.

Intravenous injection

One of the most common induction methods involves the IV injection of an anesthetic drug. Thiopental sodium, ketamine, propofol, etomidate, and oxymorphone/acepromazine are examples of inducing agents that are given intravenously. Typically, a standard dose of the agent is calculated and drawn into a syringe (or, in the case of some agents used in large animals, the agent is administered through an IV bag), then injected as needed directly into the vein, or into a butterfly catheter or indwelling catheter. The goal is for the patient to pass rapidly and safely through the first two stages of anesthesia and reach a depth that allows endotracheal intubation without resistance (stage III, plane I). A detailed outline of several induction techniques is given in Procedure 2-1. Once intubated, the animal may be maintained at a moderate or a deep level of anesthesia through the administration of an inhalation anesthetic. The use of inhalation anesthetic is not always necessary because minor surgical and short diagnostic procedures (such as porcupine quill removal or radiography) often can be performed with the patient under injectable anesthesia alone.

If a single bolus of inducing agent is given, the duration of anesthesia varies with the injectable agent used, but is usually less than 20 minutes. If necessary, anesthesia may be prolonged by repeated administration of the intravenous agent. However, with the exception of propofol and etomidate, repeated dosing is generally discouraged because it may lead to the accumulation of large amounts of anesthetic within the body and result in a prolonged recovery. If more than 20 minutes of anesthesia are required, it is usually preferable to maintain anesthesia with gas inhalation anesthetics.

Another method for administering injectable agents by the IV route is by constant infusion. A dose of the agent sufficient to maintain anesthesia for the

PROCEDURE 2-1   Intravenous Induction of Anesthesia

The method of administering an intravenous (IV) drug for the purpose of IV induction varies depending on the agent used and the veterinarian's preference. In most cases, the patient is premedicated with a tranquilizer (and in some cases, an anticholinergic). Premedication reduces the dose of anesthetic required and allows smoother induction. Whenever possible, the dose of general anesthetic should be titrated so that the patient receives only the minimum amount necessary to induce anesthesia.

1. Thiopental: To reduce the chance of sloughing from perivascular injection of a thiobarbiturate, use an indwelling catheter (see Fig. 1-3). Alternatively, skilled anesthetists may use a needle and syringe, using care to stay within the vein. Inject one half of the calculated dose over a 10- to 15-second period (bolus injection). This technique allows rapid induction of stage III anesthesia with minimal stage II excitement. If intubation is not possible after 45 seconds after injection, a second dose (one fourth of the calculated dose) may be given. This method of administration is continued until the desired depth is reached. The patient can usually be intubated within 3 minutes of the initial injection. Use caution in patients with systemic disorders (such as acidosis or hypoproteinemia) because they may require a much smaller dose than healthy patients. Reduce doses and give injections slowly in these patients.

2. Ketamine/tranquilizer mixtures: In contrast to the bolus induction technique used with barbiturates, ketamine mixtures (that is, ketamine/diazepam, ketamine/ acepromazine, ketamine/medetomidine, and ketamine/xylazine) can be injected slowly (over 30 to 60 seconds). Slow injection minimizes the toxic effects of these anesthetic agents on the cardiovascular and respiratory systems. If a bolus injection technique is preferred, one third to one half of the calculated dose of ketamine/ diazepam can be given IV over a 15- to 30-second period, with further increments every 45 seconds until the desired depth is reached.

3. Propofol can be given by slow IV injection (one third to one half of the calculated dose every 30 seconds) to induce anesthesia. More rapid induction may be useful in uncooperative patients, but is more likely to induce apnea. However, if injection of propofol is too slow, excitement may be seen.

---

entire surgical period is drawn into a large syringe and placed in a syringe pump. After an induction bolus is given, the contents of the syringe are gradually expelled by the pump into a tube connected to an IV catheter. The drug is infused at a constant rate that maintains the correct anesthetic depth. If the drug is given by constant infusion rather than by periodic boluses, a constant level of drug in the bloodstream is maintained. This method of administration is most suited to anesthetics such as propofol and analgesics such as fentanyl, which do not accumulate in body fat stores and are metabolized rapidly.

If necessary, an injectable anesthetic or analgesic can be given during a surgery to supplement inhalation anesthetics. If a patient shows a response to a painful surgical stimulus or if the patient is waking prematurely, small doses of an injectable agent can be given IV to rapidly deepen the anesthetic plane.

Intramuscular injection

Some induction agents, including ketamine and tiletamine-zolazepam (Telazol), may be administered by IM injection. This method is useful for animals in which IV injections are difficult, such as ferrets and very young puppies and kittens. Inhalant induction through the use of a mask or anesthetic chamber is an alternative way of inducing anesthesia in these animals.

Intramuscular agents are also useful in anesthesia of animals that cannot be handled easily and in which IV or mask induction is difficult (for example, aggressive domestic animals, wild animals, and captive animals in zoos). Because it is difficult to approach and handle these animals, the agent is usually administered by means of a blowpipe or tranquilizing gun or through the use of restraint equipment such as a squeeze cage or rabies pole. Agents that can be administered by this method include ketamine/medetomidine mixtures, tiletamine/zolazepam, neuroleptanalgesics, and opiates (particularly etorphine and carfentanil).

Induction by IM injection differs from IV induction in several important respects:

1. For most agents, the anesthesia dose required for induction by IM injection is 2 to 3 times the IV induction dose.
2. One disadvantage of IM induction is that the dose cannot be titrated or given "to effect." Usually the entire calculated dose is given at once.
3. Drugs administered by the IM route require several minutes to reach the brain and accumulate at a concentration high enough to induce anesthesia. IM induction of anesthesia is therefore characterized by a relatively slow onset of anesthesia compared with IV induction. Occasionally, IM injections may deposit the drug in a fascial plane between muscles, resulting in even slower or incomplete absorption.
4. IM administration is characterized by a lengthy recovery period because the animal requires considerable time to metabolize the relatively large dose of drug given by this route.

The characteristics of IM and IV anesthesia are illustrated by the use of ketamine in cats. When ketamine is given intravenously at a dose of 5 mg/kg, induction of anesthesia occurs in less than 1 minute. Alternatively, the drug can be given intramuscularly at a dose of 15 mg/kg, inducing anesthesia in 3 to 5 minutes. Recovery from IV ketamine administration is usually rapid, and healthy animals often appear fully recovered within 1 to 2 hours. In contrast, complete recovery from IM ketamine administration may require 8 to 12 hours.

Other routes of administration of injectable agents include SC, rectal, and intraperitoneal. Except for very small or difficult-to-handle patients, these routes are considered too slow or impractical for routine use.

Oral administration

Anesthesia may result when some agents (for example, ketamine) are given orally. This route of administration constitutes extra-label use of these agents. Oral administration is not used routinely, but it may be appropriate in some situations.

Typically, a single dose of the agent is drawn into a syringe and forcefully squirted into the animal's mouth. Care should be taken to avoid aspiration of the material by the patient or contact with the eyes. Alternatively, the agent can be mixed with a small amount of palatable food.

Inhalation Agents

Induction of anesthesia may be achieved through the use of rapid-acting inhalation anesthetics, such as isoflurane, halothane, or sevoflurane. Nitrous oxide is occasionally used to supplement the anesthetic effect of other inhalation agents. The gas anesthetic contained in an anesthetic machine is administered to an awake patient by means of a face mask or anesthetic chamber. Induction with inhalation agents is much more gradual than IV induction with an injectable agent.

Mask induction

The technique for mask induction is described in Procedure 2-2 and illustrated in Fig. 2-2. Mask induction is well suited for use with rapid-acting inhalation anesthetics, such as isoflurane or sevoflurane, but is more difficult to achieve with a slower-acting anesthetic, such as halothane. Mask induction may be more suitable for critical patients than induction with injectable agents because the anesthetist can quickly control the animal's depth by adjusting the vaporizer setting. If problems arise, induction can be discontinued immediately.

There are several cautions associated with the use of this technique for induction:

- One drawback of mask induction is the potential for significant operating room pollution. Waste anesthetic gas readily leaks around the mask and is

---

PROCEDURE 2-2   Mask Induction

1. Use either a malleable black rubber mask or a clear plastic mask with a rubber diaphragm for mask induction. The mask should fit tightly on the animal's face to reduce leakage of waste gas and to minimize dead space.
2. Connect the mask to the Y piece of an anesthetic machine and hold in place over the animal's muzzle (Fig. 2-2).
3. Give 100% oxygen for 2 to 3 minutes to allow the patient to adjust to the mask and to increase the amount of oxygen in the blood.
4. Set the anesthetic vaporizer to deliver 0.5% isoflurane or 1% sevoflurane. The oxygen flow rate should be set at 30 times the patient's tidal volume, or a minimum of 3 to 4 L/min (because higher flow rates help speed induction).
5. Gradually increase the concentration of anesthetic by small increments (for example, increasing the isoflurane vaporizer setting by 0.5% every 30 seconds) until an anesthetic concentration of 3% to 4% is reached for isoflurane or halothane and 8% for sevoflurane. This is higher than the expected maintenance level but allows a rapid uptake of the anesthetic and a faster induction. The slow increase in concentration helps to prevent cardiac arrhythmias and allows the animal to become accustomed to the smell of the anesthetic. Sevoflurane is less pungent than isoflurane and better accepted.
6. This method is often well accepted by cats and small dogs, although some struggling may be seen after 2 to 3 minutes when isoflurane is given, possibly corresponding to stage II excitement. Induction of stage III, plane 1, anesthesia usually requires 5 to 10 minutes, depending on the agent used.

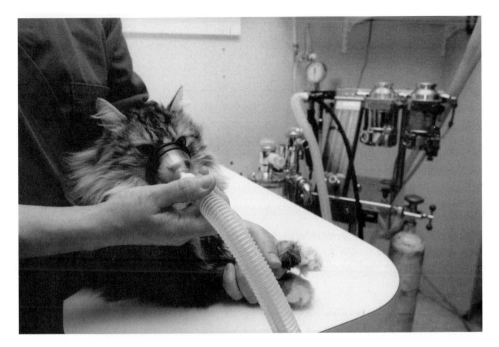

FIG. 2-2   Mask induction of a cat.

released into the room air. It is helpful to use a mask that fits snugly over the patient's face and to ensure that there is adequate room ventilation to prevent inhalation of waste gas by hospital personnel (see Chapter 5).

- Another potential drawback is the risk of stressing the patient if the animal resists the use of a mask. Struggling may cause the release of epinephrine, which predisposes the patient to potentially fatal cardiac arrhythmias. To avoid this, use mask induction only on a calm or sedated patient.
- Because of the slow induction time, mask induction may not be appropriate for patients with poor respiratory function (for example, upper airway disease or obstruction, difficult breathing due to brachycephalic conformation, diaphragmatic hernia, pleural effusion, or pulmonary edema). Rapid induction with an injectable agent and immediate endotracheal intubation are preferred in these patients. Mask induction is also unsuitable for unfasted patients and other patients at risk of vomiting during the induction procedure.
- The anesthetist must ensure that the mask does not occlude the patient's nostrils, as might happen with a cat or brachycephalic patient if the mask is too tight.

It is possible to maintain anesthesia with a mask throughout the surgical procedure. However, many anesthetists prefer to intubate the patient with an endotracheal tube after induction because this method offers protection against aspiration or airway obstruction.

Anesthetic chamber induction

Induction of anesthesia also can be achieved through the use of an anesthetic chamber (Procedure 2-3 and Fig. 2-3). A see-through sturdy container with a tight-fitting lid and ports for entry of fresh gas and exit of excess gas is required. Anesthetic chambers allow the induction of even the most uncooperative animal, but they are also associated with several problems:

- The technique is obviously suited for use only in small patients.
- One major disadvantage to this technique is the difficulty in monitoring the patient's heart rate, respirations, and other vital signs while it is in the chamber.

PROCEDURE 2-3   Induction of Anesthesia with an Anesthetic Chamber

1. To induce anesthesia using an anesthetic chamber, place the conscious animal inside the chamber, which contains ordinary room air. The chamber should be large enough for the patient to lie down with its neck extended. If possible, eye lubrication should be applied to the patient's eyes before it is placed in the induction chamber.
2. Deliver oxygen gas combined with an inhalation anesthetic to the chamber by means of an air inlet. Typically, a high concentration of anesthetic (isoflurane, 4% to 5% or sevoflurane, 8%) and a high flow rate of oxygen (3 to 5 L/min) are used.
3. Observe the behavior of the patient and remove the patient from the chamber when the patient loses its ability to stand (loss of righting reflex). This can be tested by rocking the chamber gently.
4. If the patient is too lightly anesthetized to be intubated immediately after being removed from the chamber, use a mask to induce a deeper level of anesthesia.

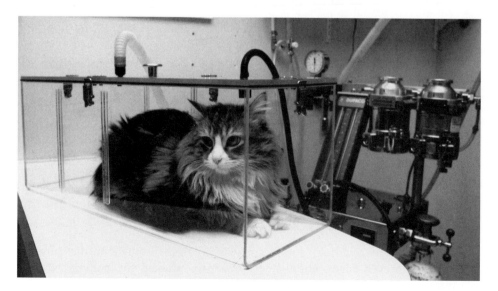

FIG. 2-3 Induction chamber.

- As with mask induction, there is some risk of regurgitation or vomiting, especially in the nonfasted patient. Because the airway is unprotected, aspiration of stomach contents may occur.
- There is considerable risk of exposure of hospital personnel to waste anesthetic gas, particularly when removing the patient from the chamber. The chamber must be equipped with a scavenger, and the anesthetic gas should be evacuated before the chamber is opened so that waste gas exposure can be avoided.

Monitoring during the Induction Period

Regardless of the induction method chosen, monitoring of the patient is of paramount importance throughout the induction period. The heart rate, pulse strength, respiratory rate and depth, mucous membrane color, and CRT should be checked frequently by the anesthetist to ensure patient safety. The animal's reflexes and jaw tone should also be monitored because they indicate the depth of anesthesia. Endotracheal intubation may be attempted after the patient shows no signs of resistance, gagging, or swallowing when the tongue is grasped and the mouth is opened.

ENDOTRACHEAL INTUBATION

Once anesthesia is induced in the patient, the anesthetist may choose to place a breathing tube (called an *endotracheal tube*) in the patient's airway. This tube conducts air directly from the oral cavity to the trachea, bypassing the nasal passages and pharynx (Fig. 2-4).

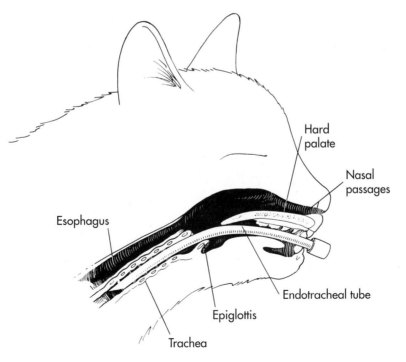

FIG. 2-4   Intubation of a cat, showing anatomy.

Advantages

Anesthesia with endotracheal intubation offers several advantages over anesthesia in the nonintubated animal:

- Intubation of the patient allows more efficient delivery of anesthetic gas to the animal than does a mask. Because gas flow rates can be lowered if an endotracheal tube is in place, intubation results in reduced exposure of hospital personnel to waste anesthetic gas and more economical anesthesia.
- An endotracheal tube that is the correct diameter and length for the patient will improve the efficiency of respiration by reducing the amount of anatomic dead space within the respiratory passages. *Anatomic dead space* describes those portions of the breathing passages that contain air but in which no gas exchange can occur (that is, the mouth, nasal passages, pharynx, trachea, and bronchi). With the anatomic dead space minimized, the endotracheal tube ensures that a larger proportion of the gas delivered to the patient reaches the exchange surface in the alveoli.
- Intubation allows the anesthetist to deliver oxygen directly to the patient when respiration must be assisted. Forced delivery of oxygen (with or without an inhalation anesthetic) to a patient can be achieved by squeezing the reservoir bag of the anesthetic machine or using the ventilator. This means of delivering oxygen to the patient is called *intermittent positive pressure ventilation (IPPV)* and is discussed in Chapter 7. Positive pressure ventilation through an endotracheal tube is necessary in animals that have been given neuromuscular blocking agents. This type of ventilation support is also helpful for patients that are having trouble breathing adequately during anesthesia and is essential for patients in respiratory or cardiac arrest. For this reason it is advisable to have a laryngoscope and an endotracheal tube of correct size readily available for all anesthetized patients, even if endotracheal intubation is not planned.
- The presence of an endotracheal tube with an inflated cuff reduces the risk of aspiration of vomitus, blood, saliva, or other material that may be present in the oral cavity or breathing passages. This material may accumulate during any procedure; however, the risk of aspiration is particularly high during oral surgery or dentistry and in patients that have not been fasted. Because of the usefulness of an endotracheal tube in maintaining a patent airway, it is customary to leave it in place throughout anesthesia and into the recovery period, until the animal regains the swallowing reflex.

Problems

There are several problems and hazards associated with endotracheal intubation:

- As discussed in Chapter 1, intubation may stimulate the activity of the vagus nerve and cause an increase in parasympathetic tone, particularly in dogs. This in turn may cause bradycardia, hypotension (low blood pressure), and cardiac arrhythmias. Occasionally, cardiac arrest may occur, particularly in an animal with preexisting cardiovascular disease. Atropine given in the preanesthetic period is helpful in preventing parasympathetic stimulation.
- Some species and breeds are difficult to intubate. Brachycephalic dogs, for example, have a large amount of redundant tissue within the oral cavity. This tissue falls over the back of the pharynx when the animal's mouth is opened,

obscuring the entrance to the trachea (the glottis). Despite this difficulty, these animals must be intubated; otherwise, it may be impossible to maintain an open airway during anesthesia. The use of a laryngoscope is helpful to visualize the oropharynx in these patients (see Chapter 4). Laryngoscopes provide a light source and can be used to manipulate tissues so that the airway is better exposed and easier to intubate. If a laryngoscope is used, intubation is less traumatic and incorrect placement of the tube in the esophagus is less likely.

- Overzealous efforts to intubate an animal may damage the larynx, pharynx, or soft palate. Particular care should be used when intubating cats, which have a narrow glottis that is easily traumatized. If the tissues of the larynx are irritated during intubation, reflex closure of the laryngeal cartilages may occur (called *laryngospasm*). This condition may result in blockage of the airway, which must be relieved or asphyxiation will result. To prevent laryngospasm, the anesthetist should avoid trauma to the laryngeal area during intubation. In cats it is also common procedure to spray the larynx with lidocaine to help desensitize the laryngeal tissues and reduce the risk of laryngospasm. Treatment of laryngospasm is discussed in Chapter 6.

- Certain food animal species and exotic and laboratory animal species are difficult to intubate because the mouth cannot be opened wide enough to allow the anesthetist to see the opening to the larynx. In some of these species "blind" intubation is possible, and in others intubation may be accomplished by palpation. In this technique, the anesthetist inserts a hand into the patient's mouth and feels the opening to the larynx, then passes the tube through the larynx into the trachea.

- Many commercially available tubes are designed for human use and are too long for veterinary patients, particularly cats. This can lead to two different problems: (1) If an excessively long tube is used, a large portion may extend forward past the animal's incisors, increasing the amount of mechanical dead space (Fig. 2-5). Mechanical dead space is the space in the breathing system occupied by gases that are breathed in and out without any change in composition. If the endotracheal tube is too long, air in the tube constitutes mechanical dead space because it will not reach the patient's lungs on inspiration, nor will it enter the breathing circuit on expiration. (2) Alternatively, a tube that is too long may be inserted too far into the breathing passages so that it enters a bronchus. This will result in the ventilation of only one lung (Fig. 2-6). If a tube of the correct length is used, one end should be at the level of the incisor teeth, and the other end should lie midway between the larynx and the thoracic inlet. One way to ensure that the length of the tube is correct is to ensure that it is shorter than the distance between the nose and the tip of the patient's shoulder or the thoracic inlet. If a tube of the appropriate length is unavailable, an endotracheal tube can be trimmed, with care being taken to avoid cutting into the cuff inflation apparatus.

- Pressure necrosis may result if the cuff of the endotracheal tube is excessively inflated. Procedure 2-4 (endotracheal intubation) describes the procedure for infusing the correct amount of air into the cuff. Cats are particularly sensitive to pressure necrosis from endotracheal tubes, and it is sometimes recommended that noncuffed tubes or tubes with low-pressure cuffs be used with this species.

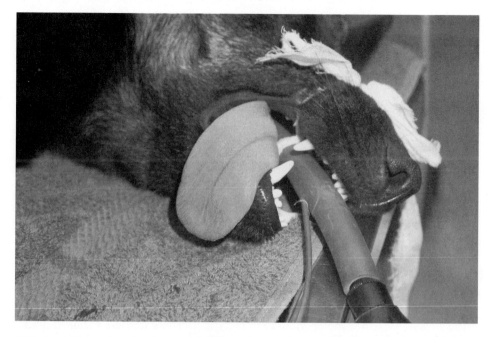

FIG. 2-5 Excessive dead space (endotracheal tube too long or not advanced sufficiently).

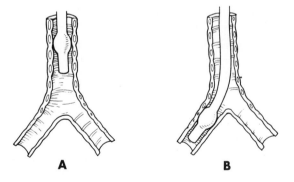

FIG. 2-6 Placement of endotracheal tube in trachea. A, Correct placement. B, Endotracheal tube advanced into bronchus (incorrect placement).

Some anesthetists suggest that if tubes with high-pressure cuffs are used, the cuff should be inflated for no longer than 30 minutes before being deflated and moved to a new location in the trachea. Others suggest that there is more risk to the patient through accidental extubation, inadvertent esophageal intubation, or damage to the tracheal mucosa caused by moving the tube in the trachea.

Text continued on p. 74

PROCEDURE 2-4   Endotracheal Intubation

1. Gather all necessary materials together before inducing the patient. Select several endotracheal tubes of varying sizes and check them for holes, loose connectors, and excessive wear. Test the cuff of each tube to make sure it remains inflated when air is introduced. Record the amount of air required to inflate the cuff.

2. Determine the length of the tube required by measuring the distance from the incisor teeth to the thoracic inlet. Estimate the diameter of the tube required by palpating the trachea (see Chapter 4).

3. Lubricate the tube with a sterile lubricant such as water soluble jelly. The jelly should not be allowed to dry on the tube. In cats, use a lubricant containing a local anesthetic such as lidocaine to decrease the incidence of laryngospasm. When a cat is anesthetized, it is also customary to spray a topical anesthetic on the laryngeal opening. Commercial laryngeal sprays are available, or 1% lidocaine (no epinephrine) may be drawn into a tuberculin syringe and aerosolized through a 26-gauge needle. Benzocaine was previously used for this purpose but its use has been discontinued because of its tendency to induce methemoglobinemia. In addition to spraying the laryngeal opening, two to four drops of lidocaine can also be dropped on the arytenoids, with a tomcat catheter on a TB syringe. Whatever agent is used, administer only a small amount of topical anesthetic (0.1 ml) because larger doses can be absorbed and lead to toxic plasma levels, especially in kittens. After spraying, delay the intubation 1 to 2 minutes to allow the local anesthetic to take effect.

4. When the animal reaches an appropriate plane of anesthesia (no response to toe pinch), open the mouth to allow intubation. An animal showing signs of resistance (such as gagging, struggling, or swallowing) is too lightly anesthetized to be intubated and the anesthetist should allow more time, or if necessary give additional anesthetic. The animal is usually restrained in sternal recumbency, although intubation in lateral or dorsal recumbency is preferred by some anesthetists. Extend the neck and raise the head so that the head and neck are in a straight line (Fig. 2-7). The animal's trunk should be propped upright and not allowed to sag laterally. Hold the upper jaw stationary, with the lips pulled dorsally, and push the lower jaw down by pulling the animal's tongue forward and down. It is advisable to use a mouth gag to reduce the chance of being inadvertently bitten by the patient. The tongue may be held out by either the assistant or the person intubating the animal. Open the mouth wide enough to allow the anesthetist to clearly see the epiglottis, which normally lies over the entrance to the trachea (Fig. 2-8). The restrainer should not push on the animal's ventral neck and head region because this may obscure the laryngeal anatomy, making intubation difficult. Frequently, the epiglottis is found behind the soft palate, which must be gently disengaged with a laryngoscope or the tip of the tube.

5. A laryngoscope is often used to assist intubation. This instrument consists of a handle containing batteries, a smooth blade (which may be curved or straight), and a light source (either a small bulb lamp or a fiber optic source). Laryngoscopes facilitate intubation by illuminating the pharyngeal area and by moving the epiglottis aside, exposing the glottis and vocal cords. The laryngoscope blade is first used to disengage the soft palate from the epiglottis. It is then gently placed at the back of the tongue, adjacent to the base of the epiglottis (in the case of a curved

Continued

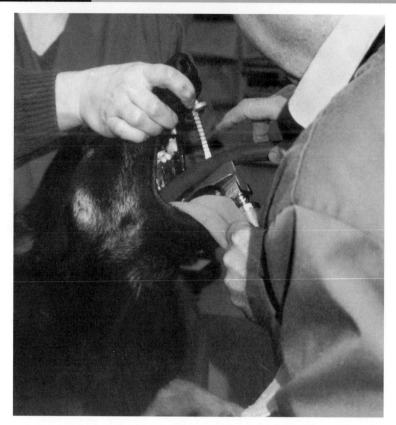

FIG. 2-7   Position of animal for intubation.

laryngoscope blade such as the Macintosh blade in Fig. 2-8) or on the tip of the epiglottis itself (straight laryngoscope blade such as the Miller or Michael's blade). This pulls the epiglottis forward and down, allowing the anesthetist to view the entrance to the trachea.

As an alternative to a laryngoscope, some anesthetists use the index finger of one hand to depress the epiglottis and guide the endotracheal tube into the trachea. This method of intubation carries some risk of being bitten by the patient if anesthetic depth is not sufficient. It is also possible to blindly place a dog by passing the tube into the mouth (which is held open with a mouth gag) while extending the tongue with the other hand. In this method, the tube is passed along the roof of the mouth, over the epiglottis, and into the entrance to the trachea. Significant trauma to pharyngeal and laryngeal tissues is possible with this technique, and esophageal intubation is common. This method is not advisable in cats because of the deep position of the larynx in the neck and their greater tendency to develop laryngospasm, compared to dogs. Whichever method is chosen, care should be taken to avoid touching the larynx before intubation.

PROCEDURE 2-4   **Endotracheal Intubation—cont'd**

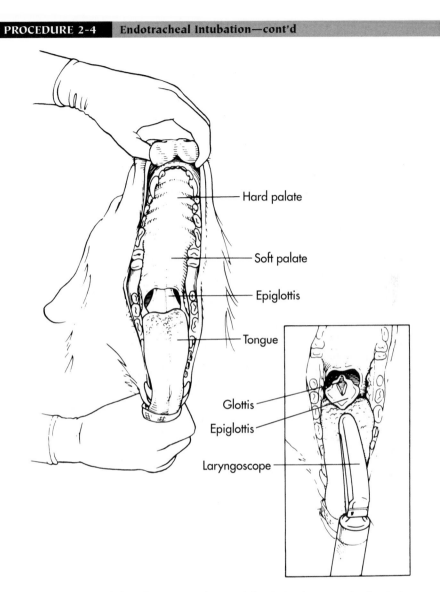

Hard palate

Soft palate

Epiglottis

Tongue

Glottis

Epiglottis

Laryngoscope

FIG. 2-8 Anatomy of the pharynx. When epiglottis is depressed, glottis is exposed. Endotracheal tube is advanced through glottis.

6. Insert the endotracheal tube past the vocal folds and into the trachea. This may be difficult in cats because the vocal cords are often positioned such that they close off the glottis. Intubation in cats is best accomplished by timing the advancement of the tube to coincide with exhalation (when the vocal cords separate and the glottis is open). The endotracheal tube should not be forced through the vocal cords, but gently rotated, if resistance is encountered. The tube should be advanced such that the curve of the tube matches that of the patient's neck. *Continued*

PROCEDURE 2-4   Endotracheal Intubation—cont'd

When a small tube is advanced, problems may arise because of bending of the tube during insertion. A thin steel or wooden rod may be inserted into the tube to act as a stylet and prevent bending (Fig. 2-9). The stylet should not protrude beyond the end of the tube because it may traumatize the laryngeal tissues.

7. Ensure that the tube enters the trachea and not the esophagus. The entrance to the esophagus lies just dorsal to the entrance to the trachea and, although difficult to see, it easily accommodates an endotracheal tube. Accidental intubation of the esophagus results in delivery of anesthetic and oxygen to the stomach rather than to the lungs, and the patient is unlikely to remain anesthetized if this occurs. Esophageal intubation can usually be avoided if the anesthetist visualizes the entrance to the trachea throughout the intubation procedure and ensures that the tube clearly enters that location.

Once the endotracheal tube is in place, confirm its presence within the trachea (rather than the esophagus). This can be done in one of several ways:
- The mouth can be opened and the entrance to the trachea observed. The tube can be seen to emerge from the glottis if it is in the correct location.
- A cough may be heard as the tube is inserted. The cough reflex is a normal response to endotracheal intubation, particularly at a light plane of anesthesia. It usually indicates that the tube is entering the correct passageway to the trachea.
- During expiration, the animal's breath can be felt as it exits the endotracheal tube. If the tube is in the trachea, a tuft of hair placed at the end of the

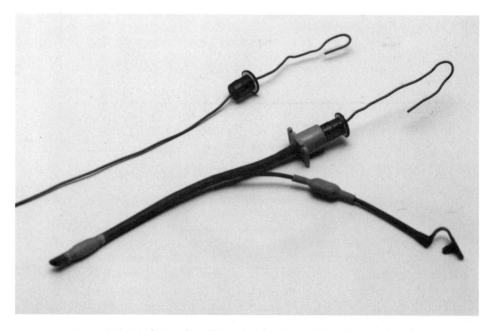

FIG. 2-9   Stylet and endotracheal tube (with stylet in place).

PROCEDURE 2-4   Endotracheal Intubation—cont'd

endotracheal tube will also move with the animal's exhalations. Either way, the anesthetist is assured that the tube has been placed in the breathing passages and not in the esophagus.
- Once the tube is connected to an anesthetic machine, the reservoir bag and unidirectional valves should move appropriately and in synchrony with the animal's inspiration and expiration if the tube is correctly placed.
- The anesthetist may palpate the animal's cervical region, ensuring that only one firm tubular structure is present, which is the trachea containing the endotracheal tube (the esophagus normally cannot be palpated). Palpation of two firm tubular structures usually indicates that the endotracheal tube is in the esophagus, and the trachea and the tube are being palpated separately.
- Vocalization is impossible if an endotracheal tube is correctly placed. Growling or whining usually indicates that the tube is in the esophagus and must be removed and reinserted in the correct location.

8. Secure the endotracheal tube in place using a piece of gauze tied around the tube and behind the animal's head (cats and brachycephalic dogs) or on top of its nose (most dogs, Fig. 2-10). In horses, the gauze is tied around the lower jaw. Alternatively, the tube can be taped in place. In all species, the tongue can be pulled out of the mouth to allow monitoring of the lingual pulse and pulse oximetry.
9. Inflate the cuff of the endotracheal tube using small increments of air. If a high-volume, low-pressure cuff is used, the cuff is overinflated if the anesthetist feels any

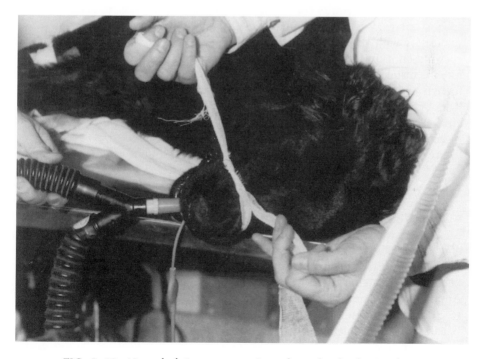

FIG. 2-10   Use of plain gauze to tie endotracheal tube in place.

Continued

back pressure. Then, check for leakage of anesthetic gas around the cuff. This is done by gently squeezing the reservoir bag. If only a tiny hiss is heard at 20-cm H_2O pressure, the cuff is adequately inflated. If there is a loud hiss, indicating that air is leaking around the tube, more air should be infused into the cuff or a larger size endotracheal tube used. If no hiss is heard, consider deflating the cuff slightly, as it may be exerting excessive pressure on the tracheal mucosa. Note that the cuff inflation should be checked again after 15 to 30 minutes of anesthesia, because tracheal diameter may have increased as a result of muscle relaxation, and further inflation may be required.

Endotracheal tubes are further discussed in Chapter 4. Details of the intubation procedure are given in Procedure 2-4 and illustrated in Figs. 2-7, 2-8, 2-9, and 2-10.

- Endotracheal tubes may become obstructed by saliva, mucus, blood, or foreign material such as gauze. This material may also occlude the distal end of the tube after use, making this a hazard for the next patient if the tube is not cleaned properly. Obstruction may also occur if the tube is kinked or twisted or if the end is occluded against the wall of the trachea. If the endotracheal tube is obstructed for any of these reasons, the patient will not receive oxygen, resulting in a serious anesthetic emergency.

- Intubated animals require careful monitoring during recovery to ensure that the tube is removed when the animal begins to swallow. If the patient regains consciousness with the tube in place, the tube may be damaged by the patient's chewing on it. In fact, patients have been known to chew tubes in half and aspirate the distal portion into the airway. Obviously, the presence of such a tracheal foreign body would be difficult to explain to the owner.

- Although endotracheal tubes used in human anesthesia are routinely discarded after a single use, it is common in veterinary practice for tubes to be used on several patients. Tubes must therefore be thoroughly disinfected between patients to prevent the spread of infectious diseases such as tracheobronchitis ("kennel cough"). However, the disinfection procedure may also pose a problem to the patient. If endotracheal tubes are soaked in a disinfectant solution for too long or in a solution that is too concentrated, the rubber will become impregnated with the disinfectant. When next used, the disinfectant still in the endotracheal tube may irritate the tracheal mucosa. This can result in the patient coughing after anesthesia or may even cause the tracheal mucosa to slough.

- Despite all precautions, an animal may cough for a day or two after anesthesia because of minor irritation from the tube's presence in the trachea and larynx. Animal owners should be warned that it is common for animals to cough for 1 to 2 days after anesthesia if an endotracheal tube is used.

Because of the problems associated with the use of endotracheal tubes and for reasons of convenience, not all animals undergo endotracheal intubation during anesthesia. If an endotracheal tube is not used, the inhalation agent is delivered by mask throughout the procedure. Also, animals lightly anesthetized with IM or IV agents for the performance of short procedures may not require the use of an endotracheal tube if the animal maintains the ability to swallow throughout the anesthesia and can breathe adequately. There should be no sounds indicating airway obstruction (such as fluid sounds in the airway), and the chest wall should move normally. Despite these exceptions, intubation is recommended for safety reasons if inhalation anesthetics are used or if a lengthy procedure is performed with the patient under injectable anesthesia.

MAINTENANCE OF ANESTHESIA

After successful induction of anesthesia, the animal enters a period in which anesthetic depth is adequate for surgical procedures. During this maintenance period, the anesthetist has two important tasks. First, the animal must be monitored closely to ensure that the vital signs (particularly heart rate and respiration) remain within acceptable limits. Second, the anesthetist must maintain the animal at an appropriate anesthetic depth (that is, one that is neither too light nor too deep). The importance of these two tasks can hardly be overemphasized. Failure to maintain an adequate depth of anesthesia may result in the animal's perception of pain and premature arousal from anesthesia. On the other hand, maintaining an animal at an excessive depth of anesthesia may lead to a slow recovery or an anesthetic overdose. Attention to vital signs is even more crucial because failure to monitor and maintain vital signs within acceptable limits may result in death or permanent brain damage.

The key to effective and safe anesthesia during the maintenance period is adequate monitoring. The word *monitor* comes from the Latin *monere*, which means "to warn." The anesthetist who closely monitors the animal under anesthesia will usually receive ample warning of problems as they arise. Although continuous monitoring of the anesthetized patient by a veterinary technician is not practical in many veterinary clinics, an attempt should be made to observe and evaluate the healthy anesthetized patient at least once every 3 to 5 minutes. This allows rapid but thorough assessment of depth, cardiovascular and ventilatory status, oxygenation, and other variables (Box 2-1). High-risk patients should be checked at more frequent intervals or, if possible, monitored continuously.

BOX 2-1 *Variables to Be Assessed at Least Every 5 Minutes Throughout Anesthesia*

- Respiration rate, depth, and character (assess both reservoir bag movement and chest movements)
- Mucous membrane color and capillary refill time (CRT)
- Heart rate
- Pulse strength and rate
- Jaw tone, eye position, and palpebral reflex activity
- Oxygen flow rate and oxygen tank pressure
- IV catheter placement and fluid administration rate
- Patient's temperature (may be adequate to palpate paws and ears)

Although the anesthetist must observe both vital signs and reflexes, it is important to differentiate between the two. The term *vital sign* refers to those variables
that indicate the response of the animal's homeostatic mechanisms to anesthesia,
including heart rate, respiration rate, CRT, and temperature. The patient's vital
signs indicate how well the patient is maintaining basic circulatory and respiratory
function during anesthesia. The term *reflex* refers to an involuntary response to a
stimulus (such as a pinprick or tap). Reflex responses give the anesthetist valuable
information on the depth of anesthesia but do not convey information on the
patient's homeostatic mechanisms.

Monitoring Vital Signs

Vital signs can be monitored by the anesthetist's senses (that is, touch, hearing, and
sight) or through the use of electronic devices such as an electrocardiogram (ECG)
machine or pulse oximeter. This section describes the variables that can be
monitored by the anesthetist without special instrumentation.

Vital signs that should be monitored during anesthesia include heart rate and
rhythm, pulse pressure, CRT, mucous membrane color, blood loss, respiratory rate
and depth, and temperature. Other vital signs that may be of interest but that
require special monitors (discussed in the next section) include blood oxygenation,
expired carbon dioxide (CO_2), ECG, and blood pressure.

Heart rate and rhythm

The minimum acceptable heart rate for anesthetized patients is 60 beats per
minute (bpm) in the dog and 100 bpm in the cat. Lower heart rates may indicate
excessive anesthetic depth or some other problem and should be brought to the
veterinarian's attention immediately. Heart rates of 60 to 120 bpm are common
during anesthesia (compared with 60 to 180 bpm in the healthy awake dog and 110
to 220 bpm in the healthy awake cat). The decreased heart rate normally seen in
an anesthetized animal is the result of the depressant effect of most anesthetics on
heart rate and myocardial function. A few drugs (for example, atropine, ketamine,
and tiletamine) have the opposite effect and can elevate heart rates.

Cardiac rhythm also may be affected by anesthetic agents, particularly halothane,
medetomidine, and xylazine. Disturbances in cardiac rhythm should be brought to
the attention of the veterinarian for assessment.

Cardiac monitoring may be achieved in several ways, including direct palpation
of the chest wall or pulse, auscultation of the chest with a stethoscope, use of an
ECG or cardiac monitor, and use of an esophageal stethoscope. Several types of
heart monitors are available that detect the patient's pulse or ECG and transmit
information to the anesthetist by an audible beep, a flash of light, or a digital readout.
Some monitors can be adjusted to sound an alarm when the heart rate moves above
or below limits set by the anesthetist.

Use of an esophageal stethoscope allows auscultation of the heart even if the
patient's chest area is covered with surgical drapes and conventional auscultation is
difficult. The esophageal stethoscope consists of a thin, flexible tube attached to a
regular stethoscope (Fig. 2-11). The tube is lubricated with a small amount of water
or lubricating jelly and is inserted through the oral cavity into the patient's esophagus.
The tube is advanced until an audible heartbeat is detected through the earpieces

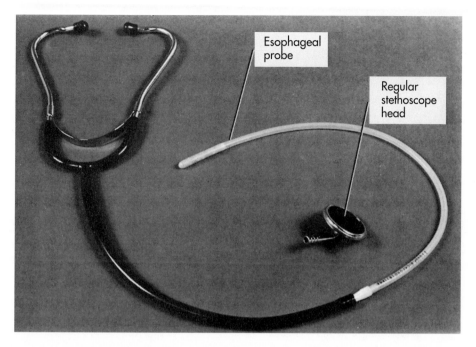

FIG. 2-11   Esophageal stethoscope. (*From Warren RG: Small animal anesthesia,*
St Louis, 1983, Mosby.)

or through an attached audio monitor. Some esophageal stethoscope probes contain
ECG leads or a temperature monitor. Insertion of the esophageal stethoscope is
usually delayed until after the endotracheal tube is in place to minimize the danger
of the stethoscope accidentally entering the trachea.

The presence of a beating heart does not necessarily imply that circulation is
adequate. Heartbeat should be assessed in conjunction with pulse strength, CRT,
mucous membrane color, and (if available) measured blood pressure values.

Capillary refill time

The CRT is the rate of return of color to a mucous membrane after the application
of gentle digital pressure (Fig. 2-12). The CRT reflects the perfusion of the tissues
with blood. Pressure on the mucous membranes compresses the small capillaries
and blocks blood flow to that area. When the pressure is released, the capillaries
rapidly refill with blood and the color returns, provided the heart is able to generate
sufficient blood pressure. However, a short CRT is not an infallible indication that
the circulation is adequate (and in fact, a normal CRT may be observed shortly
after euthanasia in some animals).

A prolonged CRT (more than 2 seconds) indicates that tissue perfusion is not
optimal and that tissues in the area tested have reduced blood supply. This may be
due to vasoconstriction (blood vessels are reduced in diameter, often because of the
release of epinephrine). Alternatively, poor perfusion may be the result of low blood

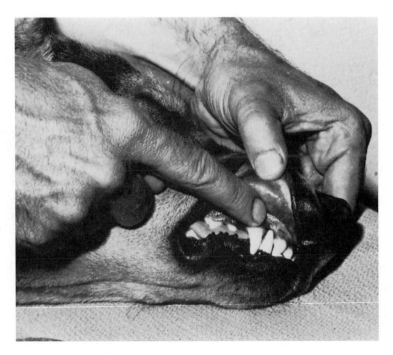

FIG. 2-12   Assessing gingiva for capillary refill time and mucous membrane color. (*From Warren RG:* Small animal anesthesia, *St Louis, 1983, Mosby.*)

pressure caused by drugs (IV opioids, acepromazine, medetomidine, inhalation agents), hypothermia, cardiac failure, excessive anesthetic depth, or shock. Another indicator of poor tissue perfusion is reduced temperature of the affected part.

Mucous membrane color

The most convenient location for observing mucous membrane color is the gingiva (see Fig. 2-12). In the case of dogs with pigmented gingiva, other sites may be used including the tongue, conjunctiva of the lower eyelid, or the mucous membrane lining the prepuce or vulva. Pale mucous membranes may indicate blood loss or anemia or may result from poor perfusion (as may occur with prolonged anesthesia). Purple or blue discoloration of mucous membranes, a condition called *cyanosis,* indicates either stagnant blood flow or a shortage of oxygen in the tissues. Cyanosis during anesthesia may be the result of respiratory failure or upper airway obstruction and must be addressed immediately.

Pulse strength

Blood pressure is the force exerted by flowing blood on arterial walls. Although the technician can only obtain an accurate reading of blood pressure through the use of special instruments, it is possible to roughly estimate blood pressure by palpating a major artery and determining the strength of the pulse. The pulse can be detected at any one of several locations, including the lingual (Fig. 2-13), femoral,

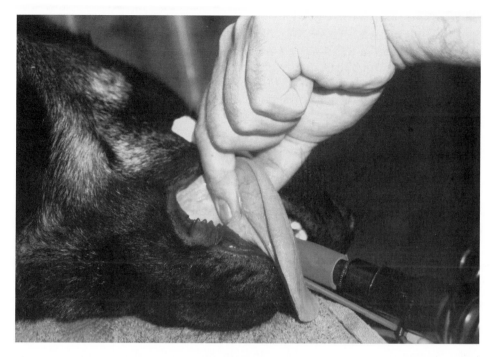

FIG. 2-13 Palpation of the lingual artery.

carotid, and dorsal pedal arteries. The pulse should be strong and synchronized with the heartbeat. Unfortunately, natural variation in pulse strength among healthy animals somewhat limits the usefulness of this method of blood pressure monitoring.

Blood pressure is important to the anesthetist because it is relatively easy to measure and when used with other variables, it can reflect the adequacy of blood circulation throughout the body. Blood pressure that is below normal limits is called *hypotension,* and blood pressure that is above normal limits is termed *hypertension.* Hypotension during anesthesia may indicate any of the following:

- *Excessive anesthetic depth.* Blood pressure is influenced by general anesthetics, such that increasing the depth of inhalation anesthesia may lead to a fall in blood pressure due to decreased cardiac output and/or vasodilation.
- *Excessive vasodilation.* Certain preanesthetic drugs (notably, acepromazine) may reduce blood pressure by causing the blood vessels to dilate. Animals that are dehydrated or hypotensive before anesthesia (for example, animals in shock) are at particular risk of having a further drop in blood pressure when given these agents.
- *Cardiac insufficiency,* often due to preexisting heart disease.
- *Excessive blood loss,* leading to hypovolemia.

Accurate monitoring of blood pressure requires the use of instruments and is discussed on p. 83.

Blood loss

Blood loss, if excessive, predisposes the patient to shock and anesthetic complications. Blood loss in major surgery may be estimated by counting used sponges. One fully soaked 3×3 inch sponge holds 5 to 6 ml of blood. The true amount of blood lost may be up to twice this figure because it is difficult to measure the blood that has clotted, been retained by surgical drapes, or pooled at the surgery site.

A healthy animal may tolerate a loss of up to 15% of its blood volume without serious circulatory effects. This is approximately 13 ml/kg in dogs and cats.

Respiration rate and depth

Respiration rate may be monitored by observing movements of the reservoir bag or of the animal's chest. Normal respiration rate in a conscious animal is 10 to 30 breaths per minute in the dog and 25 to 40 breaths per minute in the cat. At a moderate depth of anesthesia, the normal rate is 8 to 20 breaths per minute, although rates up to 50 breaths per minute may be seen. During the maintenance period, respiratory rates less than 8 breaths per minute may indicate excessive anesthetic depth and should be reported to the veterinarian.

The anesthetist must monitor not only the respiratory rate, but also the depth and character of the breathing. At deeper planes of anesthesia, there is normally a decrease in both the respiratory rate and the volume of air taken with each breath (tidal volume). This decrease in respiratory rate and volume is called *hypoventilation*. Tidal volume decreases by at least 25% in most anesthetized animals, largely because most preanesthetic and general anesthetic drugs decrease the expansion of the intercostal muscles on inspiration. As the animal's breaths become more shallow (that is, as tidal volume decreases), some alveoli in the lung may not receive amounts of air adequate for normal gas exchange. As a result the alveoli will partially collapse, leading to a condition called *atelectasis*. This is most pronounced in the "down" lung of a patient that is lying on its side. In its early stages, atelectasis can be reversed by gentle inflation of the lungs by the anesthetist. In this procedure, called *bagging*, the reservoir bag of the anesthetic machine is carefully squeezed, forcing air into the patient's breathing passages. When bagging a patient, the anesthetist should closely observe the animal's chest to ensure that it rises only slightly. This prevents overinflation of the lungs. Some anesthetists routinely bag every patient under inhalation anesthesia once every 5 minutes. Alternatively, hypoventilation and atelectasis may be prevented by mechanical ventilation of the patient through the use of a ventilator (see Chapter 7).

In contrast to the hypoventilation observed in many anesthetized patients, the anesthetist may occasionally note rapid or deep respirations in some anesthetized patients. An increase in respiratory rate is called *tachypnea*, whereas an increase in depth is termed *hyperventilation*. Tachypnea must be differentiated from panting, in which the breathing is rapid but shallow and air intake is through the open mouth. Panting is a common side effect of some opioid drugs, particularly oxymorphone.

True hyperventilation and tachypnea have many possible causes. They are a physiologic response to increased CO_2 in the blood or metabolic acidosis. When an anesthetic machine is used, hyperventilation may indicate that the CO_2 is not being adequately removed from the breathing circuit by the CO_2 absorber. Rapid respirations may also result from an underlying disease, such as pulmonary edema. Hyperventilation is also commonly seen as a response to a mild surgical stimulus. For example, it is often apparent when the surgeon pulls on the suspensory ligament of the ovary during an ovariohysterectomy. An elevated respiratory rate may also indicate a progression from moderate to light anesthesia and is one of the first signs of arousal from anesthesia. Some patients (particularly obese dogs) breathe rapidly even at a moderate depth of anesthesia.

Not only the respiratory rate and depth but also the type of respiration may be significant. The anesthetized animal's breathing should be smooth and regular, with both thoracic and diaphragmatic components. Gasping, difficult, or labored breathing must be brought to the veterinarian's attention.

The time relationship between inspiration and expiration may vary also. Normal inspiration lasts 1 to 1.5 seconds, and expiration lasts at least 2 to 3 seconds. Expiration is usually followed by a pause before the next inspiration begins. Animals anesthetized with ketamine may exhibit an *apneustic* respiratory pattern, in which inspiration is followed by a prolonged pause before expiration.

Auscultation of the chest may yield useful information, not only about cardiac function but also about respiratory function. Normal respiratory sounds are almost inaudible in the dog and cat. Harsh noises, whistles, or squeaks may indicate narrow or obstructed airways or the presence of fluid in the airways or alveoli and should be brought to the veterinarian's attention.

As evident from this discussion, the rate, depth, and type of respirations must be closely monitored by the anesthetist. A change in any of these variables may be the first warning of a change in anesthetic depth or of the onset of an anesthetic problem.

Thermoregulation

Hypothermia is probably the most common anesthetic complication in veterinary patients. Although body temperature does not change minute by minute, there is often an overall drop of temperature with time during anesthesia. Temperature loss is greatest in the first 20 minutes, and the anesthetist should be concerned with preventing temperature loss from the moment of induction. Prolonged general anesthesia may reduce the patient's temperature by 3° C or more. Several factors contribute to this effect:

- Animals are routinely shaved before surgery, and the skin may be washed with antiseptic and alcohol solutions that cool by evaporation.
- The anesthetized animal cannot generate heat by shivering or muscle activity.
- The metabolic rate of an anesthetized animal is less than that of a conscious animal, resulting in less heat generation.
- During the course of surgery, a body cavity may be opened and the viscera exposed to air at room temperature.
- Several preanesthetic and general anesthetic agents cause vasodilation, resulting in an increased rate of heat loss.
- Pediatric and geriatric animals are less able to maintain thermoregulation and are therefore predisposed to hypothermia.

There are several potential problems associated with hypothermia during the maintenance and recovery periods.

- Hypothermic animals require less anesthetic than other patients and are easily overdosed. The requirement for halothane drops by 5% per degree Celsius drop in body temperature.
- Hypothermia slows the rate at which liver enzymes metabolize anesthetic drugs, allowing the drugs to remain active in the body for a longer time. Prolonged recovery is common in hypothermic patients.
- Shivering will increase the patient's oxygen demands during the recovery period by as much as 600%. This can cause significant complications in the patient unable to respond to this increase in demand (as may be the case in a patient with cardiopulmonary disease).

To avoid these problems, the anesthetist should endeavor to monitor the patient's temperature and to maintain it as much as possible within the normal range for that species.

During anesthesia, rectal temperature should be monitored every 30 minutes. If the rectum is covered by surgery drapes or is otherwise inaccessible to the anesthetist, a rough estimate of body temperature can be obtained by touching the patient's paws or ears. Temperature also may be measured with special thermometers designed for use in the ear canal or esophagus.

Prevention of hypothermia may involve such measures as administering warm IV fluids (rather than fluids at room temperature or refrigerated fluids) and the use of a circulating warm water heating pad (Fig. 2-14), hot water bottles wrapped in towels, bubble packing, heated rice socks or oat bags, and foil wraps. It is also important to ensure a comfortable air temperature in the operating room itself. Patients should not be placed on a stainless steel table or trough unless an insulating layer of newspaper, towels, or a heating pad is provided. Electric heating pads should be avoided because burns are sometimes associated with their use. Burns may also result from the use of overheated oat bags, hot water bottles, and other heat sources.

Hyperthermia (increased body temperature) is occasionally seen in anesthetized small animals, particularly in susceptible dogs anesthetized with ketamine, halothane, or succinylcholine. Although rare, this syndrome, called *malignant hyperthermia*, may be fatal if not promptly relieved through the application of cold wet towels and the use of drugs such as dantrolene.

Use of Instruments to Monitor Vital Signs

Although a competent technician can safely monitor most patients without the use of specialized instruments, the use of monitoring devices may be of significant benefit. Instruments offer continuous monitoring, whereas the technician in a busy veterinary practice is seldom able to sit with the patient throughout the anesthetic period. Instruments also allow precise quantitative measurement of variables that are difficult to determine by observations alone, such as blood pressure and the percent of oxygen saturation in the patient's hemoglobin.

On the other hand, electronic monitoring, although convenient, should not be relied on to give a complete picture of patient status. Instruments are subject to power failure, interference from artifacts, and a loss of contact with the patient. Instrumentation cannot replace the presence of a skilled and conscientious anesthetist.

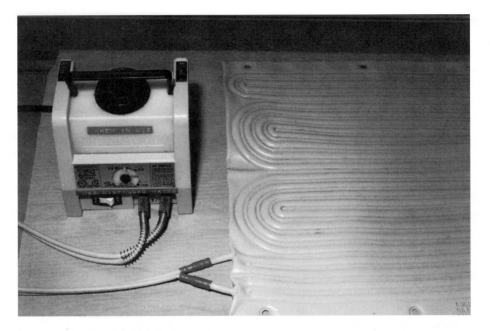

FIG. 2-14   Circulating warm water heating pad.

This section describes the instruments that can be used to monitor the following variables: blood pressure (Doppler flow probe or oscillometer), central venous pressure, blood gases (Pao_2 and $Paco_2$), Sao_2 (pulse oximetry), expired CO_2 (capnography), and electrocardiography.

Blood pressure

As described in the previous section, the anesthetist can make a rough estimate of blood pressure through manual palpation of a peripheral pulse. Blood pressure monitors allow more accurate determination of blood pressure.[*]

Several terms are used to describe various types of arterial blood pressure. *Systolic pressure* is produced by the contraction of the ventricles and propels blood through the aorta and major arteries. It is the highest pressure that is exerted throughout the cardiac cycle. *Diastolic pressure* is the pressure that remains when the heart is in its resting phase, between contractions. It is the lowest pressure that is exerted throughout the cardiac cycle.

Mean arterial pressure (MAP) is the average pressure through the cardiac cycle. It is the most important pressure from the anesthetist's standpoint because it is the best indicator of blood perfusion of the internal organs. MAP is automatically calculated by some instruments or can be mathematically derived as follows:

$$MAP = \text{diastolic pressure} + \frac{(\text{systolic pressure} - \text{diastolic pressure})}{3}$$

[*]It should be recognized that the term *blood pressure* refers only to arterial blood pressure. The pressure of blood in the veins is measured by other techniques (see section on central venous pressure).

Pulse pressure, the pressure detected by manual palpation, is the difference between systolic pressure and diastolic pressure. An animal with a systolic pressure of 180 and a diastolic pressure of 140 will have a pulse that feels similar to that of an animal with a systolic pressure of 140 and a diastolic pressure of 100.

Caution must be used when interpreting pulse pressure because fingers are not as sensitive as transducers, and pulse pressure does not always correlate well with blood pressure. For example, a systolic blood pressure of 100 mm Hg and a diastolic pressure of 30 mm Hg results in a pulse pressure difference of 70 mm Hg. Subjectively this might be considered a good blood pressure, but the MAP in this patient is approximately 55 mm Hg, which means that the driving pressure for perfusing tissues is lower than normal (a mean blood pressure of 60 or more is considered ideal). By comparison, a systolic pressure of 100 mm Hg and a diastolic pressure of 70 mm Hg results in a pulse pressure difference of only 30 mm Hg, and it will not feel as "strong" as the pulse pressure difference of 70 mm Hg. However, in this case the MAP is about 80 mm Hg, which provides adequate perfusion of tissues and organs. All instruments that monitor blood pressure are able to measure systolic blood pressure, and some are able to measure diastolic pressure and MAP as well.

Normal systolic pressure in the dog and cat is approximately 120 mm Hg (range from 90 to 160 mm Hg), and normal diastolic pressure is 80 mm Hg (range from 50 to 90 mm Hg). This can be indicated as systolic/diastolic, in this case 120/80. Normal MAP is 90 to 100 mm Hg in the awake animal and 70 to 90 mm Hg during anesthesia. These values are approximate because they vary with patient age, species, breed, and instrumentation used. When blood pressures are determined, it is often more useful to monitor trends rather than single values.

Blood pressure does not equal blood flow. In fact, very high systolic pressures often indicate constricted blood vessels, as in a patient that has received epinephrine. Blood flow to the tissues is usually decreased in this case.

Measurement of blood pressure is a valuable tool for the anesthetist.* It is useful for indicating anesthetic depth because it falls with increasing depth of anesthesia. It also indicates cardiac function and even more important, organ perfusion. If MAP falls below 70 mm Hg, blood flow to internal organs is reduced, and tissues may become hypoxic. The kidneys are particularly sensitive to reduced perfusion because of a fall in MAP during anesthesia, and kidney failure is occasionally seen after anesthesia, particularly in geriatric patients or those receiving nonsteroidal antiinflammatory drugs (see Chapter 8).

Although a modest drop in blood pressure is acceptable during anesthesia, every effort should be made to maintain the MAP at 70 mm Hg or greater. Hypotension is among the most common adverse effects of general anesthesia. See Box 2-2 for strategies to prevent hypotension.

There are two methods of monitoring blood pressure by means of instruments: direct monitoring and indirect monitoring. In direct blood pressure monitoring, the

---

*Blood pressure monitoring is also useful in awake patients as a means of detecting systemic hypertension (particularly in animals with renal failure, hyperthyroidism, diabetes mellitus, or hyperadrenocorticism) or hypotension (common in animals that are dehydrated, in shock, or suffering from heart disease or hypoadrenocorticism).

BOX 2-2 *Prevention of Hypotension during Anesthesia*

- Use caution when administering drugs with marked cardiovascular effects (acepromazine, medetomidine, xylazine), particularly in animals with preexisting hypotension.
- Avoid excessive anesthetic depth. For surgical procedures that require significant analgesia (for example, orthopedic surgeries) use analgesic before or during anesthesia to reduce the amount of inhalation anesthetic required.
- Avoid bradycardia during anesthesia.
- Administer IV fluids during anesthesia at a rate adequate to support tissue perfusion. Consider colloids if needed to maintain arterial pressure and/or tissue perfusion.
- Maintain acid/base and electrolyte values within normal limits.
- Consider the use of drugs: ephedrine: 0.1-0.2 mg/kg IV, dobutamine or dopamine 2-10 mg/kg/min.

Courtesy Dr. Peter Hellyer.

reading is obtained by means of a catheter inserted into an artery. In the case of indirect blood pressure monitoring, a probe is placed on the outside surface of the animal (usually on a leg or the tail), and a cuff is used to compress an artery.

Direct blood pressure monitoring is infrequently performed in veterinary practice, although it is common in research and referral institutions. An indwelling catheter is placed in the femoral or dorsal pedal artery by means of a surgical cutdown or percutaneous insertion technique. The catheter is connected by a length of fluid-filled tubing to a manometer or pressure transducer to display the measured pressure. There is some risk of hematoma formation and infection with this method, but readings are continuous and more accurate than those obtained by indirect methods.

In private practice, blood pressure is more commonly determined by indirect methods, which are noninvasive and less technically difficult than direct monitoring. Various types of equipment are used to occlude blood flow through an artery and detect the pressure at which some blood flow resumes (the systolic blood pressure), the pressure where normal flow is reestablished (the diastolic pressure), or the average pressure (MAP). These pressures are detected in several ways:

1. The noise made by the returning blood flow may be auscultated with a stethoscope. This method is used to determine systolic and diastolic pressure in humans but is difficult to do accurately in a dog or cat.
2. A Doppler flow probe detects an ultrasound echo from red blood cells passing through the vessel, and thereby determines systolic pressure (Fig. 2-15).
3. An oscillometer can detect the distention of the limb because of the increased volume of blood pulsing through the artery and limb with each heartbeat (Fig. 2-16). Systolic pressure, diastolic pressure, and MAP can all be determined by this method.

Doppler blood pressure monitors

The Doppler flow probe (see Fig. 2-15) is the most affordable blood pressure monitoring device that can be used on veterinary patients. (Procedure 2-5 describes the technique for measuring blood pressure with a Doppler device.) The Doppler probe emits a series of high-frequency sound waves. When the sound waves encounter a pulsating artery, the frequency is changed. This is detected by the instrument, which converts the sound wave into a "swishing" sound audible to the attendant.

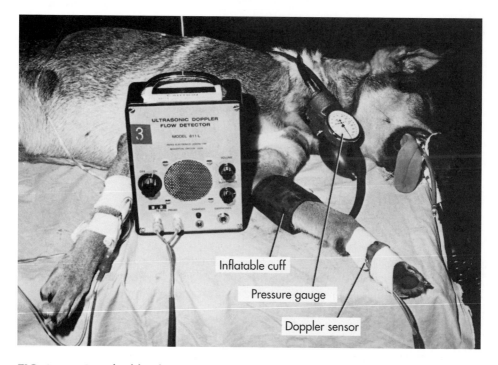

FIG. 2-15   Doppler blood pressure monitor. (*From Warren RG:* Small animal anesthesia, *St Louis, 1983, Mosby.*)

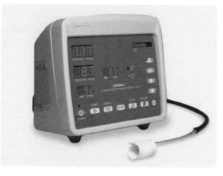

FIG. 2-16   Oscillometer blood pressure monitor.

To determine systolic pressure, a probe and a cuff are placed around the patient's leg or tail. When the cuff is inflated, an artery lying beneath the cuff is compressed. If the cuff applies a pressure that is higher than the systolic blood pressure, blood flow through the artery stops. As a result, no sound is detected by the sensor. When the cuff pressure is slowly released, blood flow will resume when the cuff pressure equals the systolic blood pressure. This blood flow will be picked up by the sensor probe and converted into an audible sound.

PROCEDURE 2-5	Measuring Indirect Blood Pressure with a Doppler Probe

1. Clip any hair from the area where the probe will be placed.
2. Apply ultrasound gel to the concave portion of the probe.
3. Select a cuff that has a width 40% of the circumference of the limb that is used for the reading (wrap IV tubing around the limb to measure). Place the cuff snugly over the limb or tail, proximal to where the probe will be placed.
4. Place the probe over the area to be evaluated, where a pulse can be felt (coccygeal, metacarpal, or metatarsal artery) and tape in place. Do not apply the tape tightly, or the artery will collapse and no readings can be taken.
5. Turn on the amplifier. If a pulsation or chirp is heard, the probe is over an artery. If no sound is heard, reposition.
6. Attach the manometer and bulb to the cuff tubing.
7. Inflate the cuff until no sound is heard.
8. The pressure gauge should be placed at the level of the right atrium; otherwise, incorrect pressure readings will be taken. For every 2 cm that the gauge is above or below the right atrium, 1 mm Hg should be added or subtracted, respectively.
9. Slowly release pressure from the cuff until the first "swishing" sound is heard. This sound is due to blood circulating past the sensor, and the manometer reading at this point is the systolic pressure.
10. Five readings are taken. The highest and lowest are discarded and the remaining readings are averaged to find the value of the systolic pressure.

Like most instruments, the Doppler system is subject to technical errors and limitations such as the following:
- Doppler monitors underestimate the systolic blood pressure in cats, and a correction factor of 14 mm Hg should be added to the systolic pressure indicated.
- The use of a cuff that is too large or too small will give false readings. The width of the cuff should be no more than 40% of the circumference of the leg around which the cuff is being wrapped.
- The sensor probe must be placed with the concave portion of the probe lying on the patient's skin.
- Only ultrasound gel should be used on the probe to augment sound wave transmission. Lubricating jelly and gels containing electrolytic substances (such as those used for ECG leads) should not be used. After use, the probe should be cleaned with gauze dampened with tap water (not alcohol or disinfectant) to prevent the gel from drying on the probe.
- Doppler monitors indicate only systolic blood pressure. Diastolic pressure and MAP cannot be measured by most Doppler systems.
- Readings are intermittent, and the device is labor intensive in that there is no automatic readout.

Oscillometer blood pressure monitors

Blood pressure can also be measured with an oscillometer, which consists of a cuff/ detector unit connected to a computerized monitor (see Fig. 2-16). Oscillometers measure blood pressure by detecting oscillations within the cuff bladder, which is placed around the leg or tail. These oscillations are caused by the pulsation of an artery beneath the cuff, which changes the volume of the limb slightly. As a computer inflates and deflates the cuff, it measures the change in intracuff pressure as it reflects the size of the limb changes with each pulse. It then calculates the systolic, mean, and diastolic pressures from these cuff pressure changes.

Oscillometers are more expensive than Doppler devices but offer two significant advantages: they work automatically and do not require an attendant to inflate or deflate the cuff, and they allow determination of diastolic pressure and MAP. However, readings are more accurate in large and medium patients than in small patients (less than 10 kg) because the instrument has difficulty in detecting the pulsations of small arteries. They are also inaccurate in animals with significant hypotension or fast heart rates. As with Doppler monitors, values for systolic pressure are 10 to 15 mm Hg lower than those obtained by direct blood pressure monitoring.

Central venous pressure

Just as blood pressure in an artery can be measured, it is possible to measure blood pressure in a large central vein such as the anterior vena cava. This value, the central venous pressure (CVP), allows the veterinarian to assess how well blood is returning to the heart and also the ability of the heart to receive and pump blood. This value is extremely helpful in monitoring animals for right-sided heart failure because it measures the backup of blood in the vena cava that results from this condition. It is also useful in preventing overhydration in animals receiving IV fluids, because CVP values rise as blood volume increases.

CVP can be directly measured by inserting a long catheter percutaneously or by cutting down into the jugular vein. The catheter is advanced into the anterior vena cava and toward the heart so that the tip of the catheter lies close to the right atrium. The catheter is connected to a water manometer to obtain a measurement. The manometer should be positioned so that "0" on the manometer is level with the right atrium (halfway between shoulder and sternum in sternal patients, and level with the sternum in laterally recumbent patients). If the catheter is correctly positioned, the meniscus of the fluid in the manometer should rise and fall with each breath. Normal CVP in dogs and cats is less than 8 cm H_2O pressure. Pressures over 12 to 15 cm H_2O (taken during exhalation) are considered elevated. As with arterial blood pressure, it is usually more valuable to monitor trends over time rather than base an assessment on a single reading.

Blood gases

Among the most important tasks of the anesthetist is to ensure that the patient's blood gases are normal. This means that the patient is sufficiently oxygenated, that carbon dioxide levels are within acceptable limits, and that respiratory acidosis is minimized. Each of these variables depends on respiratory function, which can be roughly evaluated by observation of the rate, depth, and character of the patient's respirations. However, this method of monitoring may give an inaccurate impression of the patient's respiratory function: ventilation may appear normal, yet the animal may have significant respiratory depression.

Fortunately, a more accurate assessment of respiratory function is possible through the use of several techniques, including the use of blood gas analysis (Pao_2, $Paco_2$ measurement), capnography, and pulse oximetry. These measurements indicate how well the patient is obtaining oxygen and delivering it to the tissues and how efficiently the lungs are eliminating carbon dioxide.

Before examination of the ways in which oxygen, carbon dioxide, and blood pH are measured, it may be useful to review how oxygen and carbon dioxide are carried in the bloodstream.

Oxygen. Oxygen is carried through the blood in two forms: as a free molecule dissolved in plasma (measured by the oxygen partial pressure in the arteries, abbreviated Pao_2) and chemically combined with hemoglobin in red blood cells (measured as the percentage of hemoglobin saturated with oxygen, Sao_2). Each 100 ml of oxygenated blood contains about 20 ml of oxygen: 0.3 ml dissolved in plasma and 19.7 ml joined to hemoglobin.

Both Pao_2 and Sao_2 can be measured, although by different instruments. Blood gas analyzers measure Pao_2; pulse oximeters measure Sao_2. Both indicate the degree of oxygenation of a patient (how well the lungs deliver oxygen to the blood). Most anesthetized animals show a greatly elevated Pao_2 (up to 500 mm Hg compared with the normal 90 to 115 mm Hg for an awake patient breathing room air) because they are breathing almost 100% oxygen from the anesthetic machine, whereas the nonanesthetized animal breathes approximately 21% oxygen in room air. Similarly, Sao_2 readings on anesthetized animals breathing pure oxygen are usually high (97% to 99%).

Low Pao_2 and Sao_2 values are sometimes observed during anesthesia. Pao_2 values below 60 mm Hg indicate significant hypoxia and the need for oxygen supplementation and possibly ventilation assistance to maintain minimal oxygen delivery to the tissues. Similarly, an Sao_2 reading below 90% suggests hypoxia, which should be immediately investigated and corrected.

Carbon dioxide. Carbon dioxide (CO_2) is transported through the blood in three ways. About 30% of the CO_2 joins with hemoglobin in the red blood cells. Approximately 10% is dissolved in plasma and can be measured as $Paco_2$ (the CO_2 partial pressure in the arteries). The remainder reacts with water to form carbonic acid, which is quickly converted into bicarbonate and hydrogen ions according to the reaction:

$$CO_2 + H_2O \rightarrow H_2CO_3 \rightarrow HCO_3^- + H^+$$

The anesthetist can evaluate how well the patient is eliminating CO_2 by measuring $Paco_2$ through blood gas determination. $Paco_2$ is often elevated during anesthesia (45 to 60 mm Hg compared with less than 45 mm Hg in the awake patient) because the respiratory depression produced by most anesthetics causes the body to retain CO_2. In other words, the patient does not breathe often enough or deeply enough to eliminate the normal amount of CO_2. A $Paco_2$ greater than 60 mm Hg usually indicates that the patient is hypoventilating. If this happens, the anesthetist needs to determine if the patient is in trouble by assessing the oxygenation, cardiac rhythm, blood pressure, and anesthetic depth. It may be necessary to assist ventilation by compressing the reservoir bag or through the use of a ventilator (see Chapter 7).

Because of high CO_2 levels, anesthetized patients may also become mildly acidotic (that is, excess hydrogen ions are produced from CO_2 according to the previous equation). Blood pH in anesthetized animals usually reflects this mild respiratory acidosis and is commonly 7.20 to 7.30, compared with the normal animal's blood pH of 7.35 to 7.45. Blood pH measurement can be performed at the same time blood gas determinations are made to help the anesthetist determine the acid-base status of the body and the adequacy of the patient's respiration.

Determination of Pao_2 and $Paco_2$. Blood gas levels, although useful, are not commonly measured in practice. Sample collection may be difficult because blood intended for blood gas analysis should be obtained from an artery if possible (as opposed to routine blood samples, which are taken from a vein). In certain situations, a venous sample may be used. For example, the lingual vein has extensive anastomoses with arteries in the tongue, and the blood gas values obtained from lingual vein samples are close to arterial values.

Once obtained, the blood sample must be stored on ice, and values should be measured within 2 hours. Many veterinary biochemistry laboratories and some veterinary hospitals are equipped to perform these tests, and some human hospital laboratories may be willing to accept samples from nonhuman patients. Portable analyzers have recently been introduced to the veterinary market.

Determination of Sao_2. As with Pao_2, the patient's Sao_2 (that is, the amount of oxygen bound to hemoglobin, expressed as a percentage of the total capacity) indicates its level of oxygenation. Sao_2 can be measured with a pulse oximeter. This piece of equipment is reasonably inexpensive, noninvasive, portable, and easy to use. Pulse oximeters are equipped with a probe or clip that is placed across a thin strip of the patient's tissue (Fig. 2-17). In anesthetized animals the tongue is commonly used, but the probe may also be applied to the shaved pinna, rectal mucosa, toe web, gingiva, underside of the base of the tail, vulvar fold, Achilles tendon, lip, or any other area that is thin, hairless, and nonpigmented. Many commercially available pulse oximeters continuously measure not only the Sao_2 but also the heart rate. Some units also display the ECG and expired CO_2 level.

Normal Sao_2 values should be above 95%, which is equivalent to a Pao_2 of 85 to 100 mm Hg.* If Sao_2 values drop to 90% (equivalent to a Pao_2 of 60 mm Hg), the patient is borderline hypoxic and the anesthetist should investigate. If the pulse oximeter reading falls to less than 85% for more than 30 seconds, serious hypoxia is present and must be addressed.

Pulse oximeters and blood gas analyzers allow early recognition of situations in which the patient is poorly oxygenated. A pulse oximeter reading of 90% to 95% indicates that the patient's hemoglobin is not fully saturated with oxygen and that a respiratory or cardiovascular problem may be present. The patient will not become hypoxic until the reading falls to 90% or less, and it is hoped that the anesthetist will be able to correct the problem before this occurs. Without the use of pulse oximetry or blood gases, early hypoxia is difficult to detect because cyanosis only becomes apparent if Sao_2 values fall below 85% saturation.

---

*For Sao_2 values between 75% and 90%, the Pao_2 in mm Hg is approximately equal to the Sao_2 value minus 30.

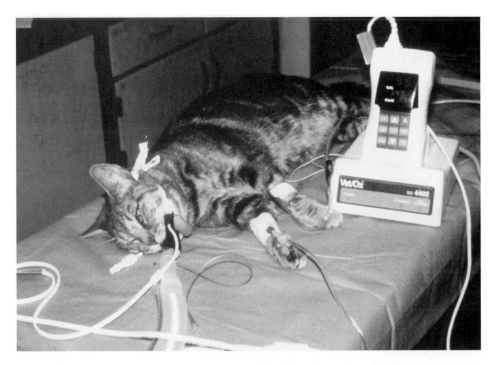

FIG. 2-17   Pulse oximeter monitoring cat through a lingual probe. (*Photo courtesy Dr. Jeff Ko.*)

If pulse oximeter or blood gas readings are abnormally low during anesthesia, the anesthetist should consider the following questions:

- Is the instrument working correctly? Readings may be affected by factors such as probe placement, external light sources, and motion.
- Some anesthetic agents (especially alpha-2 agonists such as medetomidine) cause vasoconstriction and decreased peripheral perfusion, which may significantly lower SaO_2 values. Regardless of the anesthetic agents used, perfusion of an extremity such as the tongue may decrease gradually with time and give artificially reduced SaO_2 readings. If this is the case, readings may improve if the probe is moved to a different location. If higher readings cannot be obtained, the patient should be evaluated for hypothermia, hypotension, anemia, and other causes of reduced perfusion.
- Is adequate oxygen being delivered to the patient? Inadequate oxygen delivery may result from esophageal intubation, an oxygen flow rate that is too low, an empty oxygen tank, endotracheal tube blockage or disconnection, or respiratory failure.
- Is oxygen being transferred from the alveoli to the blood? This process may be impeded by inadequate ventilation or preexisting lung disease.
- Is circulation adequate? Bradycardia or severe arrhythmias may decrease oxygenation.

Regardless of the cause, patients with subnormal PaO_2 or SaO_2 readings may require supplemental oxygen delivery or ventilation through bagging or the use of a ventilator.

Pulse oximeters can be used not only on anesthetized patients but also on animals that are in intensive care because of trauma, heart failure, respiratory difficulty, or unconsciousness. Their chief limitation is the difficulty of finding a suitable probe site in alert and mobile patients.

Capnography. Capnography is a method of monitoring the amount of CO_2 in the air that is breathed in and out by the patient (Fig. 2-18). Capnography* is a noninvasive, continuous, and practical method of monitoring ventilation in anesthetized patients.

There are two methods of sampling for capnography, either of which is appropriate for veterinary patients. Either a monitor sensor is placed between the endotracheal tube and the anesthetic circuit (mainstream capnography) or the monitor samples airway gas through a small tube attached to the junction of the endotracheal tube and the anesthetic circuit (side stream capnography). In both systems, the instrument measures the CO_2 in the air that passes the monitor on both inspiration

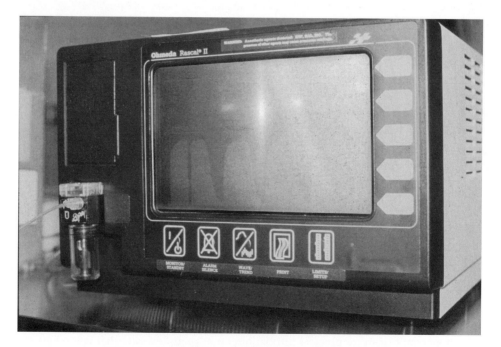

FIG. 2-18   Capnograph. (*Photo courtesy Dr. Jeff Ko.*)

---

*The term *capnography* refers to measurement of CO_2 throughout the breathing cycle. The term *capnometry* refers to measurement only of the CO_2 level at its peak (end expiration). Some instruments *(capnometers)* display only the highest CO_2 level on expiration, called the *ETCO$_2$*, whereas others *(capnographs)* display the entire wave form.

and expiration and displays this information in graph form (Fig. 2-19) or as a readout. During inspiration, the amount of CO_2 should be close to zero unless there is some rebreathing taking place or the CO_2 absorber is not working properly (A to B on the graph). During expiration, the CO_2 content of the air rises (B to C) and should reach approximately 35 to 40 mm Hg at the end of expiration when the last volume of alveolar gas is exhaled (C to D). This value is called the *end tidal carbon dioxide (ETco₂)* and is important because it closely approximates $Paco_2$. The CO_2 level then falls as expiration ends and inspiration begins (D to E).

The ETco₂ is of great significance to the anesthetist. The normal exhaled ETco₂ is 32 to 35 mm Hg in the cat and 35 to 46 mm Hg in the dog. Hypercapnia (that is, higher than normal CO_2) is present if the ETco₂ is greater than 40 mm Hg. Hypocapnia (that is, lower than normal CO_2) is present if the ETco₂ is less than 30 mm Hg.

Low values for ETco₂ may occur with rapid respiratory rates, overzealous assisted ventilation, hypothermia, or if excessive dead air space dilutes the exhaled alveolar gas. Low values may also be seen if the endotracheal tube is in the esophagus or bronchus or if the capnometer has been disconnected from the endotracheal tube. Cardiac failure causes a sudden drop in ETco₂ because ETco₂ is directly correlated to cardiac output. Capnometers are useful for monitoring cardiac resuscitation efforts, because ETco₂ values should rapidly rise when effective cardiopulmonary resuscitation (CPR) is instituted.

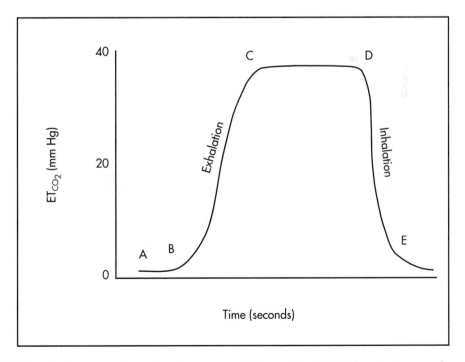

FIG. 2-19 Capnograph tracing (capnogram). (*From Wright B, Hellyer P:* Compendium 18[10]:1083-1097, 1996.)

Elevated CO_2 values may occur at any point in the graph and indicate that CO_2 is being retained by the patient. Elevated values during the inspiratory phase (see Fig. 2-19, *A* and *B*) may occur if excessive CO_2 is being breathed in by the patient (for example, if the CO_2 absorber is depleted). Elevated CO_2 during the expiratory plateau is most commonly due to hypoventilation (see Fig. 2-19, *C* and *D*). If this is the case, $ETCO_2$ should rapidly fall when ventilation is assisted by bagging or a mechanical ventilator.

It can be seen that there may be a variety of reasons for hypercapnia or hypocapnia, including metabolic, ventilatory, and circulatory abnormalities. Some of these need to be quickly corrected, whereas others may be self-limiting. It should be noted that erroneous readings sometimes arise, and it is important for the anesthesia technician to work with the veterinarian to properly identify problems and correct them when necessary.

Electrocardiography

Electrocardiography allows the anesthetist to monitor heart rate and rhythm on a continuous or intermittent basis. Although the alert anesthetist may detect arrhythmias by careful auscultation and palpation of the pulse, the ECG allows precise characterization of these abnormalities. It is extremely useful for monitoring not only anesthetized animals, but also animals in cardiac arrest, because the ECG pattern can be used to guide treatment (see p. 270 in Chapter 6). Veterinary technicians should be familiar with the procedure for setting up an ECG machine and leads, as outlined in veterinary nursing references.

The term *cardiac arrhythmia* (or *cardiac dysrhythmia*) includes any pattern of electrical activity that differs from the healthy awake animal. The ECG reveals arrhythmias that vary in significance from innocuous to life threatening. Some arrhythmias may be well tolerated by young healthy patients but may be significant problems in animals with preexisting heart disease and in geriatric patients.

The anesthetist should be able to recognize the most common ECG patterns that signify an impending problem or emergency. These include the following:

* *Tachycardia.* Anesthetized animals exhibiting heart rates greater than 200 bpm in a cat, 180 bpm in a small dog, and 160 bpm in a large dog should be reported to the veterinarian. Tachycardia may result from the use of drugs (for example, ketamine, atropine, or epinephrine) or may be a response to surgical stimulation. If surgical stimulation is the cause, it does not necessarily indicate insufficient anesthetic depth unless accompanied by rapid respiration, spontaneous movement, or active reflexes. Tachycardia may also arise because of an anesthetic-related problem, such as hypoxia, hypotension, or excessive CO_2 levels in the blood. Tachycardia may also be due to preexisting conditions such as hyperthyroidism, anemia, circulatory shock, septicemia, cardiac disease, or (in the awake patient) excitement. Treatment depends on the cause but may include application of direct digital pressure to the eyeballs or the use of drugs that slow the heart, such as propranolol.

* *Bradycardia.* Heart rates of less than 60 bpm in a large dog, 70 bpm in a small dog, and 100 bpm in a cat should be reported to the veterinarian. Like tachycardia, bradycardia may be the result of drug administration (for example, xylazine, medetomidine, or opioids given without atropine) or may indicate a problem

with anesthesia (for example, excessive anesthetic depth, hypoxia, or hypothermia). Treatment, if necessary, may include administration of appropriate reversal agents (atipamezole, naloxone) or atropine. Animals with normal blood pressure and Sao$_2$ probably have adequate tissue perfusion, and treatment may be unnecessary, but this decision lies with the veterinarian.

- *Heart block.* The presence of a heart block indicates that the electrical impulse that causes the heart to beat is not being transmitted efficiently throughout the heart. In first-degree heart block the interval between the P wave and QRS complex is prolonged, but each P wave is followed by a QRS complex. In second-degree heart block (Fig. 2-20), some P waves (atrial contractions) are not followed by QRS complexes (ventricular contractions). In third-degree heart block (Fig. 2-21), the atrial and ventricular contractions occur independently, and the normal pattern of a P wave followed by a QRS complex is absent. Both second- and third-degree heart blocks decrease the efficiency of cardiac contractions They are commonly seen after the administration of alpha-2 agonist agents such as medetomidine. Other causes include high vagal tone, hyperkalemia, and cardiac disease.

- *Premature ventricular contractions (PVCs, also called VPCs).* A PVC is an impulse that arises from a focus in ventricular muscle and represents an ineffective and uncoordinated contraction (Fig. 2-22). These often appear as bizarre, wide QRS complexes on the ECG tracing. Isolated PVCs are commonly seen in anesthetized animals, especially those induced with barbiturates or maintained with halothane,

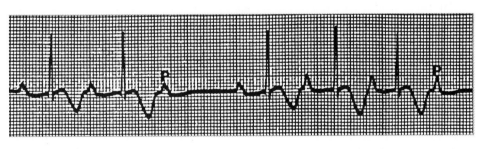

FIG. 2-20   ECG tracing showing second-degree heart block. (*From Glaze K: Vet Tech 18[1]:25-33, 1997.*)

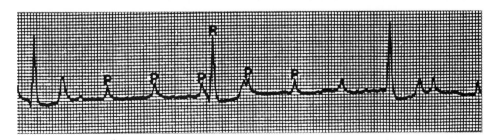

FIG. 2-21   ECG tracing showing third-degree heart block. (*From Glaze K: Vet Tech 18[1]:25-33, 1997.*)

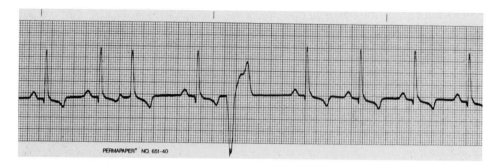

FIG. 2-22   Premature ventricular contractions. (*From Kittleson MD, Kienle RD: Small animal cardiovascular medicine, St Louis, 1998, Mosby.*)

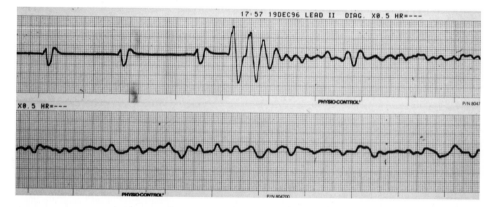

FIG. 2-23   Ventricular fibrillation. (*From Kittleson MD, Kienle RD: Small animal cardiovascular medicine, St Louis, 1998, Mosby.*)

and do not always require treatment. Hypoxia is another common cause of PVCs in anesthetized animals, and in some cases they may be eliminated by increasing the delivery of oxygen to the patient. PVCs may also occur in animals with cardiac disease, gastric torsion, trauma to the heart, or acid-base or electrolyte disorders. Epinephrine is a potent stimulus of PVCs, and they are common in animals given epinephrine injections and in animals that release epinephrine from their adrenal glands as a result of fear, pain, or excitement. This is one reason why it is unwise to forcibly restrain a struggling animal during induction, because the release of epinephrine may potentiate severe and even fatal arrhythmias (particularly in patients given halothane or other arrhythmogenic agents).

TABLE 2-2			

Indicators of Anesthetic Depth

| | ANESTHETIC DEPTH | | |
SIGN	LIGHT	MEDIUM	DEEP
Spontaneous movement	Maybe	No	No
Swallowing	Maybe	No	No
Vaporizer setting	Low	Medium (1.1-1.5 MAC)	High
Muscle tone	Normal	Moderate	None
Palpebral reflex	Active	Moderate	None
Eyeball position	Central	Ventromedial	Central
Pupillary light reflex	Present	May be present	Absent
Shivering	Maybe	No	No
Heart rate	Often elevated	Variable	Often decreased
Respiratory rate	Often elevated	8-30 breaths/min	Often decreased

Modified from Haskins SC: *Vet Clin North Am Small Anim Pract* 22(2):432-434, 1992.
MAC, Minimum alveolar concentration.

The appearance of frequent PVCs in an ECG tracing (more than 15 per minute or more than 3 in a row) or PVCs seen in conjunction with falling blood pressure indicates that the heart is significantly compromised and should be brought to the attention of the veterinarian. Intravenous lidocaine is the most common treatment for severe PVCs.

- *Fibrillation.* Fibrillation is the contraction of small muscle bundles within the ventricles or atria. Ventricular fibrillation indicates that cardiac arrest is imminent. Ventricular fibrillation appears on an ECG tracing as an irregular undulating line, with complete absence of recognizable QRS complexes (Fig. 2-23).

The ECG records electrical activity of the heart but is not a sure indicator of mechanical function. It is possible for an animal to have a normal ECG even though heart contractions have ceased (a state that is called *electromechanical dissociation*).

Reflexes and Other Indicators of Anesthetic Depth

The anesthetist should have at all times an accurate assessment of the patient's depth of anesthesia. Anesthetic depth is a complex interaction between the action of the anesthetics and the patient's physiologic responses. Body temperature, ventilation, blood pH, and blood pressure all have a potent influence on the way in which an anesthetic affects the animal. It is therefore important to monitor the whole animal, assessing the apparent depth in light of the animal's vital signs.

Anesthetic depth is indicated in several ways. Reflex activity, muscle relaxation, heart and respiratory rates, pupil size, and eye rotation are all useful guides in determining how deeply or lightly the patient is anesthetized (Table 2-2). For some anesthetics (particularly cyclohexamine agents such as ketamine) it may be difficult for the anesthetist to determine the level of anesthetic depth; however, the following guidelines are useful for anesthesia induced by most general anesthetic agents.

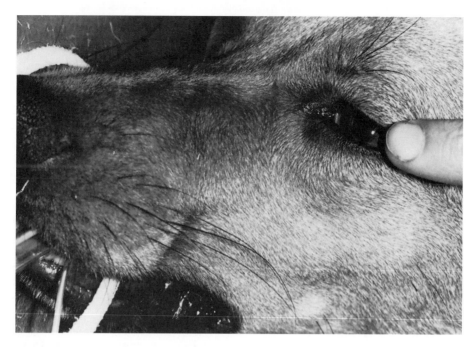

FIG. 2-24   Assessment of the palpebral reflex. (*From Warren RG:* Small animal anesthesia, *St Louis, 1983, Mosby.*)

Reflex activity

All healthy, conscious animals demonstrate predictable reflex responses to certain types of stimuli. One example is the cough reflex, in which the animal responds to the presence of foreign material in the airways by forceful coughing. Reflex responses help protect the animal from injury (in the case of the cough reflex, by clearing upper airway obstructions and preventing aspiration of injurious materials). These protective reflexes are progressively depressed at increasing depths of anesthesia, such that an animal in stage III, plane 3 (or deeper anesthesia) may have few reflex responses or none. The reflexes most commonly monitored in veterinary anesthesia include the palpebral, swallowing, pedal, ear flick, corneal, and laryngeal reflexes.

Palpebral reflex

The palpebral reflex (blink reflex) can be tested by lightly tapping the medial or lateral canthus of the eye and observing whether the animal blinks in response (Fig. 2-24). Some anesthetists prefer to test this reflex by lightly stroking the hairs of the upper eyelid. In the conscious animal, this reflex helps protect the eye from injury. Most animals retain the palpebral reflex throughout stages I and II and partially through stage III, although individual and species variations exist. The stage at which the palpebral reflex is lost also varies among different anesthetic agents: at a surgical plane of anesthesia, it is usually present in barbiturate anesthesia, occasionally present in methoxyflurane anesthesia, but seldom present in halothane anesthesia (in dogs).

As with most reflexes, loss of the palpebral reflex indicates an increase in anesthetic depth, whereas return of the reflex usually indicates imminent arousal from anesthesia.

Swallowing reflex

The swallowing reflex occurs spontaneously in awake animals and is usually stimulated by the presence of saliva or food in the pharynx. Lightly anesthetized animals swallow frequently, and this reflex can be readily monitored by observing movement in the patient's ventral neck region. The swallowing reflex is lost at a medium depth of anesthesia and is regained just before the patient recovers consciousness. The return of the swallowing reflex during recovery indicates that it is safe to remove the endotracheal tube. Animals that vomit after this point usually will swallow rather than aspirate the vomited material, and the endotracheal tube is therefore no longer needed to protect the airway. (In fact, if the endotracheal tube is not removed at this point, the patient may soon begin to chew on it.)

Pedal reflex

The pedal reflex is elicited by squeezing or pinching a digit or pad and observing whether the unconscious animal flexes the leg, withdrawing the paw from the examiner (Fig. 2-25). The pedal reflex is a good indicator of anesthetic depth in animals that have been given the general anesthetic pentobarbital. It is also a helpful indicator of depth in animals undergoing mask inductions, in which the presence of a mask makes assessment of other reflexes or jaw tone somewhat difficult. This reflex is not as useful in inhalation anesthesia because the reflex is usually absent in the maintenance period.

Ear flick reflex

The ear flick reflex (pinna reflex) is particularly useful in cats. This test consists of gently touching the hairs on the inner surface of the pinna and observing the resultant twitch of the ear. This reflex may be retained well into stage III, particularly in cats anesthetized with ketamine. This reflex may be difficult to elicit in some animals and may be easily lost if tested too frequently within a short time period.

Corneal reflex

The corneal reflex can be tested by touching the cornea with a sterile object (a drop of water or artificial tear solution is commonly used) and noting whether the animal blinks and withdraws the eye into the orbital fossa. This reflex is not commonly tested in dogs and cats unless it is necessary to determine if the patient is too deeply anesthetized. This reflex is usually present until stage III, plane 4, anesthesia.

Laryngeal reflex

The laryngeal reflex is stimulated when the larynx is touched by an object. The reflex response is an immediate closure of the epiglottis and vocal cords. This reflex normally protects the animal from aspiration of material into the trachea. The laryngeal reflex may be observed during intubation if the animal is not sufficiently anesthetized to allow the tube to be passed. It is easily elicited in cats, in which a sustained laryngeal reflex response is the cause of laryngospasm (see Chapter 6).

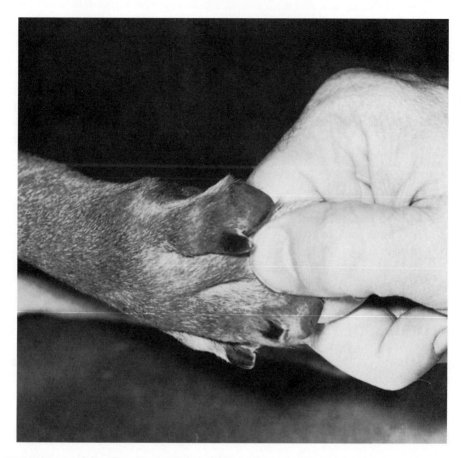

FIG. 2-25   Pedal reflex. (*From Warren RG:* Small animal anesthesia, *St Louis, 1983, Mosby.*)

Muscle tone

Muscle tone is also a useful guide to anesthetic depth. With increasing depth, skeletal muscles become more relaxed and offer little resistance to movement. Among the muscles that can be readily assessed are the muscles of mastication, which control jaw tone. Jaw tone is assessed by attempting to open the jaws wide and estimating the amount of passive resistance (Fig. 2-26). Muscle tone can also be assessed by attempting to flex and extend the foreleg at the elbow and carpus. Anal tone also indicates skeletal muscle relaxation and may be assessed by noting the size of the rectal orifice. Some degree of muscle relaxation is desirable for most procedures; however, extreme muscle relaxation resulting in a flaccid jaw tone is unnecessary and may indicate excessive anesthetic depth.

The degree of muscle relaxation observed in the patient depends not only on anesthetic depth but also on the particular drugs given to the animal, some of which promote relaxation (for example, diazepam and xylazine) and some of which increase muscle tone (for example, ketamine and tiletamine). Specific muscle-

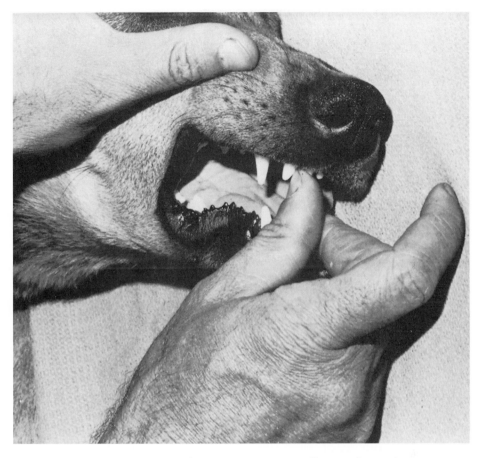

FIG. 2-26   Assessing jaw tone. (*From Warren RG:* Small animal anesthesia, *St Louis, 1983, Mosby.*)

paralyzing agents, such as atracurium, may be used in combination with general anesthetics to achieve pronounced muscle relaxation for certain procedures (see Chapter 7). This may be advantageous to the surgeon but gives the anesthetist one less parameter with which to monitor anesthetic depth.

Eye position and pupil size

Eye position, pupil size, and the pupillary response to light also may indicate anesthetic depth, although there is considerable variation among individual animals. The eyeball itself is usually central in stage I anesthesia. It becomes eccentric in stage II, making the animal appear to be looking toward its chin (Fig. 2-27). As the animal approaches a surgical plane of anesthesia, the eyeball often becomes more central, and the central position is maintained through increasing depth of anesthesia. Some anesthetics (for example, ketamine) do not cause eye rotation, even at moderate anesthetic depth.

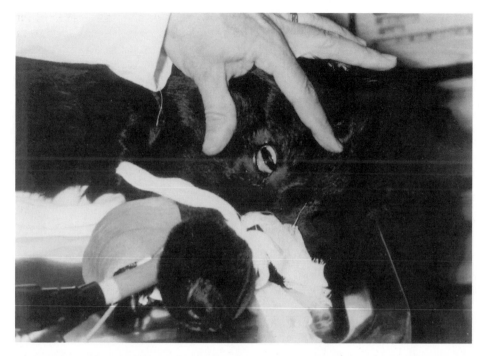

FIG. 2-27   Ventral rotation of the eyeball and prolapse of the third eyelid during anesthesia.

The size of the pupil may also reflect anesthetic depth; the anesthetized patient normally has dilated pupils (mydriasis) during stage II anesthesia, constricted pupils (miosis) when lightly anesthetized, and progressively greater pupil dilation as anesthetic depth increases. The ability of the pupil to constrict in response to light (pupillary light reflex) also diminishes with increasing depth of anesthesia and is usually absent at surgical anesthetic depth. Dilated, central pupils that are not responsive to light may indicate a dangerously deep level of anesthesia. The anesthetist should be aware, however, that atropine can cause pupil dilation, particularly in cats. This interaction may confuse the interpretation of pupil size and the pupillary light reflex.

Salivary and lacrimal secretions

The presence or absence of salivary and lacrimal secretions may give clues about anesthetic depth, particularly in an animal that has not received anticholinergics. Production of tears and saliva diminishes with increasing anesthetic depth and is totally absent in deep surgical anesthesia. Because of the relative absence of tears and the subsequent danger of corneal drying, the use of ophthalmic drops or ointment is advised for all animals undergoing general anesthesia. Atropine ointment should not be used because it causes significant pupil dilation.

Heart and respiratory rates

Heart and respiratory rates may be a valuable guide to anesthetic depth. Both variables show a tendency to decrease as the animal enters deeper levels of anesthesia and a tendency to increase with lighter anesthesia. Caution should be used in interpreting both heart rate and respiratory rate because they are subject to many influences in addition to anesthetic depth. For example, heart rate increases in response to a fall in blood pressure. Heart rate is also elevated by the perception of a painful stimulus. Some preanesthetic and anesthetic drugs (for example, ketamine and atropine) increase heart rate, whereas most other agents decrease heart rate. Heart rate also may be affected by endotracheal intubation, which may cause bradycardia. Like heart rate, respiratory rate may reflect anesthetic depth but is influenced by other variables, including the Pao_2, the $Paco_2$, and the anesthetic agent used.

Response to surgical stimulation

One other variable that may indicate anesthetic depth is the response of the animal to surgical stimulation. As previously mentioned, certain procedures, such as manipulation of viscera or pulling on the suspensory ligament of the ovary, may result in a response that indicates a perception of pain, although the perception is not usually conscious. Animals perceiving surgical stimulation may show an increase in heart rate and blood pressure. The anesthetist should not necessarily interpret these signs as an indication that the animal's anesthetic depth is inadequate unless the increase in heart rate is considerable. Minor changes in heart rate during surgery are considered normal, and, in fact, the absence of such a response may indicate an unnecessarily deep level of anesthesia. Increased respiratory rate or signs of voluntary movement by the patient, however, do indicate insufficient anesthetic depth and the perception of pain. Lacrimation, salivation, and sweating (most easily observed on the foot pads) also indicate that the patient may be perceiving a painful stimulus and that depth is inadequate.

Judging Anesthetic Depth

During the course of anesthesia, the anesthetist should monitor as many variables as possible and weigh all available evidence before judging the anesthetic depth of the patient. No one piece of information is unfailingly reliable, and it is foolish to determine the anesthetic plane by monitoring only one reflex or vital sign. In addition, each animal is unique and has an individual response to increasing anesthetic depth. For example, some dogs anesthetized with ketamine maintain the palpebral reflex throughout stage III, whereas others lose this reflex as early as stage III, plane 2. If the palpebral reflex is used as the sole criterion for judging anesthetic depth, the animal that retains that reflex into deep anesthesia may be incorrectly judged to be only lightly anesthetized. Increasing the concentration of anesthetic delivered to such a patient might easily result in dangerously deep anesthesia. Observation of the other indicators of anesthetic depth would likely give the anesthetist a more balanced view of the situation and a more accurate assessment of true anesthetic depth. Examples of the use of judgment in interpreting anesthetic depth are given in Box 2-3.

Similarly, observation of the amount of anesthetic being delivered to the patient (for example, by the vaporizer of an anesthetic machine) does not in itself indicate the patient's anesthetic depth. Although high vaporizer settings result in increased delivery of anesthetic to the patient and, subsequently, an increase in patient depth, there is tremendous variation in patient response. This variation is due in part to the patient's response to anesthetic and in part to the influence of other drugs given

BOX 2-3 *Examples of Depth Assessment*

1. A mature cat has been anesthetized with thiopental given intravenously. The anesthetist notes that the cat appears unconscious and relaxed. The pulse is strong, and the heart rate is 144 bpm. The respirations are regular, and the rate is 20 breaths per minute. The pupils are centrally positioned. The palpebral reflex is brisk, but there is no pedal or ear flick reflex. The anesthetist wishes to intubate the animal. At this depth of anesthesia, is it possible? What other tests could the anesthetist perform to determine anesthetic depth?

   Answer: The cat appears to be in stage III, plane 1 anesthesia and may be deep enough to intubate. The anesthetist should assess the jaw tone and observe whether there is any resistance when the tongue is gently pulled before assuming that intubation is possible.

2. A 13-year-old dog has been anesthetized by mask induction with isoflurane. After intubation, it is maintained on 2% isoflurane. The anesthetist wishes to ensure that the dog is sufficiently anesthetized to allow removal of a large skin tumor. The dog's respirations are shallow, with a rate of 8 breaths per minute. The heart rate is 90 bpm. There is no response to surgery, and all reflexes are absent. The pupils are central; the jaw tone is slack. Is the animal adequately anesthetized for this procedure?

   Answer: The animal is indeed adequately anesthetized and in fact may be at an excessive anesthetic depth. Respiration rate is slow and tidal volume is low. The absence of all reflexes, the central pupils, and the slack jaw tone all indicate that the animal may be in stage III, plane 3 anesthesia. At this point, the anesthetist should consider reducing the isoflurane setting to 1.5% and monitoring the animal for signs of decreased depth. After doing this, the anesthetist should carefully monitor the animal for signs of pain perception (for example, increased respiratory rate, voluntary movement, lacrimation, and sweat on the foot pads) to ensure that the vaporizer setting is high enough for adequate analgesia. Ideally, the heart rate and respiratory rate will increase slightly but not enough to indicate imminent arousal.

3. An 8-year-old dog has been anesthetized with atropine and IV ketamine/diazepam and is now under halothane anesthesia. The dog's heart rate is 100 bpm, and the respirations are 8 breaths per minute. The jaw tone appears moderate, but the pupils are central and show no response to light. No reflexes are present. Is the anesthetic depth appropriate?

   Answer: The anesthetist cannot be sure whether the anesthetic depth is appropriate or too deep because some variables indicate stage III, plane 2 (heart rate, jaw tone), but others indicate stage III, plane 3 (respiratory rate, reflexes, pupil position and response to light). The patient has been given atropine and ketamine, which may have elevated the heart rate. At this point, the anesthetist should assume the patient is excessively deep and should reduce the concentration of halothane. At the same time, the anesthetist should monitor the patient for signs of arousal.

to the animal. One animal may be maintained at stable surgical anesthesia when given a concentration of 1% halothane gas, whereas another animal may require 2% halothane and still another may be satisfactorily maintained at 0.5% halothane. The concentration of anesthetic gas received by the animal also is not necessarily the concentration indicated by the vaporizer setting; it may vary with the oxygen flow rate and quality of ventilation received by the patient (see Chapter 4). Nevertheless, a consideration of the vaporizer setting and the length of time that the animal has been anesthetized may help the anesthetist decide if an animal is anesthetized too lightly or too deeply. The basic rule is that if there is doubt about the level of anesthesia in a particular patient, one should decrease the vaporizer setting and monitor the animal closely to assess anesthetic depth.

Recording Information during Anesthesia

Complete and accurate medical records are a legal requirement in veterinary practice. Most jurisdictions require that some form of anesthetic record be maintained. In many cases, this record can be in the form of a logbook in which information is listed, such as the date, client and patient identification, preoperative physical status, nature of the procedure performed with the patient under anesthesia, and the anesthetic protocol. A brief description of the animal's response to anesthesia should also be given. The use of narcotics and other controlled drugs must be meticulously documented. Records of this type allow the veterinarian to review the total number of anesthetic procedures that have been carried out in a given period and determine the number of animals that had anesthetic complications. This information may be helpful in assessing the anesthetic protocols and procedures used by a practice.

Additionally, medical information regarding the anesthetic procedure must be written in the patient's record. This allows the veterinarian to quickly review the animal's anesthetic history and may be helpful in determining the best anesthetic protocol to use for future procedures. For example, if the record indicates that the animal has undergone anesthesia with a barbiturate agent and experienced a lengthy recovery, the veterinarian may choose to anesthetize the dog with an alternative agent in the future. On the other hand, if a geriatric dog with congestive heart failure has been recently anesthetized without incident with a particular agent, the veterinarian would be justified in using the same agent for the next anesthesia.

In some situations, an anesthesia form such as those given in Figs. 2-28 and 2-29 is used to record a detailed description of an anesthetic procedure. This type of record contains information on the patient's preoperative status (for example, temperature, pulse, and respiration and the results of diagnostic tests), the anesthetic protocol used (including fluids administered and the amounts and concentrations of drugs given), the patient's vital signs throughout anesthesia (for example, pulse, respiration, blood pressure, temperature, and lab results), the time at which anesthesia commenced and was terminated, the beginning and end of surgery, and the time required for recovery. Typically, the information is recorded chronologically to allow an overview of the patient's responses at every point throughout the procedure. Detailed records of this type are not commonly used in veterinary practice; however, they are useful in a teaching, referral, or research institution.

PATIENT POSITIONING AND COMFORT DURING ANESTHESIA

In addition to monitoring the patient's vital signs and reflexes as described, the anesthetist should ensure that the patient is not compromised by rough handling or careless positioning during the procedure. Examples of appropriate patient care during anesthesia include the following:

- During induction, the animal should be supported as it loses consciousness. Particular care should be taken to avoid striking the animal's head on the table during induction and during the animal's transfer to surgery.

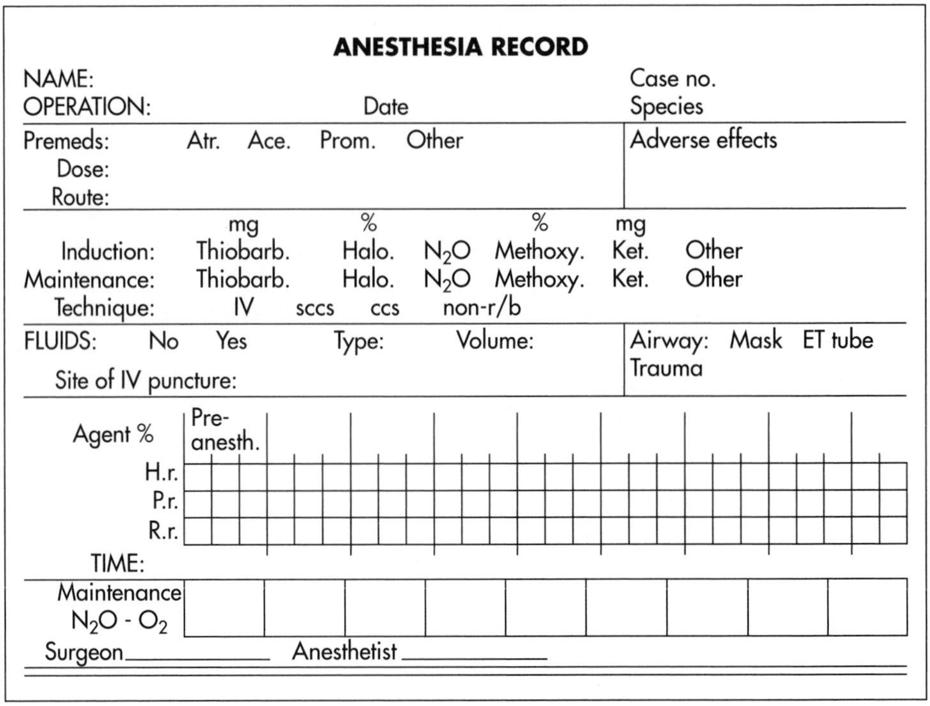

ANESTHESIA RECORD

NAME:					Case no.	
OPERATION:			Date		Species	
Premeds:	Atr.	Ace.	Prom.	Other	Adverse effects	
Dose:						
Route:						

	mg	%	%	mg	
Induction:	Thiobarb.	Halo.	N₂O Methoxy.	Ket. Other	
Maintenance:	Thiobarb.	Halo.	N₂O Methoxy.	Ket. Other	
Technique:	IV sccs ccs	non-r/b			

FLUIDS: No Yes	Type: Volume:	Airway: Mask ET tube	
Site of IV puncture:		Trauma	

Agent %	Pre-anesth.											
H.r.												
P.r.												
R.r.												
TIME:												
Maintenance N₂O - O₂												

Surgeon_____ Anesthetist _____

FIG. 2-28 Anesthetic record (short form). (*From Warren RG:* Small animal anesthesia, *St Louis, 1983, Mosby.*)

- If an intubated patient is to be turned over, the endotracheal tube should be temporarily disconnected from the anesthetic circuit. Rolling or twisting the animal while it is still connected to the circuit may cause the endotracheal tube to twist and collapse, resulting in an airway obstruction (Fig. 2-30), or cause the distal end of the tube to traumatize or lacerate the trachea.
- Before the surgery preparation begins, the anesthetist must ensure that the patient's endotracheal tube is correctly placed (that is, not in the esophagus) and that it is large enough to prevent significant leakage of waste gas around the tube. Once the surgical preparation starts, it is difficult to position the animal to allow reintubation without compromising aseptic technique.
- The hoses of the anesthetic machine should be supported so that there is no drag on the endotracheal tube. This could result in tracheal trauma by the tube or inadvertent removal of the tube. Care should be used to avoid positions that kink or bend the endotracheal tube, and the position of the hoses and endotracheal tube should be checked during patient transfer and after repositioning. The reservoir bag should be placed so that it is clearly visible at all times.
- When positioning the animal on the surgery table, the anesthetist should ensure that the animal assumes as normal a posture as possible. In particular, overextension or hyperflexion of the neck and limbs should be avoided because either may result in permanent neurologic injury. Hyperflexion of the neck also may lead to endotracheal tube obstruction.

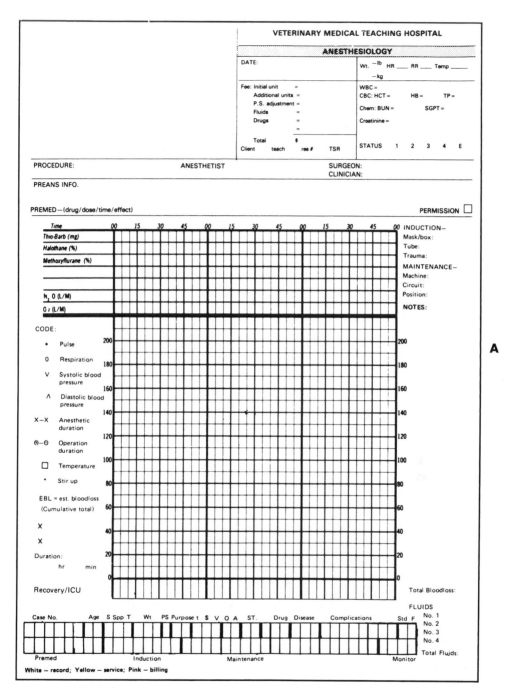

FIG. 2-29 **A,** Comprehensive anesthetic record. (*From Warren RG: Small animal anesthesia, St Louis, 1983, Mosby.*)

Continued

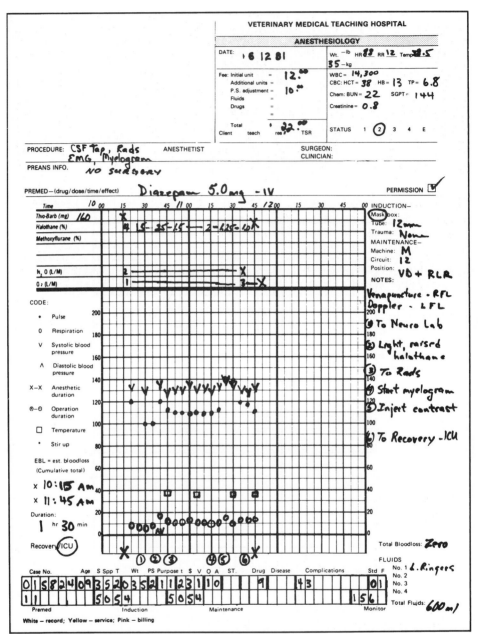

FIG. 2-29, cont'd B, Sample case. (*From Warren RG:* Small animal anesthesia, *St Louis, 1983, Mosby.*)

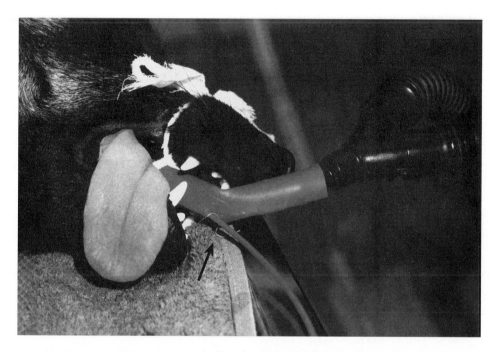

FIG. 2-30   Kinked endotracheal tube in a dog.

- Care should be taken when attaching restraining devices such as ropes or gauze ties to the patient. These devices must not be excessively tight, or blood circulation to the limbs may be compromised. Overextension of the front legs may also interfere with breathing.
- Heavy drapes or instruments must not compress the chest of small patients because this may interfere with respiration.
- The practice of tilting the surgery table allows the surgeon easier access to some abdominal organs, particularly the uterus and ovaries. However, the anesthetist should be aware that tilting the table more than 15 degrees may cause the abdominal organs to significantly compress the diaphragm, which may compromise heart and lung function. Head-down tilted positions should be avoided in animals with breathing difficulties, especially those with diaphragmatic hernia.
- If an anesthetized patient is known to have unilateral lung disease, the patient should be positioned before and after surgery with the normal side up.
- Artificial tear solution or other corneal lubricant should be instilled into the eyes of an anesthetized patient every 90 minutes. This is particularly important if an anticholinergic is used. General anesthesia decreases tear secretion for a period of up to 24 hours after anesthesia, and some dogs may need periodic application of a corneal lubricant for up to 36 hours after anesthesia. Cats maintain some tear production throughout anesthesia; however, lubrication is advisable if an anticholinergic or ketamine is given.

RECOVERY FROM GENERAL ANESTHESIA

The *recovery period* may be defined as the period between discontinuation of anesthetic administration (whether injectable or inhalation) and the time the animal is able to stand and walk without assistance. The length of the recovery period depends on many factors, including the following:

- *The length of the anesthesia.* As a general rule, the longer the period of anesthetic administration, the longer the expected recovery period.
- *The condition of the patient.* Lengthy recoveries are seen in animals that have almost any debilitating disease (particularly liver and kidney disease).
- *The type of anesthetic given and the route of administration.* Animals given inhalation agents such as isoflurane or sevoflurane typically show shorter recovery periods than do animals given injectable drugs such as barbiturates or ketamine. Lengthy recoveries are particularly common if the injectable agent is given IM rather than IV.
- *The patient's temperature.* Hypothermic patients are slow to metabolize and excrete anesthetic drugs.
- *The breed of the patient.* Certain canine breeds (for example, greyhounds, salukis, Afghan hounds, whippets, and Russian wolfhounds) are slow to recover from certain anesthetic agents, especially barbiturates.

Stages of Recovery

An animal recovering from general anesthesia gradually progresses back through the same anesthetic stages that were experienced during induction. As the animal moves from deep to moderate to light anesthesia, vital signs and reflexes change in predictable ways. Heart rate, respiratory rate, and respiratory volume increase. The pupil, which had rotated ventrally, moves back to its normal central position (although it may rotate ventrally again and return to a central position before arousal). Reflex responses, including the palpebral, pedal, and ear flick, become stronger. The animal may shiver, swallow, chew, or attempt to lick. Shortly after swallowing, the animal will normally show signs of consciousness, including voluntary movement of the head or limbs, opening the eyelids, and vocalization.

Anesthetist's Role in the Recovery Period

The recovery period is by no means a time of relaxation for the anesthetist. Anesthetic complications and death may occur during this period, even in animals that appear to have no problems during induction or maintenance. Ideally, recovery should occur in an area in which the animal can be watched on a continual basis. An emergency kit, monitoring equipment (for example, stethoscope, pulse oximeter, and thermometer), and oxygen should be readily available.

The duties of the anesthetist during the recovery period include monitoring vital signs, extubation at the appropriate time, maintenance of a patent airway after extubation, administering oxygen as necessary, reassuring the patient and providing adequate analgesia, preventing patient self-injury, administering medications as requested by the veterinarian, and general nursing care (warming the patient, ensuring patient comfort and hygiene).

Monitoring

Vital signs should be evaluated every 5 minutes during the recovery period. Particular attention should be given to mucous membrane color, capillary refill, and breathing. Periodic, hands-on evaluation is necessary; observation from across the room is not adequate. For example, a recovering animal may have significant bradycardia and respiratory depression, yet show no signs that are evident to the casual observer. Animals exhibiting abnormal vital signs or a delayed return to consciousness should be examined by the veterinarian. Conditions such as shock, hemorrhage, hypoglycemia, and hypothermia may be present and must be treated as soon as possible. It is also important that the recovering patient be closely monitored for problems such as vomiting, seizures, laryngospasm, and dyspnea. These are discussed in detail in Chapter 6.

Extubation

The endotracheal tube must be removed when the patient shows signs of imminent arousal. In dogs the appearance of the swallowing reflex (signaled by swallowing movements observed in the throat region) is most often cited as the appropriate time to remove the tube because the returning swallowing reflex will help protect the animal from aspiration if vomiting occurs. Animals that show voluntary limb or head movement or spastic movement of the tongue or animals that attempt to chew the endotracheal tube are close to consciousness and should be extubated even if swallowing has not been observed. One exception to this general rule is brachycephalic dogs: many anesthetists prefer to delay extubation in brachycephalic dogs until the dog is able to lift its head unassisted. This is because early extubation may lead to significant respiratory distress in these animals.

If a recovering patient shows signs of respiratory distress after extubation, the anesthetist must determine whether this is due to poor pulmonary function (in which case oxygen therapy may be needed) or respiratory distress due to upper airway obstruction. One helpful clue is that animals with airway obstruction may have noisy respirations, especially on inspiration. If obstruction is present, the anesthetist should reposition the patient and gently pull its tongue forward. If the obstruction persists, it may be necessary to induce and reintubate the patient. It is wise to prepare for possible respiratory distress in a brachycephalic dog by setting out a laryngoscope, an endotracheal tube, and the appropriate dose of thiopental or another inducing agent near the recovery cage of the animal in case reintubation becomes necessary.

In cats the endotracheal tube may be removed when signs of impending arousal are observed. These include swallowing, an active palpebral reflex, and voluntary limb, tail, or head movements. Delaying extubation is not advisable in cats because it may predispose the patient to laryngospasm.

In all patients, it is necessary to deflate the endotracheal tube cuff and untie any restraining gauze before removing the tube. Some anesthetists prefer to deflate the cuff and untie the gauze before signs of arousal are seen so that the tube can be quickly removed when swallowing occurs. Ideally, the tube should be removed at the end of an inspiration. When an endotracheal tube is removed after a dental surgery or prophylaxis or after any procedure in which blood or other fluid is present in the oral cavity, the cuff should be left partially inflated to prevent these fluids from entering the air passages.

After extubation, all animals should be placed in sternal recumbency with the neck extended. This position helps maintain a patent airway. Occasionally, fluid or mucus may accumulate in the pharynx or trachea and should be removed by suction. This should be done before the patient is fully awake to avoid being bitten by the recovering patient.

Administration of oxygen

If possible, oxygen should be provided for several minutes after the discontinuation of the anesthetic agent, by means of an endotracheal tube or mask. Oxygen administration may benefit the recovering patient in several ways.*

- By maintaining the patient on the breathing circuit for a short time during recovery, the anesthetist ensures that the patient is adequately oxygenated and that the anesthetic gases the patient is exhaling are being scavenged.
- Periodic bagging with pure oxygen is advisable for as long as the recovering patient is connected to the machine because this helps reinflate collapsed alveoli.
- Oxygen therapy helps to prevent hypoxemia in the cold, shivering patient.

If an anesthetic machine has been used for the procedure, it is customary to continue oxygen administration at a high flow rate (for example, 200 ml/kg/min) for 5 minutes after turning off the anesthetic vaporizer or until the animal swallows, at which time the patient must be disconnected from the machine and the endotracheal tube must be removed.

A patient that is intubated and breathing oxygen from an anesthetic machine receives close to 100% oxygen. This is beneficial for the relatively short time required for most operations, but prolonged intake of high levels of oxygen (for example, greater than 50% oxygen for more than 24 hours) can be toxic. For nonanesthetized patients, 30% to 40% oxygen is ideal. Delivered oxygen should be humidified if administration lasts more than a few hours.

If oxygen therapy is to be continued past the time when the patient is extubated, a face mask can be used, although constant supervision is necessary and some patients do not tolerate a mask. The flow rate depends on the size of the patient and how tightly the mask fits. Alternatives to a face mask include the following:

- An oxygen delivery source such as a Y piece or Bain circuit can be held close to the patient's nose.
- An Elizabethan collar can be placed around the patient's neck, with an oxygen line secured to the inside of the collar. The front is covered with cellophane, with a small ventilation hole. A flow rate of 1 L/min provides 30% to 40% oxygen.
- A lubricated soft rubber catheter (5 to 10 F) with multiple fenestrations in the distal end can be introduced into the ventral nostril. Intranasal proparacaine or 2% lidocaine can be used to desensitize the nasal tissues to allow insertion. The catheter is advanced to the level of the carnassial teeth and attached to the dorsum of the nose with an adhesive agent such as cyanoacrylate. A flow rate of 100 to 150 ml/kg provides 30% to 50% oxygen.
- Oxygen cage.

---

*Oxygen therapy may benefit not only recovering anesthetized patients, but also patients with seizures, cranial trauma, lung disease, congestive heart failure, hyperthermia, and other conditions.

Stimulation of the patient

In some cases patient recovery may be hastened by gentle stimulation. This may include talking to the patient, pinching the toes, opening the mouth, gently moving the limbs, or rubbing the chest. Stimulation of this type increases the flow of information to the reticular activation center (RAC) of the brain, which is the area responsible for maintaining consciousness in the awake animal. A lack of stimulation to the RAC may cause drowsiness in the conscious animal, and it is therefore speculated that stimulation of this area may help the animal to awaken. It is also advisable to turn the patient every 10 to 15 minutes to prevent pooling of blood in the dependent parts of the body, including the lungs. This condition is called *hypostatic congestion*. When the intubated patient is turned from one side to another, the head and neck should be turned as a single unit to minimize the chance of the endotracheal tube lacerating the trachea. The anesthetist should also be gentle when moving a patient that may be in pain because movement may add to patient discomfort.

Reassuring the patient

During the recovery period, the anesthetist should take every possible step to comfort and reassure the awakening patient. The anesthetist should bear in mind that the animal has no means of understanding the events that have led to its present disoriented state. Quiet, calm handling and reassurance are therefore essential.

The anesthetist can take several steps to minimize patient discomfort during recovery. All ties restraining the animal to the surgery table should be removed before the animal regains consciousness. The anesthetist should ensure that all accessory procedures, such as bandaging, chest tube placement, and urinary catheterization, have been completed and that the esophageal stethoscope, ECG leads, and thermometer are removed before the patient returns to consciousness. It is advisable to leave venous access (that is, indwelling catheter or butterfly) in place until the endotracheal tube has been removed and patient recovery is seen to be uneventful. These catheters allow easy administration of fluids or drugs in the event that the patient's condition requires them.

Postoperative analgesics

Analgesics should be administered as requested by the veterinarian, preferably before the animal experiences postoperative pain (see Chapter 8). If the animal has received appropriate analgesia, it should be able to sleep comfortably and demonstrate minimal signs of pain after the surgery. A change in analgesic dose or frequency, or a switch to another analgesic may be necessary if postoperative pain is apparent despite the administration of medication.

Nursing care

Nursing care of the recovering animal should include the application of heat to all hypothermic animals. This can be achieved by various means, including the use of warm towels, hot water bottles wrapped in towels, infrared heat lamps placed approximately 1 m (3 feet) from the patient, hot air dryers, rice or oat bags heated in a microwave, circulating warm water heating pads, or placing the patient in an incubator designed for human babies. Often the patient is unable to move voluntarily at this point, and the anesthetist must ensure that the patient is not burned by prolonged contact with an external heat source. Gradual rewarming is preferred to rapid rewarming because the latter may cause dilation of cutaneous vessels, leading to hypotension. The patient should be provided with ample bedding or padded material to prevent heat loss and increase patient comfort.

Preventing patient self-injury

Some animals may pass through a period of excitement (similar to stage II anesthesia) before completely regaining consciousness. As in induction, stage II recovery is characterized by vocalization, delirium, hyperventilation, head thrashing, and rapid paddling movements of the front legs. Occasionally an animal may appear to be disoriented during anesthetic recovery, and patients (particularly those recovering from ketamine anesthesia) may chew at their paws or claw their faces. Occasionally, a recumbent animal may thrash or make ineffectual attempts to stand. Animals showing these or similar signs of a "stormy recovery" usually return to normal within a short time, but close observation is necessary to prevent self-trauma or disruption of the surgical repair. Tranquilization and/or the administration of analgesics should be considered in these patients.

Anesthetized or recovering animals must never be left alone on a table or in a cage with the door open because of the danger of falling. Food and water should not be left in the animal's cage during recovery because it is not unknown for recovering animals to drown in water bowls or suffocate in food bowls. Some patients may be able to drink soon after standing; however, most have little appetite for food for several hours after recovery. Vomiting during the recovery period is common, but provided the patient is conscious, this is seldom dangerous.

Summary

The importance of nursing care during the recovery period cannot be overemphasized. Postoperative problems such as hemorrhage, the removal of sutures by the animal, aspiration of vomit and subsequent inhalation pneumonia, and burns often may be prevented if the animal is closely monitored. The anesthetist's duty toward the patient does not end until the patient is awake and standing, fully recovered from the anesthesia.

KEY POINTS

1. General anesthesia is a state of controlled and reversible unconsciousness accompanied by analgesia, amnesia, loss of motor response to stimuli, and depressed reflex responses. Ideally, respiration and circulation are not affected; however, in practice they may be impaired to a greater or lesser extent.
2. General anesthetic agents are usually administered by injection or inhalation.
3. The anesthetic period can be divided into preanesthesia, induction, maintenance, and recovery. Traditionally, anesthetic depth has been described in terms of stages and planes of anesthesia, with stage III, plane 2, being suitable for most surgical procedures.

4. Anesthetic safety is improved through the use of preanesthetic agents, use of the minimum effective dosages, selection of a protocol well suited to the patient, and by close monitoring of the patient.

5. Induction of anesthesia may be achieved by intravenous (IV) or intramuscular (IM) administration of an injectable agent or by mask or chamber administration of an inhalation agent. Regardless of the method used, the patient is often intubated immediately after induction and maintained on an inhalation agent.

6. Intubation improves the safety and efficiency of anesthesia; however, it may be associated with problems such as vagal nerve stimulation, laryngospasm, airway obstruction, and pressure necrosis of the trachea.

7. During the maintenance period, the anesthetist must monitor the animal closely to ensure that vital signs remain within acceptable limits. The anesthetist also must monitor reflex activity and other variables to ensure that the anesthetic depth is appropriate.

8. Vital signs that should be monitored by the anesthetist include heart rate and rhythm, pulse strength, capillary refill time, mucous membrane color, respiration rate and depth, and temperature.

9. Through the use of monitoring instruments, it is possible to gain accurate knowledge of the patient's blood gas levels, oxygen saturation, exhaled carbon dioxide levels, electrocardiogram (ECG), central venous pressure (CVP), and arterial blood pressure.

10. Indicators of anesthetic depth include reflexes (particularly the palpebral reflex), muscle tone, eye position, pupil size, and response to surgical stimulation. Heart rate and respiratory rate also may change as anesthetic depth is altered. The anesthetist should assess depth after considering several variables because no single indicator is unfailingly accurate.

11. The anesthetist must keep accurate medical records, the nature of which will vary depending on the clinical situation.

12. Patient comfort must be ensured throughout the procedure. This is accomplished by frequent monitoring, correct positioning, and gentle handling procedures.

13. The length of the recovery period depends on many factors, including the anesthetic protocol and the patient's condition. Return to consciousness is accompanied by increasing heart and respiratory rates, increased reflex responses, and voluntary movement.

14. During the recovery period, the anesthetist must continue to monitor the patient's vital signs, particularly temperature. It is often helpful to administer oxygen for several minutes after the anesthetic has been discontinued.

15. In dogs extubation should occur when the swallowing reflex returns. In cats extubation should occur when the patient shows signs of impending arousal, such as voluntary movements, swallowing, or active reflexes.

16. Other recovery duties may include stimulation of the patient, administration of oxygen, postoperative analgesia, and general nursing care.

1. As the depth of anesthesia increases, there will be a continued depression of cardiovascular and respiratory function.
   True   False
2. The surgical plane of anesthesia is generally considered to be:
   a. Stage III, plane 1
   b. Stage III, plane 2
   c. Stage III, plane 3
   d. Stage III, plane 4
3. Breath holding, vocalization, and involuntary movement of the limbs are most likely an indication that the animal is in what stage/plane of anesthesia?
   a. Stage I
   b. Stage II
   c. Stage III, plane 1
   d. Stage III, plane 2
4. Anatomic dead space is considered to be the:
   a. Air within the circuit
   b. Air within the digestive tract
   c. Air within the trachea and other airways
   d. Air within the alveoli
5. The minimum acceptable heart rate for an anesthetized large breed dog is

   _____ bpm.
   a. 60
   b. 70
   c. 80
   d. 100
6. If the ECG is normal, the heart must be beating normally.
   True   False

7. In general, a respiratory rate of less than _____ breaths per minute in an anesthetized dog should be reported to the veterinarian.
   a. 4
   b. 8
   c. 12
   d. 16
8. Tachypnea is:
   a. An increase in respiratory depth (tidal volume)
   b. An increase in respiratory rate
   c. A decrease in respiratory depth (tidal volume)
   d. A decrease in respiratory rate
9. The term *atelectasis* refers to:
   a. Increased fluid in the alveoli
   b. Hyperinflation of the alveoli
   c. Collapsed alveoli
   d. A decrease in the perfusion of blood around the alveoli

10. A patient that has been anesthetized will often have a:
    a. Mild metabolic acidosis
    b. Mild metabolic alkalosis
    c. Mild respiratory acidosis
    d. Mild respiratory alkalosis
11. An animal that is in a surgical plane of anesthesia should not respond in any way to any procedure that is being done to it (for example, pulling on viscera should not change heart rate).
    True   False
12. A 20-kg dog has been anesthetized by mask induction with isoflurane and after intubation is maintained on 2% isoflurane with a flow rate of 2 L of oxygen per minute. The heart rate is 80 bpm, respiratory rate is 8 breaths per minute and shallow, the jaw tone is relaxed, and all reflexes are absent. This animal is most likely in what stage of anesthesia?
    a. Stage III, plane 1
    b. Stage III, plane 2
    c. Stage III, plane 3
    d. Stage III, plane 4
13. After an anesthetic procedure, when is it best to extubate a dog?
    a. Right after you turn off the vaporizer
    b. About 10 minutes after turning off the vaporizer
    c. When the animal begins to swallow
    d. Any time that is convenient
14. Hypostatic congestion may be present at the end of the anesthetic protocol. This term refers to the:
    a. Accumulation of mucus in the trachea
    b. Pooling of blood in the lungs
    c. Leakage of fluid into the chest
    d. Pooling of ingesta in one area of the gastrointestinal tract
15. Pulse oximetry allows accurate determination of:
    a. Arterial blood pressure
    b. Pulse pressure
    c. Pao_2
    d. Percent saturation of hemoglobin by oxygen
    e. Blood gas values

For the following questions, more than one answer may be correct.

16. Pale mucous membranes may be an indication of:
    a. Blood loss
    b. Anemia
    c. Decreased perfusion
    d. Hypertension
17. An endotracheal tube is used to:
    a. Decrease dead space
    b. Allow for a patent airway
    c. Protect the patient from aspiration of vomitus
    d. Allow the anesthetist to ventilate the patient

18. Problems associated with endotracheal intubation include:
    a. Decreased dead space
    b. Pressure necrosis of the tracheal mucosa
    c. Intubation of a bronchus
    d. Spread of infectious disease
19. An animal under stage III, plane 2, anesthesia would exhibit which of the following signs?
    a. Very brisk palpebral reflex
    b. Regular respiration
    c. Relaxed skeletal muscle tone
    d. Very dilated pupils
20. As you place an endotracheal tube into an animal, what clinical signs will indicate to you that the endotracheal tube is in the trachea?
    a. The animal may cough as you insert the tube down the trachea.
    b. You can feel only one tube in the neck region.
    c. The reservoir bag of the anesthetic machine expands when the patient exhales.
    d. When you compress the reservoir bag, the stomach rises.

ANSWERS FOR CHAPTER 2

1. True	**2.** b	**3.** b	**4.** c	**5.** a
6. False	**7.** b	**8.** b	**9.** c	**10.** c
11. False	**12.** c	**13.** c	**14.** b	**15.** d
16. a, b, c	**17.** a, b, c, d	**18.** b, c, d	**19.** b, c	**20.** a, b, c

Selected Readings

Camps-Palau MA, Marks SL, Cornick JL: Small animal oxygen therapy, *Compendium* 21(7):587-597, 1999.
Carr AP: Measuring blood pressure in dogs and cats, *Vet Med* 3:135-144, 2001.
Edwards NJ: *ECG manual for the veterinary technician,* Philadelphia, 1993, WB Saunders.
Grosenbaugh DA, Muir WW: Blood pressure monitoring, *Vet Med* 1:48-59, 1998.
Haskins SC: General guidelines for judging anesthetic depth, *Vet Clin North Am Small Anim Pract* 22(2):432-434, 1992.
Haskins SC: Opinions in small animal anesthesia, *Vet Clin North Am Small Anim Pract* 22(2):326-469, 1992.
Lee L: Recovery complications in small animal anesthesia, *Vet Tech* 13(5):327-335, 1992.
Muir WW III, Hubbell JAE, Skarda RT, et al: *Handbook of veterinary anesthesia,* ed 3, St Louis, 2000, Mosby.
Paddleford RR: *Manual of small animal anesthesia,* New York, 1988, Churchill Livingstone.
Rivera A, Rudloff E, Kirby R: Monitoring in the intensive care unit, *Vet Tech* 17(1):27-43, 1996.
Short CE: *Principles and practice of veterinary anesthesia,* Baltimore, 1987, Williams & Wilkins.
Wright B, Hellyer P: Respiratory monitoring during anesthesia: pulse oximetry and capnography, *Compendium* 18(10):1083-1097, 1996.

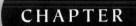

CHAPTER 3

Anesthetic Agents and Techniques

PERFORMANCE OBJECTIVES

After completion of this chapter, the reader will be able to:
- Define the terms *dissociative anesthesia, apneustic respiration, volatile anesthetic, sponge effect, second gas effect, diffusion hypoxia, analeptic agent,* and *reversing agent.*
- Describe the advantages and disadvantages associated with the use of injectable anesthetic agents.
- Describe the advantages and disadvantages associated with the use of inhalation anesthetic agents.
- List the injectable anesthetic drugs that may be used as general anesthetics and be familiar with the following information regarding each agent: method of administration, mode of action, effect on the heart and respiration, route of elimination from the body, and adverse effects.
- List the inhalation anesthetic agents commonly used in veterinary medicine and the advantages and disadvantages of each agent.
- Describe the pharmacologic properties of isoflurane, sevoflurane, halothane, methoxyflurane, and nitrous oxide.
- Describe the uptake, distribution, and elimination of the commonly used inhalation anesthetic agents.
- Define and explain the significance of minimum alveolar concentration, vapor pressure, solubility (partition) coefficient, and rubber solubility.
- Describe the use of nitrous oxide in veterinary anesthesia and the potential hazards associated with nitrous oxide anesthesia.

As described in Chapter 2, general anesthesia may be achieved through the administration of one or more potent anesthetic agents. These agents can be divided into two broad classes: injectable drugs (including barbiturates, cyclohexamines, neuroleptanalgesics, propofol, and etomidate) and inhalation agents (including halothane, isoflurane, sevoflurane, desflurane, methoxyflurane, and nitrous oxide) (see Fig. 2-1). The pharmacologic and physiologic effects of general anesthetics are described in detail in this chapter.

COMPARISON OF INHALATION AND INJECTABLE ANESTHESIA

Although both inhalation and injectable agents are commonly used in veterinary practice, inhalation anesthesia is considered to have a greater margin of safety. The advantages of inhalation anesthesia include the following.

119

- When an inhalation agent is used, the depth of anesthesia can be readily altered by the anesthetist. Inhalation agents continuously enter and leave the body via the respiratory system, which allows the concentration of anesthetic in the blood (and thus the brain) to be changed rapidly. If the patient appears too awake, the concentration of anesthetic delivered by the anesthetic machine to the animal can be increased, resulting in a deeper level of anesthesia. If the anesthetist wants to bring the patient to a lighter depth of anesthesia or to initiate recovery, the anesthetist can discontinue administration of the inhalation agent by turning off the anesthetic vaporizer. In contrast, the depth of the anesthesia produced by an injectable agent cannot be readily altered except by injection of additional drug to increase anesthetic depth or by the use of a reversing agent (in the case of opioids and alpha-2 agonists).
- The elimination of inhalation agents, particularly isoflurane and sevoflurane, occurs mainly through the lungs. This is in contrast to the elimination of injectable agents, which is achieved in three ways: by redistribution of the drug within the body, by liver metabolism, and by renal excretion. Patient recovery from an injectable agent generally depends more on the patient's hepatic and renal function than is the case with an inhalation anesthetic. These factors are not always significant in a young, healthy patient; however, they are often of concern to the veterinarian choosing an anesthetic protocol for a patient with preexisting problems.
- Inhalation anesthesia allows the constant delivery of a high concentration of oxygen (close to 100%) to the patient. In contrast, animals under injectable anesthesia breathe room air containing approximately 20% oxygen unless they receive supplemental oxygen by mask or endotracheal tube.
- Most patients under inhalation anesthesia are intubated, and mechanical ventilation with the anesthetic machine is relatively easy. This increases the safety of the anesthetic procedure because the anesthetist can respond promptly in case of hypoventilation or respiratory arrest. The endotracheal tube also reduces the risk of aspiration or airway obstruction.

The disadvantages of inhalation anesthesia compared with injectable anesthesia are the following:

- Inhalation anesthesia requires an anesthetic machine for delivery of anesthetic and oxygen to the patient. Injectable anesthetics do not require the use of this equipment and in the short run may be simpler and more economical to use. Once the equipment has been purchased, however, the cost of using an inhalation agent is comparable to that of injectable agents.
- Induction of anesthesia with inhalation agents alone is slow compared with induction with injectable agents.
- Inhalation anesthesia has the potential for the escape of waste anesthetic gas into room air. Waste gas exhaled by the patient or leaked from anesthetic equipment results in operating room pollution. Personnel inhaling high levels of waste gas may be at increased risk for reproductive disorders and other health problems (see Chapter 5).

Many years of experience in veterinary anesthesia have shown that both injectable and inhalation anesthetics are effective and can be used with a wide margin of safety. It should be emphasized, however, that both injectable and inhalation agents have an overall depressant effect on the cardiovascular, respiratory, and thermoregulatory systems. Constant vigilance on the part of the anesthetist is necessary to prevent and to respond to anesthetic complications that may arise from the use of any agent.

INJECTABLE ANESTHETICS

Injectable agents are commonly used to induce anesthesia in small and large animals. The characteristics of an ideal injectable agent for induction of anesthesia include the following:

- Rapid onset and recovery
- Lack of tissue toxicity
- Lack of adverse cardiovascular and respiratory effects
- Rapid metabolism even in animals with deficient liver and kidney function
- Provides analgesia
- Provides muscle relaxation

The following injectable anesthetics are used in small animal anesthesia:

- Barbiturates (including thiopental sodium, methohexital, and pentobarbital)
- Cyclohexamines (including ketamine and tiletamine)
- Neuroleptanalgesic agents (the combination of an opioid, such as morphine, butorphanol, or oxymorphone, with a tranquilizing agent)
- Propofol
- Etomidate
- Guaifenesin

Recommended dosages for these agents are given in Table 3-1. Dosages are approximate and should be adjusted according to the patient's age, physical status, and the veterinarian's recommendations. If possible, injectable agents should be titrated and given to effect, instead of the calculated dose being given as a single bolus.

Barbiturates
Classes of barbiturates

Barbiturates, particularly thiopental, are commonly used to induce anesthesia in dogs and cats. Their low cost and familiarity of use contribute to their continued popularity. Better alternatives exist for debilitated or high-risk patients, but barbiturates offer a good margin of safety for most animals.

All barbiturates in clinical use are derivatives of barbituric acid. Three classes of barbiturates are used in veterinary anesthesia: ultrashort-acting barbiturates (for example, methohexital), short-acting barbiturates (for example, thiopental), and intermediate-acting barbiturates (for example, pentobarbital). A fourth class of barbiturates, the long-acting barbiturates such as phenobarbital, is used as sedatives and anticonvulsants but not as anesthetics in clinical practice.

These classes of barbiturate drugs vary in lipid solubility, distribution within the body, rapidity of action, and duration of effect. Intermediate-acting barbiturates such as pentobarbital are relatively slow to take effect because they have low lipid solubility. The length of anesthesia and the recovery time are also prolonged compared with other barbiturate agents because intermediate-acting barbiturates such as pentobarbital rely on liver metabolism (which is relatively slow) for the termination of effects. In contrast, short-acting barbiturates such as thiopental and ultrashort-acting barbiturates such as methohexital have a rapid effect and brief duration of

TABLE 3-1		
Suggested Dosage Ranges of Injectable Anesthetic Agents		
DRUG	PURPOSE	DOSE
Thiopental sodium	Intravenous induction 2% solution (20 mg/ml)	Dog: 10-12.5 mg/kg with premedication Cat: 10 mg/kg with premedication
Methohexital	Intravenous induction 1% solution (10 mg/ml)	5 mg/kg with premedication
Pentobarbital	Intravenous anesthesia	10-20 mg/kg with premedication 22-33 mg/kg without premedication
Ketamine/diazepam (a 50-50 mixture of 5 mg/ml diazepam and 100 mg/ml ketamine)	Intravenous induction (cats and dogs)	0.1-0.14 ml/kg with premedication
Ketamine (following acepromazine and atropine premedication)	Cats only: Intramuscular (minor procedures) Intramuscular (major procedures)	10-30 mg/kg 30-45 mg/kg
Propofol	Intravenous induction Maintenance of anesthesia	3-8 mg/kg 0.5-1 mg/kg every 3-5 min or continuous infusion 0.3-0.5 mg/kg/min
Etomidate	Intravenous induction	0.5-2 mg/kg
Tiletamine/zolazepam	Intravenous induction Intramuscular use	1-2 mg/kg 4-8 mg/kg

Modified from *Veterinary teaching hospital undergraduate manual*, Guelph, Ontario, Canada, 1992, Ontario Veterinary College.

action, and recovery time is relatively short. These agents are highly lipid soluble, and the termination of their effects is achieved by redistribution of the drug from the brain to muscle and fat.

Distribution and elimination of barbiturates

To understand the mode of action of specific barbiturate agents, it is necessary to have some knowledge of the distribution and elimination of these drugs within the body. Thiopental, the most commonly used barbiturate agent, is always given by intravenous (IV) injection. Within seconds of injection it is dispersed throughout the body via the bloodstream. Large amounts of the drug rapidly reach the brain because of the excellent blood supply this organ receives. Thiopental is highly lipid soluble, and the high lipid content of the brain enhances its entry into brain tissue. The rapid absorption of thiopental into the brain explains why an animal loses consciousness within 30 seconds of injection. Pentobarbital is less lipid soluble than thiopental and requires several minutes to reach its full effect.

All barbiturate agents produce their effects by depressing the reticular-activating center of the brain, causing a loss of consciousness. This effect is terminated when the agent leaves the brain and is redistributed elsewhere in the body.

Tissues such as muscle and fat have proportionately less blood flow than the brain, and barbiturate levels in these tissues rise more slowly than in the brain (Fig. 3-1). Gradually, as the drug enters muscle and fat, the level of thiopental in the blood begins to fall. Once the thiopental concentration in the blood falls below that in the brain tissue, the drug begins to leave the brain and reenter the circulation, where it continues to be redistributed to muscle, fat, and other body tissues. (The drug leaves the brain because barbiturates, like all drugs, diffuse from areas of high concentration to areas of low concentration.) The animal will show signs of recovery as the concentration of thiopental in the brain decreases, although the drug is still present in other tissues. Over the next few hours, the barbiturate is gradually released from the muscle and fat and is eliminated from the body by liver metabolism and excretion of the metabolites in urine.

Because barbiturates are stored in the body and then are slowly metabolized over time, it is inadvisable to administer these drugs on a continuous or repeated basis during the course of a surgical procedure. This could lead to an overdose or prolonged recovery.

The variation in lipid solubility of various barbiturate agents helps explain differences in the duration of anesthesia for these agents. The rapid recovery of healthy

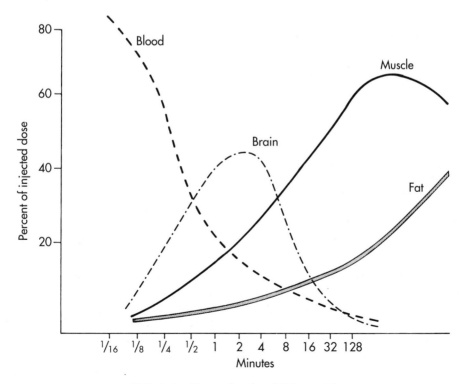

FIG. 3-1   Tissue levels of thiopental.

animals from anesthesia with thiopental or methohexital is the result of the high lipid solubility and rapid redistribution of these agents into muscle and body fat. Pentobarbital is less soluble in lipids and as a result remains in circulation rather than being redistributed to body fat. Sustained blood levels of pentobarbital result in a sustained high concentration of the drug in the brain and a long duration of action.

Use in practice

The convenience, relative safety, low cost of barbiturates, and the rapid induction that these drugs permit have led to their extensive use (particularly thiopental) in small animal anesthesia. Thiopental and methohexital are used as induction agents to allow endotracheal intubation. After intubation, anesthesia is usually maintained with an inhalation anesthetic such as halothane or isoflurane. Thiopental may also be used as the sole agent of anesthesia for brief procedures. Endotracheal intubation is strongly advised for all patients anesthetized with barbiturates, even for brief periods, to prevent aspiration of fluid or vomitus and to allow the anesthetist to support ventilation if necessary.

Because of the potential depressant effects of barbiturates on the cardiovascular and respiratory systems and because of the variation in dose requirements among patients, these drugs are normally administered to effect (that is, only the amount necessary to induce anesthesia is given). Most commonly, half of the calculated dosage is given as a bolus, and the effect of this bolus is observed before additional drug is administered. (Induction with thiopental is described in detail in Procedure 2-1.)

Effect on vital systems

Barbiturates may have significant adverse effects on ventilatory and cardiovascular function. In fact, concentrated barbiturate solutions are commonly used as euthanasia agents, a fact that illustrates the potential depressant effects of these drugs on cardiopulmonary function. Once injected into an animal, there is no way to retrieve or chemically reverse a barbiturate drug. Barbiturate overdoses are treated by ventilatory and cardiovascular support, diuresis with IV fluids, and intensive nursing care.

Respiratory depression. Barbiturates may profoundly depress respiration. This effect is evident immediately after IV administration of thiopental for anesthetic induction, when a brief period of apnea (cessation of breathing) is common. This is seen especially after rapid injection or administration of high doses. Apnea results from direct depression of the respiratory center in the medulla, which is the area of the brain that controls respiration. In the awake animal, the respiratory center responds to rising levels of carbon dioxide (CO_2) in the blood by sending out impulses to the muscles that initiate inspiration. Barbiturates cause the respiratory center to become relatively insensitive to increased blood CO_2 levels, and as a result fewer nervous impulses are sent to the respiratory muscles. Respiratory rate decreases, and if the concentration of the drug in the brain is high, respiration may cease for a short time. Breathing resumes when the concentration of the drug in the plasma and brain decreases sufficiently such that the ventilatory control centers in the brain are not as depressed or when decreased oxygen in the bloodstream stimulates breathing. Most healthy patients are not adversely affected by a brief period of apnea; however, the patient's mucous membrane color and heart rate should be closely monitored to ensure that circulation is maintained. Mucous membranes should remain pink, the heartbeat should be regular, and the pulse should be strong throughout the induction period. A pulse oximeter can also be used to monitor oxygenation levels. If spontaneous respiration does not resume within 1 to 2 minutes, or if cardiovascular function appears to be threatened, ventilatory support may be necessary. This can be provided by intubation and bagging or through the use of a mechanical ventilator (see Chapter 7). Other induction agents (ketamine, propofol) also cause respiratory depression after IV injection and have the same requirement for close monitoring.

During anesthesia induced with a longer-acting agent such as pentobarbital, the most common effect on respiration is a persistent reduction in tidal volume (that is, shallow breaths). The effect may be short-lived, or the patient's respirations may appear shallow throughout the anesthetic period. Patients with reduced tidal volume are predisposed to respiratory acidosis and poor tissue oxygenation, particularly if barbiturates are used as the sole agent of anesthesia and oxygen delivery through an anesthetic machine is unavailable.

Respiratory depression is also a potential problem when barbiturates are used in cesarean deliveries. Barbiturates, like most anesthetic agents, readily cross the placenta and enter the fetal circulation. If they are still present in the neonatal brain, barbiturates may interfere with the puppy's or kitten's ability to breathe immediately after delivery. In fact, the newborn animal is more susceptible than the mother to the effect of barbiturates, and respiration may be completely inhibited by doses of barbiturates that do not even cause anesthesia in the mother. Neonatal survival rates are particularly poor when an intermediate-acting barbiturate, such as pentobarbital, is part of the anesthetic protocol for a cesarean delivery.

Respiratory depression is not the only effect of barbiturates on the respiratory system; coughing and laryngospasm are also seen. These effects are thought to result from excessive salivation and may be minimized by the preanesthetic use of an anticholinergic such as atropine.

Cardiac depression. Although less commonly seen than respiratory depression, cardiac effects may be significant in barbiturate anesthesia, particularly in the first 10 minutes after IV injection. It has been shown in the dog that barbiturates cause a dose-dependent decrease in cardiac output and blood pressure. Thiopental and other anesthetics (notably, halothane) also increase the heart's sensitivity to the action of epinephrine. This hormone is released by the adrenal gland, particularly in patients that are excited or stressed. Circulating epinephrine may have profound effects on the heart, causing potentially dangerous arrhythmias. It is not uncommon for cardiac arrhythmias such as ventricular premature contractions (VPCs) to occur during the induction period because of the combined effect of barbiturates, epinephrine, and hypoxia. Occasionally, a condition termed *bigeminy* is seen, in which each normal beat is followed by a single abnormal beat. These cardiac arrhythmias are not clinically significant in most patients; however, cardiac arrest has been reported, especially in animals that are stressed during induction. Barbiturate anesthesia should be used with caution in animals with known cardiac disease because a dose of barbiturate that is well tolerated by a healthy heart may severely stress a diseased heart.

Adverse effects on the heart can be minimized by ensuring that barbiturates are given slowly (over 10 to 15 seconds in the case of thiopental) and that dilute concentrations are used (for example, 2% or 2.5%). Preoxygenating a patient for 3 to 5 minutes before inducing anesthesia with a barbiturate also helps to reduce the adverse cardiac effects of these drugs. Another strategy is to combine thiopental with the antiarrhythmic drug lidocaine (4 mg/kg) with the two drugs given alternately into an IV catheter (with separate syringes for the two drugs). Lidocaine (one fourth the total dose) is given first, followed by one fourth the calculated dose of thiopental, and this pattern is slowly repeated until the patient reaches the appropriate stage of anesthesia.

If cardiac arrhythmias occur, it is often helpful to give the patient two to three breaths of oxygen (by squeezing the reservoir bag of the anesthetic machine).

Other effects. In addition to the cardiovascular and respiratory problems previously outlined, barbiturates may exhibit exaggerated and potentially dangerous potency in some animals. Classes of patients that are particularly sensitive to barbiturates include hypoproteinemic animals, acidotic animals, and very lean animals.

Effect on hypoproteinemic animals. Barbiturates are normally found in the blood in two forms: free drug and drug bound to plasma proteins. Only the free (unbound) molecules of barbiturate are able to enter the brain to induce the anesthetic effect because the molecules bound to proteins are unable to cross cell membranes. In hypoproteinemic animals (that is, those with total plasma protein less than 3 g/dl, often as a result of renal, hepatic, or intestinal disease) there is less plasma protein to bind barbiturate molecules. Consequently, there is relatively more barbiturate in the active, unbound form. The potency of barbiturates within the body is therefore increased in animals with low plasma protein levels. Dosages of barbiturates suitable for healthy animals may cause prolonged unconsciousness or death in these patients.

Effect on acidotic animals. The potency of barbiturates depends on blood pH because these drugs have a greater effect if blood pH is low (acidosis). Caution should therefore be used when administering barbiturates to animals with metabolic or respiratory acidosis. A normal dose of barbiturates can produce high drug levels in the brain and an exaggerated response in these animals. Therefore the dose of barbiturates required to anesthetize acidotic animals may be significantly less than that required to anesthetize healthy animals.

Effect on sighthounds. Because of the high lipid solubility of barbiturates, these agents have increased potency and duration of action in very thin animals, including sighthounds (Afghan hounds, whippets, salukis, borzoi, and greyhounds). Distribution of thiopental into body fat cannot readily occur in such lean animals, and therefore drug levels in the brain remain high. Hepatic metabolism of barbiturates may also be slow in sighthounds, further delaying clearance from the body. For these reasons, thiopental and pentobarbital are not recommended for use in sighthounds, although methohexital is considered relatively safe.

Effect on critically ill animals. Animals with hepatic or renal disease and animals with hypothermia may exhibit prolonged recovery or hangover from thiopental and other barbiturates because metabolism and excretion are delayed. Barbiturates also show greater potency in animals that have hypotension or shock. The body responds to lowered blood pressure by reducing the blood flow to nonessential tissues (such as fat) and increasing blood flow to the brain and heart. Animals in shock can be expected to show greatly increased sensitivity to barbiturates because the normal redistribution of these agents from the brain to body fat stores does not occur.

Tissue irritation. Barbiturate solutions are strongly alkaline (pH 9.5 to 10.5) and may cause significant tissue damage if injected perivascularly or into an artery, particularly if the concentration of barbiturate exceeds 2.5%. Perivascular injection of concentrated barbiturate solutions may be followed within 48 hours by local swelling, pain, necrosis, and even tissue sloughing. The irritation caused by perivascular barbiturate injections may cause the animal to chew at the area, thereby increasing tissue damage. Tissue sloughs are slow to heal and usually result in permanent scarring.

A dilute solution of barbiturate should be used (in the case of thiopental used in cats or dogs, 2% to 2.5%) to avoid tissue irritation. As an additional precaution, barbiturates are often administered through an IV catheter or butterfly. If perivascular injection occurs, the area should be immediately infiltrated with saline (in a volume equal to the volume of barbiturate injected) to dilute the barbiturate and reduce its irritating effect. Many veterinarians add 2% lidocaine without epinephrine to the saline to give a local analgesic effect.

Excitement during induction or recovery. Perivascular injection or too slow administration of some barbiturates may result in stage II excitement during induction. This occurs because the amount of barbiturate injected IV (and therefore, the amount reaching the brain) is insufficient to produce a deeper level of anesthesia. If excitement is observed, it is necessary to immediately administer more barbiturate to induce a deeper stage of anesthesia.

The use of barbiturates, particularly pentobarbital, is also associated with a high incidence of excitement during the recovery period. Paddling and vocalization are commonly seen but may be relieved by administration of IV diazepam. Use of preanesthetic tranquilizers or opioids is helpful in reducing the incidence and severity of excitement in the recovery period.

Loss of potency. Thiobarbiturate agents are unstable in solution. These drugs are purchased in powdered form and are reconstituted by adding sterile saline or water. Once reconstituted, thiopental has a short shelf life (that is, a maximum of 2 weeks if refrigerated, less at room temperature). A solution should not be used if a precipitate is present.

Interaction with other drugs. Barbiturates enhance the neuromuscular blocking effect of muscle relaxants (see Chapter 7). Chronic administration of barbiturates (for example, phenobarbital given daily to an epileptic dog or cat) increases the activity of some hepatic enzymes. This may lead to more rapid clearance and therefore shorter duration of effect of drugs that are metabolized in the liver such as diazepam and opioids.

Record-keeping requirements

Prolonged use of barbiturates is associated with drug dependence in humans, and for this reason most countries have enacted laws regulating the purchase, storage, and use of these agents. Careful record keeping is essential to comply with these regulations.

Commonly used barbiturate drugs

The characteristics of commonly used barbiturate agents are summarized in Table 3-2.

Thiopental. Thiopental (Pentothal, Thiopentone) is among the most commonly used induction agents in small animal anesthesia and has also found widespread use as the sole anesthetic for brief procedures. It is classified as a short-acting barbiturate because the onset of action after injection is rapid (30 to 60 seconds) and duration of anesthesia is brief (10 to 20 minutes). Complete recovery usually occurs within 1 to 2 hours. Thiopental has a wide margin of safety in healthy patients.

Thiopental is supplied as crystalline powder in multidose vials. Sterile water or saline is added to the vial, making a 2% or 2.5% (20 mg/ml or 25 mg/ml) solution for small animals and a 5% (50 mg/ml) solution for large animals. All vials should be labeled with the percent concentration and date of reconstitution because solutions remain stable for a limited time and there is no bacteriostatic agent present. Care should be taken to avoid injecting air into prepared solutions because this may cause premature precipitation of the barbiturate.

Premedication with a tranquilizer/opioid/anticholinergic combination is common before thiopental administration. This provides better muscle relaxation, smoother recovery, and some analgesia.

The dosage of thiopental used for induction varies from 6 to 20 mg/kg, depending on concurrent use of other agents and the depth of anesthesia required. Dosages are commonly reduced by up to 80% in debilitated animals or in animals that have been heavily sedated. One method for IV induction with thiopental is described in Procedure 2-1. Thiopental can also be combined with lidocaine as described previously or with diazepam (10 mg/kg thiopental and 0.2 mg/kg diazepam in separate syringes, with one quarter of the dose of each drug given alternately, allowing 30 seconds between each injection). Thiopental has also been mixed with propofol (see p. 138). Whether given alone or in combination with other drugs, thiopental is always given "to effect." Repeated administration is cumulative, and recovery can be greatly prolonged if anesthesia is maintained for more than 30 minutes. For this reason it is not advisable to maintain anesthesia with repeated thiopental injections.

Methohexital. Methohexital is an ultrashort-acting methylated oxybarbiturate similar to thiopental in that the onset of action is rapid (15 to 60 seconds), duration of anesthesia is brief (5 to 10 minutes), and recovery is usually prompt. In fact, animals induced with methohexital and subsequently connected to an anesthetic machine may show signs of recovery before the inhalation anesthetic has had time to take effect. The rapid induction achieved with this agent is useful when anesthetizing a patient with a full stomach, because the anesthetist can intubate rapidly, decreasing the risk of aspiration of vomitus.

As with thiobarbiturates, methohexital is provided as a powder that must be reconstituted. A 1% solution is commonly used in small animals. The reconstituted drug has a shelf life of 6 weeks and does not require refrigeration.

Methohexital is significantly more expensive than thiopental. The cost of drug required to anesthetize a 20-kg dog with thiopental is under $1.00, whereas for methohexital the cost would be approximately $7.50.

Methohexital is administered in a manner similar to that of thiobarbiturates. In the premedicated patient, one third to one half of the calculated dose is given intra-

TABLE 3-2

Characteristics of Commonly Used Barbiturate Agents

GENERIC NAME	TRADE NAME	CLASSIFICATION	TIME TO ONSET OF ANESTHESIA	DURATION OF ACTION	RECOVERY TIME	METHOD OF ELIMINATION
Pentobarbital	Nembutal Somnotol	Short-acting	Several minutes	30 minutes-2 hours	6-24 hours	Liver metabolism
Thiopental sodium	Pentothal	Ultrashort-acting	30-60 seconds	10-20 minutes	1-2 hours	Redistribution followed by liver metabolism
Methohexital	Brevital	Ultrashort-acting	15-60 seconds	5-10 minutes	30 minutes	Redistribution followed by rapid liver metabolism

venously over 10 seconds. One injection is usually sufficient to allow intubation, but additional drug should be given in 30 seconds if an adequate plane of anesthesia is not reached. Further delay will result in a poor induction because of the rapid redistribution of the drug.

Methohexital is used most commonly in sighthounds because it produces faster recoveries and less hangover than thiopental. Liver metabolism of methohexital is much faster than other barbiturates; therefore repeated administration is not cumulative.

Although methohexital is a useful drug for veterinary anesthesia, it should be used with caution. Methohexital can cause profound respiratory depression, and the lethal dose is only 2 to 3 times the anesthetic dose. Methohexital is also associated with excitement and seizures during induction (if given too slowly) or during recovery. Premedication with a tranquilizer helps to prevent seizures and is always recommended. Postoperative seizures may be controlled with IV diazepam. Animals with preexisting central nervous system (CNS) disease, including epilepsy, should not receive methohexital.

Pentobarbital. Pentobarbital is classified as a short-acting barbiturate. The onset of action is 30 to 60 seconds after IV injection, although the full effect may not be seen for several minutes. The anesthetic effect lasts 30 minutes to 2 hours, depending on dosage and species.

Pentobarbital is supplied as a 5%, 6% or 6.5% solution (50 mg/ml, 60 mg/ml, and 65 mg/ml, respectively). It is commonly diluted with sterile water or saline to a 2% or 3% solution for use in dogs and cats. The dosage used in dogs varies from 5 to 30 mg/kg, depending on concurrent use of other general anesthetic agents or preanesthetics. This agent must be used with caution because it has a narrow margin of safety; the euthanasia dose in healthy animals is only 40 to 60 mg/kg, which is approximately double the dose used for surgical anesthesia.

Pentobarbital, like all barbiturates, is given to effect. One half of the calculated dose is given over 3 to 5 seconds, and the animal is observed for at least 2 to 5 minutes before additional drug is given. Small increments can be given until surgical anesthesia is achieved (usually 5 to 10 minutes after the initial injection). The animal should be intubated to preserve a patent airway and to allow oxygen administration if necessary. Additional drug can be given to prolong anesthesia; however, repeated dosages may be associated with excitement during the recovery period and with an extended recovery time.

Animals anesthetized with pentobarbital will initially appear unable to raise their head. As more pentobarbital is given, the jaw and tongue become completely relaxed, but a pedal reflex is still present, indicating a light plane of anesthesia. As the animal achieves a moderate depth of anesthesia, the pedal reflex becomes sluggish. If the pedal reflex is lost, the animal likely requires intubation and respiratory support.

Although pentobarbital is most commonly administered intravenously, intramuscular (IM) pentobarbital has been used as a premedication or sedative. It is also administered by intraperitoneal injection (particularly to rodents, see Chapter 9); however, its potency and duration of effect are variable when given by this route.

Before the introduction of inhalation agents such as methoxyflurane and halothane, pentobarbital was commonly used as the sole anesthetic agent for procedures such as ovariohysterectomy in the dog. However, there are several problems associated with the use of pentobarbital in small animal anesthesia:
• Pentobarbital provides minimal muscle relaxation or analgesia.

- If pentobarbital anesthesia is performed without the benefit of intubation and the administration of oxygen, the patient may have significant respiratory depression resulting in hypercapnia (that is, elevated blood CO_2) and respiratory acidosis.
- Anesthetic depth is difficult to control, except by injecting more agent.
- Recovery depends on adequate liver and kidney function. Recovery may be prolonged, particularly in cats, foals, and calves, which lack the necessary liver enzymes to metabolize the drug quickly. Excitement during induction and recovery is common in both cats and dogs anesthetized with pentobarbital.

Because of these disadvantages, the use of this agent for major surgical procedures is now uncommon in veterinary practice. It is still used occasionally in research, either as a sole anesthetic or in combination with nitrous oxide and a neuroleptanalgesic as part of a balanced anesthesia technique.

Pentobarbital is an effective agent for control of seizures. It is used in the treatment of medical conditions such as status epilepticus due to epilepsy, strychnine poisoning, and other causes (2 to 5 mg/kg loading dose, followed by 1 to 2 mg/kg/hr infusion).

Cyclohexamines

With the introduction of the injectable anesthetic phencyclidine in the late 1950s, a new class of injectable anesthetic drugs, the cyclohexamines, became available to veterinarians. Although phencyclidine is not used in veterinary medicine because of its abuse potential, its derivatives, ketamine hydrochloride and tiletamine hydrochloride, are used to induce anesthesia in many species.

Mechanism of action

The mechanism of action of the cyclohexamines appears to be a disruption of nerve conduction pathways within the cerebrum and stimulation of the reticular activating center of the brain. Unlike most general anesthetics, which cause CNS depression, cyclohexamines cause selective CNS stimulation, possibly because of a suppression of inhibitory neurons by these drugs. This results in a distinctive type of trancelike anesthesia termed *dissociative anesthesia* or *catalepsy*, in which the animal appears awake but immobile and unaware of its surroundings (Fig. 3-2). Characteristics of dissociative anesthesia include the following:

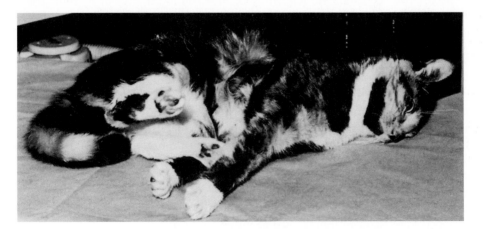

FIG. 3-2 Catalepsy induced by cyclohexamine agents.

- Reflex responses (palpebral, laryngeal) are exaggerated rather than depressed. For example, animals under dissociative anesthesia usually have a brisk palpebral reflex. Because reflex activity is preserved, even at moderate anesthetic depth, it may be difficult to determine anesthetic depth in patients under cyclohexamine anesthesia. Patients that show signs of purposeful movement are likely too light, whereas those with very depressed respiration are too deep. The anesthetist may have some difficulty in determining where an individual patient lies between these two extremes.
- Pharyngeal and laryngeal reflexes, although weak, may persist throughout anesthesia. However, the use of an endotracheal tube is still advisable to ensure patient safety. This is particularly true if a dental prophylaxis or other oral procedure is planned because blood, saliva, irrigating solutions, and other liquids present in the oral cavity may be easily aspirated if an endotracheal tube is not in place.
- Animals anesthetized with these agents may show marked sensitivity to sound, light, and other sensory stimuli. These agents are used in combination with other drugs, particularly diazepam, to avoid excitement and improve muscle relaxation.
- Muscle tone is increased, almost to the point of rigidity. The animal assumes a stiff posture, with outstretched front limbs and extended neck. Spontaneous, random movements of the head and neck may be seen even when the animal is deeply anesthetized. This is in marked contrast to the muscle relaxation that is seen with inhalation agents. The concurrent use of a tranquilizing agent such as diazepam, acepromazine, medetomidine, or xylazine helps prevent excessive muscle rigidity, improves ease of intubation, and produces a more sleeplike state.
- Although dissociative anesthetics provide significant analgesia to the skin and limbs, visceral analgesia is poor. Because the analgesia provided by these agents is not adequate to relieve acute visceral pain, they should not be used as the sole anesthetic agent for abdominal surgery (including ovariohysterectomy), thoracic surgery, or orthopedic manipulations. A patient given a dissociative anesthetic may be able to perceive pain but is unable to visibly respond to it, although growling may be heard if an endotracheal tube is not in place. It is the veterinarian's obligation to ensure that pain is not perceived, through the use of supplementary anesthetic agents and/or analgesics (for example, opioids or inhalation anesthetics) for all major surgical procedures.
- Dissociative agents are eliminated by metabolism in the liver or by renal excretion. These drugs may have an exaggerated effect on animals with reduced liver or kidney function.

Use in practice

Unlike thiopental, cyclohexamines may be given by either the IM or IV routes in some species. The versatility and wide margin of safety of cyclohexamine drugs has led to their widespread acceptance in veterinary anesthesia, particularly for use in cats. When given in combination with a tranquilizer (for example, diazepam, xylazine, medetomidine, acepromazine, or zolazepam), they are useful for brief procedures, such as feline castrations, or as a means of induction before intubation and inhalation anesthesia. They are also useful for chemical restraint of intractable cats, allowing examinations and minor treatments without endangering hospital personnel. In dogs, cyclohexamine-tranquilizer combinations (ketamine/diazepam or tiletamine/zolazepam) are also commonly used as induction agents.

One limitation of cyclohexamine use in veterinary practice is the lack of an effective reversing agent. Such an agent would be helpful in speeding recovery and controlling postanesthesia excitement.

Effect on vital systems

Dissociative anesthetics have the following effects on the vital functions of anesthetized animals:

Cardiac effects. Unlike most anesthetics, cyclohexamines do not decrease heart rate or depress myocardial function. In fact, most animals exhibit tachycardia and vasoconstriction; both systolic and diastolic blood pressures are often increased. These effects arise because cyclohexamines cause the release of epinephrine, which stimulates sympathetic activity. These cardiovascular effects are not usually harmful to the animal; however, cyclohexamines should be used with caution in animals with cardiac arrhythmias or preexisting cardiac disease (for example, cats with hyperthyroidism or cardiomyopathy). Ketamine and xylazine used in combination (particularly at high doses) are associated with significant risk of cardiovascular problems. Because both ketamine and atropine may induce tachycardia, some anesthetists prefer to use glycopyrrolate rather than atropine if an anticholinergic is required, because glycopyrrolate does not produce the same degree of tachycardia as does atropine.

Effect on respiration. Animals anesthetized with cyclohexamines exhibit apneustic respiration, a peculiar type of breathing pattern in which the patient holds its breath for several seconds at the end of the inspiratory phase, which is followed by a short, quick expiratory phase. Respiratory rate and tidal volume may be reduced, although tissue oxygenation is usually adequate. Some animals appear to hold their breath when anesthetized with ketamine, but they often can be stimulated to exhale by tapping the nose or gently stroking the thorax.

Other effects

Cyclohexamines have many other effects, including the following:

Tissue irritation. Ketamine and tiletamine are irritating to tissues, and many animals show transitory signs of discomfort when these drugs are given IM. However, these agents do not cause tissue necrosis.

Effect on salivation. Cyclohexamine agents may cause increased salivation. A low dose of anticholinergic (glycopyrrolate or atropine) may be given before use of a cyclohexamine agent to prevent profuse salivation and the resultant risk of aspiration.

Effect on CSF and intraocular pressure. Cyclohexamines may increase cerebrospinal fluid (CSF) pressure, and although this effect is not hazardous to most healthy patients, the drug is contraindicated in patients with cranial trauma, inflammation of the CNS, or intracranial tumors. Cyclohexamines also increase intraocular pressure, and their use is contraindicated for some ocular surgeries.

Effect on the eyes. Unlike conventional anesthesia, the dissociative state produced by cyclohexamine agents does not result in closure of the eyelids or eyeball rotation. The eye normally remains open, with a central and dilated pupil. The use of ophthalmic lubricant is advised to prevent corneal drying. Another unusual characteristic of dissociative anesthetics is their tendency to induce nystagmus, a repetitive side-to-side motion of the eyeball. Ketamine-induced nystagmus is more commonly seen in cats than in dogs. This condition is harmless and resolves on recovery from anesthesia.

CNS activity. Animals recovering from cyclohexamine anesthesia often show an exaggerated response to touch, light, or sound, and seizurelike activity may be observed. Diazepam (0.5 to 1 mg/kg) may be given IV (or, if IV injection is impossible, by the IM or rectal route) to reduce seizure activity. Reduction of light, sound, and other stimuli is also helpful. Some animals recovering from dissociative anesthesia may attempt to paw their faces or demonstrate other bizarre behavior, possibly a result of hallucinations induced by cyclohexamine agents. Recovering patients should be closely monitored to prevent self-injury, and it is advisable that recovery takes place in a hospital cage rather than in the owner's home.

Personality changes have been reported in animals after recovery from ketamine anesthesia. Fortunately, these usually resolve spontaneously after a few days or weeks.

Because CNS stimulation is seen with cyclohexamine agents, these drugs are contraindicated in animals with a history of epilepsy or other seizure disorders. Cyclohexamines should be avoided in animals that have ingested strychnine, metaldehyde, marijuana or other street drugs, organophosphates, and other toxins that affect the CNS. Cyclohexamines should also be used with caution in animals undergoing procedures involving the neurologic system, including CSF taps and myelograms, because the animal is at increased risk for postoperative seizures immediately after these procedures.

Ketamine

Ketamine (Ketaset, Ketalean, Vetalar) is the most commonly used induction agent in North American small animal practice and can be used to anesthetize not only cats and dogs but also birds, horses, and exotic species. Currently, ketamine is licensed only for use in cats. It is most commonly supplied as a 100-mg/ml solution. The cost of induction of a 20-kg dog with ketamine/diazepam is approximately twice that of thiopental induction. In 1999 ketamine was classified as a Schedule III controlled substance in the United States. It is presently classified as a prescription drug in Canada.

Ketamine has a rapid onset of action after IV or IM administration. This is a result of its high lipid solubility, which allows quick entry into brain tissue. Cats may lose their righting reflex within 90 seconds of IV administration and within 2 to 4 minutes of an IM injection of ketamine.

IV administration has several advantages over IM administration. Induction and recovery are more rapid and the dose is much less if the IV route is used. The anesthetist must ensure that the dose of ketamine is correct for the route of administration used: if the IM dose is inadvertently given by the IV route, serious overdose and death may result. Ketamine is given only by the IV route in dogs because IM ketamine may cause excitement and seizure activity. In cats, the primary use of IM injections is for restraint of fractious animals, in which IV injections are problematic.

Ketamine can also be administered orally to fractious cats, although this is an off-label use. For a 5-kg cat, 100 mg of ketamine is drawn into a syringe, and a feline urethral catheter is attached. This is inserted through the cage bars, and the drug is squirted into the cat's mouth. The oral ketamine takes effect in 5 to 10 minutes. If the eyes are accidentally sprayed with ketamine, they should be flushed with saline after the animal is anesthetized.

Although ketamine can be administered repeatedly to maintain anesthesia, this should be done with caution. After repeated injections, large amounts of the drug accumulate in the tissues, increasing the risk of seizure activity during recovery and significantly prolonging the recovery period.

Recovery from ketamine anesthesia normally occurs within 2 to 6 hours in healthy patients, depending on the dosage given and the administration route. Unlike barbiturates, redistribution to body fat does not occur with cyclohexamines: recovery occurs as the drug gradually leaves the brain and is metabolized and excreted. Dogs appear to have faster recoveries than cats, probably because of differences in the method of ketamine metabolism and excretion. Elimination of ketamine depends on hepatic metabolism in the dog, but in the cat it is primarily excreted through the kidney. It follows that ketamine should be used with caution in dogs with hepatic disease and in cats with compromised renal function or urinary obstruction.

Ketamine-tranquilizer mixtures

Ketamine is usually administered in combination with a tranquilizer, such as diazepam, xylazine, medetomidine, guaifenesin (in large animals), or acepro-mazine. The tranquilizer may be given as a premedication or mixed with ketamine and administered simultaneously. The use of a tranquilizer reduces the dose of ketamine required, may increase analgesia (if alpha-2 agonists are used), aids muscle relaxation, and allows smoother recovery than the use of ketamine alone. As previously mentioned, administration of an anticholinergic is helpful in preventing excessive salivation.

Ketamine-diazepam mixtures. These are popular for IV induction of cats and dogs (including sighthounds) and are formulated by combining equal volumes of diazepam (5 mg/ml) and ketamine (100 mg/ml). The resulting mixture may show precipitation if stored for a prolonged period. After premedication with an opioid and/or atropine, ketamine-diazepam is given by IV administration at a dosage rate of 1 ml/7 kg. The animal loses consciousness within 30 to 90 seconds and remains sufficiently deep for intubation or minor surgery for 5 to 10 minutes. This is followed by a 30- to 60-minute recovery period.

The combination of ketamine and diazepam has several advantages, including minimal depressant effects on the heart, good muscle relaxation, superior recovery, and some analgesia. Respiratory depression, however, may be greater than that seen with ketamine alone.

Ketamine-diazepam does not work well when given by the IM route in either cats or dogs, because diazepam is poorly absorbed after IM injection. However, another benzodiazepine agent, midazolam, is water soluble and may be combined with ketamine in a manner similar to diazepam for use in minor procedures (midazolam 0.3 mg/kg and ketamine 10 mg/kg). The midazolam-ketamine mixture is well absorbed after IM administration in cats.

Ketamine-xylazine mixtures. These are used primarily for feline and equine anes-thesia. This combination is associated with significant cardiovascular and respiratory side effects in small animals, including hypoventilation, hypertension, and decreased cardiac output. This combination causes even more significant cardiovascular prob-lems in dogs and should not be used in that species. Horses do not show significant cardiovascular abnormalities with this combination. Ketamine-xylazine may be given either IM or IV in cats, which is a significant advantage of this combination. IM ketamine-xylazine may be safer than IV use and is a particularly convenient anesthetic combination for use in uncooperative cats. In cats, the combination induces profound catalepsy with excellent muscle relaxation and some analgesia (although the analgesia is inadequate for major surgery and probably lasts 15 minutes or less).

Because of the potentially adverse effect of xylazine on the cardiovascular and respiratory systems in small animals, this anesthetic combination does not offer the safety of ketamine-diazepam mixtures. Oxygen supplementation is advised during the maintenance period. Patients recovering from ketamine-xylazine anesthesia should be closely monitored because anesthetic complications and even death may result from cardiovascular collapse and respiratory depression long after the surgical procedure is finished.

The combination of ketamine and xylazine is associated with an increased risk of aspiration of vomitus because xylazine acts as an emetic in cats, and the swallowing reflexes may not be maintained adequately. This risk may be alleviated somewhat by premedicating the patient with atropine and xylazine and allowing 10 or 15 minutes for emesis to occur before anesthesia is induced by the administration of ketamine.

In contrast to the situation in small animals, ketamine-xylazine provides excellent analgesia, muscle relaxation and sedation in horse with minimal cardiovascular side effects (see Chapter 10).

Ketamine-medetomidine mixtures. Ketamine can be given with medetomidine, either combined in a syringe or separately (medetomidine first, ketamine 10 to 15 minutes later). IM administration is preferred to IV administration because cardiovascular side effects are less pronounced with the IM route. Bradycardia and heart block may be seen, and high doses may be associated with seizures during the recovery period. Reversal of medetomidine with atipamezole should be delayed for at least 1 hour after administration of the ketamine-medetomidine combination to avoid rough recoveries. The anesthetist should anticipate that by reversing the medetomidine, there is the likelihood that the analgesia provided by the medetomidine will also be reversed, and the patient may become acutely painful.

Ketamine-acepromazine mixtures. These are given commonly to cats using either the IV or IM route. Acepromazine (0.05 to 0.1 mg/kg) and atropine (to reduce salivation) may be given as a premedication, followed 15 minutes later by ketamine (10 to 15 mg/kg); or the three drugs can be mixed together in a syringe. There is less respiratory depression and fewer cardiovascular side effects with this combination than with ketamine-xylazine. Muscle relaxation, however, is limited. As with other ketamine-tranquilizer combinations, the anesthesia produced is not sufficient for major surgery unless supplemented with an opioid agent or inhalation anesthetic.

Tiletamine

Tiletamine is a newer dissociative agent with effects similar to ketamine. Tiletamine is sold only in combination with zolazepam, which is a benzodiazepine agent closely related to diazepam. The use of zolazepam in combination with tiletamine reduces the risk of seizures during recovery and helps promote skeletal muscle relaxation. The product (Telazol) is sold as a powder, which contains 50 mg/ml of each drug.

It can be reconstituted with sterile water, saline, or 5% dextrose solution and is stable for 4 days at room temperature and 14 days if refrigerated. Telazol is a class III controlled substance in the United States. It is currently unavailable in Canada.

Tiletamine-zolazepam is useful as an induction agent in healthy dogs and cats, particularly in animals with aggressive temperaments. It can be used as a sole agent of anesthesia (after premedication) or supplemented with inhalation anesthetics. The dosage used is frequently lower than that recommended by the manufacturer.

The combination of tiletamine and zolazepam is similar in effect to ketamine-diazepam but offers the following advantages:

- Tiletamine appears to cause less pronounced apneustic respiration than ketamine. However, respiratory depression may be significant, particularly if a high dose is used or tiletamine is used in combination with other sedatives or anesthetics.
- Tiletamine-zolazepam may be administered by the IM, IV, or subcutaneous (SC) route, although currently in the United States, it is approved only for IM use in dogs and cats.
- Tiletamine-zolazepam is effective in many species of wildlife, and in some species it is the drug of choice for capture and immobilization.

Because it can be given by a variety of routes including IM or SC, tiletamine-zolazepam is particularly useful for chemical restraint of aggressive dogs and cats. A mixture of 3 mg/kg tiletamine and 0.4 mg/kg butorphanol given IM (or 2 mg/kg tiletamine and 0.2 mg/kg butorphanol given IV) provides adequate restraint for examination and minor procedures in dogs. In fractious cats, a dose of 2.5 mg/kg tiletamine can be given SC. Onset of anesthesia is 2 to 5 minutes after IM injection (slightly longer after SC injection), and duration of anesthesia is 20 to 30 minutes. As with ketamine, IM injection may be painful.

IV induction is usually preceded by acepromazine/opioid premedication. A dose of 4 mg/kg is drawn up and one third of the dose is given every 60 seconds until the animal can be intubated. Injection should be slow and given "to effect" only.

Tiletamine-zolazepam can be given orally to dogs at a dose of 20 mg/kg. It is usually combined with acepromazine to enhance sedation.

Many reflexes are maintained throughout tiletamine-zolazepam anesthesia (including the palpebral, corneal, laryngeal, pedal, and pinna reflexes), and depth of anesthesia may be difficult to judge. As with ketamine, there is some analgesia, but visceral analgesia is inadequate for major abdominal surgery unless supplemented with other agents. Tachycardia and cardiac arrhythmias may be present in light anesthesia, and cardiac output is significantly reduced at high doses (more than 20 mg/kg IM). Like ketamine, tiletamine induces marked increase in salivation and respiratory secretions unless the patient is premedicated with an anticholinergic agent.

One disadvantage of tiletamine-zolazepam is the long and difficult recoveries seen in some animals. As with ketamine, ataxia and increased sensitivity to stimuli are commonly observed during the recovery period. Tremors, muscle rigidity, seizure activity, and hyperthermia can also be seen, especially in dogs given tiletamine-zolazepam at label doses by the IM route. IV diazepam administration may be helpful in affected animals. In cats, recovery may be prolonged (up to 5 hours after IM injection), particularly if high doses are administered. Because the drug is metabolized by the liver and excreted via the kidneys, prolonged recovery should be expected in animals with liver or kidney dysfunction.

Tiletamine-zolazepam should be avoided in patients with American Society of Anesthesiologists (ASA) status of III or greater and in animals with CNS signs, hyperthyroidism, cardiac disease, pancreatic or renal disease, pregnancy, glaucoma, or penetrating eye injuries.

Neuroleptanalgesia

As outlined in Chapter 1, the combination of an opioid and a tranquilizing agent can be used to induce the state of profound sedation termed *neuroleptanalgesia*. The same combination of drugs can be used to induce general anesthesia of dogs when given by IV injection. Neuroleptanalgesia combinations are not suitable for routine induction of anesthesia in healthy young dogs, because true anesthesia is unlikely to occur in these patients unless the neuroleptanalgesia is supplemented with nitrous oxide, isoflurane, or another anesthetic agent. However, neuroleptanalgesics may have a profound effect in high-risk or debilitated dogs (including those with hepatic, renal, and CNS disorders) and are a useful and safe alternative to barbiturates or ketamine induction in these animals. Neuroleptanalgesics are seldom used to induce anesthesia in cats because of unacceptable side effects (excitement, mania).

The opioid agents most commonly used for neuroleptanalgesia are morphine, meperidine, butorphanol, hydromorphone, and oxymorphone. These are combined with a tranquilizer such as acepromazine, diazepam, droperidol, or medetomidine.

Induction with opioid-tranquilizer combinations provides a wide margin of safety in most patients, although care must be taken to administer the drugs slowly. If opioid-tranquilizer combinations are rapidly injected, CNS stimulation may be seen. The anesthetist using neuroleptanalgesics must also be prepared to intubate and ventilate the patient's lungs if necessary because respiratory depression may be profound.

Several procedures have been described for induction of anesthesia with neuroleptanalgesics. These include the following:
- Administration of atropine and acepromazine 15 minutes before slow IV injection of the opioid.
- Administration of atropine, followed 15 minutes later by slow IV administration of a tranquilizer-opioid mixture. If diazepam is selected as the tranquilizing agent, the opioid should be given first, followed 1 to 2 minutes later by diazepam. If diazepam is given before the opioid agent has taken effect, excitement may be seen (especially in spaniel and setter breeds). In young dogs, acepromazine offers more reliable sedation than diazepam and can be given at the same time as the opioid.
- Administration of atropine and acepromazine, followed 15 minutes later by rapid administration of IV fluids containing the opioid agent. Administration of the fluids may be discontinued when the desired level of anesthesia is reached.
- IM administration of a mixture of acepromazine and an opioid (usually oxymorphone or meperidine).

The regimens just mentioned can be safely carried out without atropine, provided the heart rate is carefully monitored. If bradycardia is noted, atropine or glycopyrrolate should be administered.

Propofol

Propofol (Diprivan, Rapinovet) is a recently introduced induction agent that may be used as the sole agent for brief procedures or for anesthetic induction before intubation and inhalant anesthesia. It is a substituted phenol with a chemical structure unlike that of other anesthetic or preanesthetic agents. Propofol has a neutral pH and is provided as an oil-in-water emulsion with a concentration of 10 mg/ml. Although this agent has a milky appearance, it can be safely administered IV.

Propofol can be diluted with saline or 5% dextrose in water for use in small dogs and cats. Dilution allows more accurate dosing and helps to prevent respiratory and cardiovascular side effects. The manufacturer recommends that propofol not be diluted to a concentration less than 0.2% (2 mg/ml). It should not be mixed with other fluids or drugs.

Injections should be given by the IV route only, over a period of 20 to 60 seconds until the desired anesthetic depth is reached. (IM injections may cause mild sedation and ataxia but do not induce anesthesia because the drug is metabolized too rapidly.) One effective induction method is to give one third to one half of the calculated dose as an initial bolus. This is followed by smaller amounts administered every 30 seconds until the desired plane of anesthesia is reached. The dose of propofol needed for a patient and the duration of anesthesia depend on the type of premedication used; however, when given at a dose rate of 6 mg/kg IV, onset of anesthesia is usually less than 60 seconds and duration of anesthesia is 5 to 10 minutes.

Propofol can also be combined half and half with 2.5% thiopental by volume and used for induction of dogs. The amounts of drug required to permit intubation are less than those needed when each drug is administered alone. Recovery quality and recovery times are reported to be similar to those of propofol alone and superior to those of thiopental. Because the dose of propofol is less, the combination with thiopental offers significant cost savings.

One unique feature of propofol is that anesthesia may be readily maintained in dogs for longer periods by administering additional drug. Unlike cyclohexamines or barbiturates, propofol can be given repeatedly to a canine patient without concern that recovery will be prolonged or of a poor quality. Injections can be repeated every 3 to 5 minutes or as required, depending on the status of the patient. Alternatively, propofol can be delivered by continuous infusion. In this procedure, a small dose of propofol (0.2 to 0.4 mg/kg/min) is continuously administered to the patient by a syringe pump, syringe driver, or IV line. This method allows the anesthetist to precisely control the depth of anesthesia at a stable plane for up to several hours. Intubation and oxygenation are advisable for patients unless the period of anesthesia is anticipated to be very brief.

In dogs, recovery from propofol anesthesia is rapid and smooth, even after multiple injections. Because of the rapid recovery seen with this agent, it is useful for ambulatory surgery. Dogs that have received propofol may appear completely recovered within 20 minutes of injection. Cats recover quickly (approximately 30 minutes) after single injections but may experience longer recoveries after multiple injections.

Propofol has a rapid onset and short duration of action because it is very lipophilic, similar to the thiobarbiturates. Propofol is rapidly taken up by vessel-rich groups such as the brain, heart, liver, and kidneys but is very quickly redistributed to muscle and fat and is subsequently metabolized. Dogs have the ability to metabolize propofol 5 to 10 times faster than thiopental. This helps to account for rapid recovery and minimal hangover effects seen even after repeated injections.

Propofol has a wide margin of safety in both the dog and cat. Other characteristics include the following:

- Transient excitement and muscle tremors are seen occasionally during induction, especially if injection is slow or the animal has not been premedicated. Paddling, muscle twitching, nystagmus, and opisthotonus (extended head and front legs) have been reported. If seen, these can be treated with acepromazine (0.1 mg/kg IV, given slowly), diazepam (0.3 to 0.5 mg/kg IV), or pentobarbital (2 mg/kg).
- Overall effects on the cardiovascular system are similar to barbiturates. Episodes of tachycardia or bradycardia may occur, especially during the first 2 minutes after injection. Hypotension frequently occurs immediately after injection. It is often of short duration in animals with normal cardiovascular function, but in some patients it may be significant, prolonged, and unresponsive to the usual corrective measures such as fluid loading and administration of ionotropes such as dopamine. Propofol should not be given to animals with preexisting hypotension, such as patients in shock or those that have blood loss or dehydration.
- Propofol, like thiopental, has the potential to depress respiration, particularly after rapid IV injection. Apnea is sometimes seen, especially if the drug is given as a single bolus. Given the potential respiratory depression associated with the use of propofol, the anesthetist should titrate the dose to effect and monitor respiratory rate and depth carefully during the first 1 to 2 minutes after injection. If apnea lasts more than 1 minute or if pulse oximetry shows oxygen saturation to be less than 90%, the patient should be intubated and the lungs ventilated with oxygen. The best approach is prevention of hypoxemia by delivering oxygen to the patient (by face mask) for 3 to 5 minutes before inducing anesthesia with propofol.
- Because metabolism of propofol is rapid, propofol is relatively safe and effective in animals with liver or kidney disease.
- Atropine premedication is unnecessary. However, preanesthetic tranquilizers should be given because they decrease the dose of propofol required by as much as 75% and facilitate IV injection in fractious animals. Some premedications, however, may prolong recovery time.
- Propofol decreases intracranial and intraocular pressure.
- Propofol appears to be safe for use in sighthounds, and recovery is more rapid than with thiopental, although slower than recovery from propofol in other breeds.
- Some muscle relaxation occurs with this agent, although analgesia is poor.

One significant disadvantage of propofol is the poor storage characteristics of this agent. Because the product contains soybean oil, egg lecithin, and glycerol, it will support bacterial growth. Ampules and bottles should be handled in a strict aseptic manner, and the manufacturer recommends that unused product be discarded within 6 hours of opening to avoid contamination. (Unopened, the shelf life is approximately 3 years.) Some authorities suggest that unused propofol can be stored up to 24 hours, provided sterile technique is used for opening, dispensing, and storing the product. Refrigeration may be preferable to storage at room temperature. Unfortunately, detailed studies on the storage characteristics of propofol have not been published, but the incidence of clinic infection due to contaminated drug appears to be real but low.

The cost of propofol induction in dogs is approximately four times that of ketamine-diazepam and eight times that of thiopental.

Etomidate

Etomidate (Amidate) and the similar agent metomidate (Hypnodil) are sedative-hypnotic imidazole drugs that are occasionally used for induction of anesthesia in cats and dogs. Anesthesia with etomidate is characterized by good muscle relaxation but no analgesia. The duration of effect is short because, like propofol, metabolism of etomidate is rapid.

Etomidate is always administered IV, following premedication with an opioid or diazepam (0.25 mg/kg diazepam given IV, 30 seconds before etomidate). As with other induction agents, the dose is titrated, starting with one fourth to one half the calculated dose, depending on how rapid an induction is desired. Alternatively, etomidate can be given by infusion, at a rate of 50 to 150 μg/kg/min. The rate should be adjusted according to the nature of the procedure and the response of the patient. Like propofol, etomidate can be administered in repeated boluses to maintain anesthesia.

Etomidate has minimal effect on cardiovascular function (including heart rate, rhythm, cardiac output, and blood pressure) and is the induction agent of choice for difficult cardiac cases and animals in shock. Cerebral perfusion is better maintained than with other injectable agents. It is a mild respiratory depressant, and transient apnea may be seen following rapid injection.

Although etomidate has a wide margin of safety, it has the following potential adverse effects:

- IV injection is reported to be painful and may cause phlebitis, especially when the drug is injected into small veins. Perivascular injection may be associated with the development of sterile abscesses.
- Rapid injection of etomidate may cause red blood cell hemolysis in cats. This is clinically insignificant unless the cat has an extremely low hematocrit or the drug is given repeatedly.
- Adrenal cortical function may be depressed for several hours after etomidate administration. This is not harmful unless the drug is given for several hours or repeated over several days. Caution should be used in animals with preexisting hypoadrenocorticism (Addison's disease).
- Nausea, vomiting, and involuntary excitement may occur during induction or recovery, particularly in patients that have not been adequately premedicated.

Etomidate is also significantly more expensive than other IV induction agents. Like propofol, it does not contain a preservative, and open vials should be discarded after use.

Guaifenesin

Guaifenesin (glyceryl guaiacolate, GGE) is a muscle relaxant that is commonly given to large animals to induce anesthesia (usually in combination with ketamine, diazepam, and/or xylazine). Because concentrated solutions of this agent can cause red blood cell hemolysis, a 5% or 10% solution in dextrose is preferred. The 5% solution is prepared by adding 50 g of guaifenesin to 50 g of medical grade dextrose, which is dissolved in 1 L of very hot sterile water. If a precipitate develops, it can be dissolved by rewarming the solution.

Guaifenesin is always given by IV catheter. It is administered rapidly IV after premedication. Recovery is usually smooth.

Guaifenesin should not be used without premedication or as the sole agent, because excitement is likely to be seen during induction. Sedation and analgesia are inadequate for surgery when this agent is used alone.

Guaifenesin may decrease blood pressure, especially when used with inhalation agents. The most common sign of overdose is spasm of the extensor tendons. If this is seen, administration of guaifenesin should be discontinued, or cardiac arrest may occur.

INHALATION ANESTHETICS

Inhalation anesthesia has become so commonplace in veterinary and human anesthesia that it is difficult to imagine the impact that the introduction of the first inhalation anesthetic had on surgical practice. Before the introduction of anesthesia, every surgical procedure was associated with pain, and it was usually necessary for surgeons to work at breakneck speed while the patients were manually restrained by attendants. The introduction of diethyl ether in 1842, nitrous oxide in 1844, and chloroform in 1847 allowed the performance of safe and humane surgery, marking one of the most significant advances of medical science. Indeed, inhalation anesthesia continues to be the safest and most commonly used form of surgical anesthesia.

The inhalation anesthetics in common use in small animal practice at the present time are isoflurane, halothane, and sevoflurane. Methoxyflurane, enflurane, desflurane, and nitrous oxide are occasionally used in some practices and research institutions. Many other inhalation agents that were used in the past (including diethyl ether, chloroform, divinyl ether, and trichloroethylene) are now of historical interest only.

Characteristics of an Ideal Agent

Although each inhalation agent has desirable properties, the ideal inhalation agent does not exist. The characteristics of such an agent would include the following:

1. Minimal toxicity to the patient, particularly to the cardiovascular, respiratory, hepatic, renal, and nervous systems
2. No unwanted side effects such as postoperative seizures, nausea, or vomiting
3. Minimal toxicity of waste gas vapors to anesthetists and other operating room personnel
4. Pleasant smell and nonirritating vapor, allowing easy administration to awake animals
5. Rapid and gentle induction and recovery
6. Anesthetic depth easily controlled and quickly altered
7. No dependence on liver and kidney function for metabolism and excretion
8. Good muscle relaxation
9. Adequate postoperative analgesia
10. Low cost
11. Adequate potency to achieve surgical anesthesia
12. Handling ease safety (that is, agent should be nonflammable, nonexplosive, and chemically stable)
13. No requirement of specialized or expensive equipment

14. No reaction with anesthetic machine components, including carbon dioxide absorbent, metal, or rubber

Halothane, isoflurane, and sevoflurane approach this standard in many respects and are safe for most veterinary patients.

In choosing an inhalation agent to be used for a particular procedure, the veterinarian must consider several factors, including the availability of each agent, the special needs of the patient, the preference of the anesthetist and surgeon, and cost.

Classes of Inhalation Agents
Nitrous oxide

Nitrous oxide, introduced as an anesthetic more than 150 years ago, is still used extensively in human anesthesia and, to a lesser extent, in veterinary anesthesia as well. In contrast to the other inhalation agents (which are liquids that are poured into the anesthetic machine vaporizer), nitrous oxide is delivered from a gas cylinder attached to the anesthetic machine and does not require a vaporizer for administration. Like oxygen, it is administered with a flowmeter that controls the amount of gas reaching the breathing circuit and therefore the patient. Nitrous oxide is not a potent agent, and by itself it does not induce anesthesia in animals. However, it can be combined with other anesthetics (such as halothane). Use of this agent is discussed in detail on p. 155.

Diethyl ether

Diethyl ether (Aether) was for many years the most widely used anesthetic. Animals anesthetized with this agent normally maintain a relatively stable cardiac output and blood pressure, although heart rate may be slightly elevated. Ether does not sensitize the heart to epinephrine, and thus there is little risk of cardiac arrhythmias. It also produces good muscle relaxation and analgesia.

Despite these advantages, ether has significant drawbacks that have greatly limited its use in contemporary anesthesia. One major problem is the irritating effect of this agent on the tracheal and bronchial mucosa. This results in increased salivation and mucous secretions and an increased risk of laryngospasm and airway blockage. Induction and recovery from ether anesthesia may be prolonged, and postoperative nausea is common. In addition, ether is flammable and explosive and requires an explosion-proof refrigerator for safe storage. Devastating operating room fires have resulted from the use of ether in conjunction with oxygen.

Halogenated compounds

The most commonly used inhalation agents, halothane, sevoflurane, and isoflurane, are chemically similar and are classified as halogenated organic compounds. Other halogenated agents include methoxyflurane, enflurane, and desflurane. These agents are liquid at room temperature. They are stored inside the vaporizer of the anesthetic machine and evaporate in the oxygen that flows through the vaporizer. The resulting mixture of oxygen and anesthetic is delivered to the patient through a breathing circuit (discussed in detail in Chapter 4).

The physical properties and pharmacology of the most commonly used halogenated agents are summarized in Tables 3-3 and 3-4.

TABLE 3-3

Physical Properties of the Common Inhalation Anesthetics

	NITROUS OXIDE	HALOTHANE	METHOXYFLURANE	ISOFLURANE	SEVOFLURANE
Formula	N_2O	$CF_3CHClBr$	$CH_3OCF_2CHCl_2$	$CF_3CHClOCHF_2$	$CFH_2COCF_3CF_3$
Molecular weight	44	197	165	184	200
Date of first clinical use	1845	1956	1959	1981	
Trade name	—	Fluothane Penthrane	Metofane	Aerrane Forane SevoFlo	Ultane
Saturated vapor pressure at 750 mm Hg and 20°C	800 (psi)	243	22.5	240	160
Blood:gas solubility coefficient	0.47	2.4	13	1.4	0.6
Oil or fat solubility	1.4	224	825	60	53
Rubber solubility	1.2	120	635	62	29
MAC in dogs (%)	188	0.87	0.23	1.28	2.1-2.3
MAC in cats (%)	255	0.98	0.23	1.63	2.6
MAC in horses (%)	—	0.88	—	1.31	2.36
Metabolism (%)	—	20	50	0.2	3

Modified from Warren RG: *Small animal anesthesia,* St Louis, 1989, Mosby.

TABLE 3-4

Pharmacologic Properties of Selected Agents

PROPERTY	METHOXYFLURANE	HALOTHANE	ISOFLURANE	SEVOFLURANE
Muscle relaxation	Excellent	Fair	Good	Moderate
Effect on nondepolarizing muscle relaxants	None	Increased	Greatly increased	Probably increased
Analgesia	Excellent	Slight	Slight	Slight
Effect on respiration	Marked depression of rate and depth	Some depression	Depression	Depression
Effect on heart	Mild depression	Severe depression	Slight	Slight
Potential for causing cardiac arrhythmias	Some	Very common	None reported	None reported
Effect on blood pressure	May decrease	Decreases	Decreases	Decreases
Elimination from the body	Metabolism 50% Respiration 50%	Metabolism 20% Respiration 80%	Respiration 99%	Respiration 97%
Effect on the liver	Rare toxicity reported in humans	May rarely cause hepatitis in humans	None reported	None reported
Effect on the kidneys	Toxicity reported in humans and animals	None reported	None reported	Toxicity reported in rats
Lipid solubility	High	Moderate	Low	Low
Maintenance range	0.25%-1%	0.5%-2%	1.5%-2.5%	2.5%-4%

Modified from McKelvey D: Halothane, isoflurane, and methoxyflurane, *Vet Tech* 12(1):25, 1991.

Mechanism of Action

The mechanism of action of anesthetic molecules within the brain is poorly understood. It has been suggested that anesthetics exert their effects by enhancing the activity of gamma-aminobutyric acid (GABA), an inhibitory neurotransmitter. According to this theory, anesthesia is the result of the inhibition of nerve function, which results from increased GABA activity. Another theory suggests that anesthetics dissolve in nerve cell membranes and cause the membrane to lose its ability to conduct nerve impulses.

Effect of Inhalation Agents on Vital Systems

Although individual inhalation agents vary somewhat in their effects, the following characteristics are common to all (see also Table 3-4).

- In general, inhalation agents depress ventilation in a dose-dependent manner, by causing a decrease in tidal volume and respiratory rate. It follows that hypoventilation is a possible side effect of all inhalation agents. In addition, hypoventilation predisposes the animal to carbon dioxide retention and respiratory acidosis.
- Inhalation agents depress cardiovascular function. Although the effect on heart rate is variable, all of these agents cause vasodilation and decreased cardiac output and may decrease blood pressure and tissue perfusion. Renal perfusion and cerebral perfusion may be compromised by these agents.
- Some inhalation agents (notably halothane) cause the heart muscle to have increased sensitivity to the effects of epinephrine, which may lead to the development of cardiac arrhythmias such as tachycardia, VPCs, and ventricular fibrillation.
- Some agents (methoxyflurane, halothane) undergo some liver metabolism. Isoflurane, sevoflurane, and desflurane undergo minimal liver metabolism because they are eliminated from the body chiefly through the lungs.
- Because inhalation anesthetics may decrease blood pressure, they have a potential to decrease renal blood flow. This can be clinically significant in animals with preexisting renal disease or in animals receiving nephrotoxic drugs such as gentamicin or nonsteroidal antiinflammatory drugs (NSAIDs) (see Chapter 8).
- All inhalation anesthetics cause a dose-related, reversible depression of the CNS. Animals with head trauma or increased intracranial pressure due to brain tumors may have dangerously increased intracranial pressure when anesthetized with inhalation agents, especially if carbon dioxide levels in the blood are allowed to increase. However, inhalation anesthetics, with the exception of enflurane, are considered safe for animals with a history of epilepsy.

Despite this list of potential adverse effects, inhalation anesthesia is considered safe for most patients. However, safety depends to a large degree on the care with which these agents are administered and the vigilance of the anesthetist in monitoring their effect on the patient.

Distribution and Elimination

To understand the properties of the inhalation agents, their uptake by, distribution within, and elimination from the body must be discussed. Liquid anesthetic in the anesthetic machine is vaporized, mixed with oxygen, and delivered to the patient by mask or endotracheal tube. The anesthetic travels via the air passages to the lung alveoli, where it diffuses across the alveolar cells and enters the bloodstream. The rate of diffusion is controlled by the concentration gradient between the alveolus and the bloodstream, as well as the lipid solubility of the drug. During the induction period, the concentration of the agent in the alveolus is high, and the concentration in the blood is low. This creates a steep concentration gradient, and diffusion of anesthetic from the alveolus into the blood is rapid during this period.

As with injectable agents, inhalation agents reach body tissues by the bloodstream, and tissues with greater blood flow (brain, heart, kidney) are more quickly saturated with anesthetic than tissue with lesser blood flow such as skeletal muscle and fat. Because of their relatively high lipid solubility, inhalation agents readily leave the circulation and enter the brain, inducing anesthesia. The depth of anesthesia is determined by the partial pressure of the anesthetic agent in the brain. This in turn is related to the partial pressure of anesthetic in the blood and alveoli. Anesthesia is maintained as long as sufficient quantities of inhalation agent are delivered to the alveoli so that the blood, alveolar, and brain concentrations are maintained.

When the concentration of the inhalation agent administered is reduced or discontinued by adjusting the anesthetic machine vaporizer, the amount of anesthetic in the alveolus is reduced. Because the blood level is still high, the concentration gradient now favors the diffusion of anesthetic from the blood into the alveoli. The blood levels of the anesthetic are quickly reduced, provided the animal continues to breathe and eliminate anesthetic from the alveoli. The anesthetist can hasten the elimination of anesthetic by periodically bagging the animal with 100% oxygen. This removes anesthetic from the alveoli and reestablishes a steep concentration gradient between the alveoli and the blood. As the concentration of the anesthetic in the blood falls, the agent leaves the brain and the patient wakes up.

Some anesthetic agents (in particular, methoxyflurane) have high lipid solubility and may accumulate in body fat stores, thereby escaping elimination through the lungs at the end of anesthesia. These agents rely on liver metabolism and renal excretion for their complete elimination from the body. Slower recovery and prolonged anesthetic hangover are common with these agents.

Physical Properties

Isoflurane, halothane, methoxyflurane, and nitrous oxide differ considerably in their anesthetic effects, in part, because of differences in their physical and chemical properties. The properties of chief importance to the anesthetist include vapor pressure, solubility coefficient, minimum alveolar concentration (MAC), and rubber solubility. These agents also vary in their pharmacologic properties, including their effects on the cardiovascular, respiratory, and other vital systems. The physical properties and pharmacology of commonly used inhalation anesthetic agents are summarized in Tables 3-3 and 3-4.

Vapor pressure

The vapor pressure of an inhalation anesthetic is a measure of the tendency of a molecule to escape from the liquid phase to the vapor or gas phase. Vapor pressure is agent and temperature dependent. The vapor pressures for the commonly used inhalants are often given at temperatures of 20° C or 22° C, which is approximately room temperature. Vapor pressure is significant because it determines how readily the anesthetic liquid evaporates in the anesthetic machine vaporizer.

Agents with a high vapor pressure, such as halothane or isoflurane, are described as volatile, because they evaporate easily. In fact, both isoflurane and halothane evaporate so readily that they may reach a concentration of over 30% in the oxygen delivered to the patient, a level that could cause a fatal anesthetic overdose. A special type of vaporizer (called a *precision vaporizer*) limits the evaporation of these agents and allows their safe use for anesthesia. Vaporizers are available for each of the commonly used anesthetics, which allow only a controlled amount of anesthetic to be vaporized. For example, most precision vaporizers intended for use with isoflurane allow a maximum concentration of 5%, a level that is sufficient for all practical uses. The use of these volatile inhalation agents in a simple, nonprecision vaporizer is difficult because of the lack of control over the evaporation of the anesthetic and the increased risk of overdose. A skilled anesthetist and close monitoring of the patient and anesthetic machine are required if a nonprecision vaporizer is used (see Chapter 4).

Some agents, such as methoxyflurane, have relatively low vapor pressure and do not require the use of a precision vaporizer. At 20° C the maximum methoxyflurane concentration attainable in the anesthetic circuit is 4%. A simple, inexpensive, non-precision vaporizer, such as a glass jar with a wick, is adequate for vaporizing methoxyflurane. Precision vaporizers for methoxyflurane are available on some machines; however, they are not a requirement for safe anesthesia.

Because each type of vaporizer is designed for use with a particular agent and its specific vapor pressure, it is theoretically necessary to use a different vaporizer for each agent. In practice, the similar vapor pressures of isoflurane and halothane result in similar evaporation rates, and isoflurane may be used safely in many vaporizers designed for halothane use. A new or recently serviced halothane vapor-izer should deliver predictable levels of isoflurane within 10% of the dial setting, which is considered acceptable for anesthesia. However, the use of halothane vapor-izers for isoflurane is not recommended by anesthetic or vaporizer manufac-turers because of litigation reasons (chiefly because mistakes involving confusion or mixture of agents can occur if the anesthetic currently in the vaporizer is not clearly labeled).

Although it is unacceptable to combine halothane and isoflurane in the same vaporizer, it is acceptable to switch from one anesthetic to another during the course of surgery if the patient demonstrates an adverse reaction to the first anesthetic. In this case, separate vaporizers must be available for each anesthetic because of the difficulty in rapidly emptying the first anesthetic from the vaporizer.

Because of significant differences in vapor pressure, sevoflurane, desflurane, and methoxyflurane should not be used in a vaporizer designed for halothane or isoflurane.

Solubility coefficient

Many of the physiologic effects of inhalant anesthetics can be explained by their solubility characteristics in various biologic solvents such as blood and tissue. Solu-bility is usually expressed as a partition coefficient, and these coefficients provide information about an anesthetic's speed of induction, recovery, and potency. The blood:gas solubility coefficient (or partition coefficient) is a measure of the distri-bution of the inhalation agent between the blood and gas phases in the body. It is therefore a measure of the capacity of the blood and gas phases for an anesthetic. A low blood:gas solubility coefficient indicates that the anesthetic is less soluble in blood than an anesthetic with a higher blood:gas solubility coefficient. This is of importance to the anesthetist because the blood:gas solubility indicates the speed of induction and recovery one should expect for a given inhalant anesthetic. The lower the blood:gas solubility coefficient for an inhalant anesthetic, the faster the expected induction and recovery. An example of an agent with a low blood:gas solubility is sevoflurane, an anesthetic with very rapid induction and recovery characteristics.

In contrast, an agent with a high solubility coefficient will be extremely soluble in the blood and tissues. Because the anesthetic is rapidly absorbed into the blood and tissues (called the *sponge effect*), high levels of the anesthetic do not build up within the alveoli. As a result, agents with high solubility coefficients induce anesthesia less rapidly than do agents with low solubility coefficients. Similarly, agents with high solubility coefficients are slow to leave tissues, especially fat, and this gradual release results in a slow recovery. Methoxyflurane is an example of an agent with a high solubility coefficient and, as expected, demonstrates relatively slow induction and recovery rates.

The blood:gas solubility coefficient of an inhalant agent has a significant effect on the clinical use of the agent.

Induction. The rapid induction possible with isoflurane and sevoflurane is due to their low solubility coefficients and allows the use of these agents for mask or chamber induction. Methoxyflurane, with a high solubility coefficient, is not well suited to these induction methods.

Maintenance. Agents with low solubility coefficients also have the advantage of allowing a rapid patient response to changes in anesthetic concentration during anesthesia. Patients anesthetized with isoflurane or sevoflurane may respond within 1 minute to changes in the vaporizer setting. If an agent with a higher solubility coefficient is used (such as halothane and especially methoxyflurane), the anesthetist will observe a slower patient response to changes in the vaporizer setting.

Recovery. Patients anesthetized with agents with low solubility coefficients have a relatively fast recovery time. Patients anesthetized with sevoflurane or isoflurane are often fully awake within a few minutes after the vaporizer is turned off. Patients anesthetized with methoxyflurane often sleep quietly for 30 to 60 minutes after anesthesia.

Minimum alveolar concentration

The MAC of an anesthetic agent is the lowest concentration that produces no response in 50% of the patients exposed to a painful stimulus (for example, a clamp applied to the base of the tail or a surgical incision). Thus MAC not only is an effective anesthetic concentration, but also indicates the strength of an inhalation anesthetic. An agent with a low MAC is a more potent anesthetic than an agent with a high MAC. For example, halothane has a lower MAC than isoflurane and is, therefore, more potent; a higher concentration of isoflurane will be necessary to maintain a similar anesthetic depth.

For a given inhalation anesthetic, a vaporizer setting of approximately $1 \times MAC$ will produce light anesthesia in most patients, $1.5 \times MAC$ will produce a surgical depth of anesthesia, and $2 \times MAC$ will produce deep anesthesia. These figures are useful only as a rough guide: MAC varies with the age, metabolic activity, and body temperature of the patient. Factors such as disease, pregnancy, obesity, and treatment with other drugs may also alter the potency of an anesthetic agent in a given patient. The anesthetist should also be aware that the response to an anesthetic depends on the concentration of the anesthetic in the patient's brain, which is not necessarily the same as that indicated by the anesthetic machine vaporizer, particularly early in the induction period (see Chapter 4).

Halothane

Halothane (Fluothane), first introduced in 1956, is still one of the most commonly used inhalation agents in veterinary anesthesia. Chemically, it is classified as a halogenated hydrocarbon.

Physical and chemical properties

The chief physical and chemical properties of halothane are as follows:

- Halothane has a relatively high vapor pressure and, as such, normally requires a precision vaporizer for its safe use. Halothane delivered through a nonprecision vaporizer may readily achieve a concentration over 30%, which dangerously exceeds the normal concentration required for anesthesia (1% to 2%). Special techniques are required for use of halothane in a nonprecision vaporizer (see Chapter 4).
- Halothane has a moderately low solubility coefficient and moderate fat solubility, allowing fairly rapid induction and recovery. Delivery of halothane by mask usually results in unconsciousness and stage III anesthesia in a tranquilized animal within 10 minutes. Recovery time from anesthesia varies with length of anesthesia, patient condition, and the concurrent use of other agents; however, sternal recumbency is usually achieved in less than 1 hour after the anesthetic is discontinued. Because of its moderate lipid solubility, a portion of the anesthetic is retained within body fat stores rather than being eliminated by the lungs during recovery. The stored halothane is subsequently metabolized by the liver, with elimination of the metabolites by the kidney.
- Halothane has a moderate MAC and, in terms of anesthetic potency, is midway between methoxyflurane and isoflurane.
- Halothane has moderate rubber solubility. This is of concern to the anesthetist because hoses, reservoir bags, and other anesthetic machine parts contain rubber and may absorb halothane during the course of anesthesia. Release of the agent from machine parts may delay patient recovery after the vaporizer has been turned off.
- Halothane is somewhat unstable and for commercial use is mixed with the preservative thymol. The presence of a preservative may cause a buildup of residue within the vaporizer, turning the liquid in the vaporizer yellow. The residue may cause Teflon moving parts in some vaporizers to stick, and periodic cleaning and recalibration is recommended.

Pharmacologic effects

Halothane is a relatively safe agent for veterinary use; however, it does have the following adverse effects on organ function:

- Halothane sensitizes the heart to the action of catecholamines (such as epinephrine) and thus may induce arrhythmias. Arrhythmias may be treated by increasing patient oxygenation and ensuring that anesthetic depth is adequate. If this does not alleviate the arrhythmia, the patient may be given IV lidocaine or switched to another anesthetic, if available.

- Halothane increases vagal tone, and bradycardia may result.
- Halothane has a mild depressant effect on myocardial cells, decreasing myocardial contraction and cardiac output. This effect is dose dependent (that is, the higher the concentration, the greater the effect).
- Halothane decreases peripheral resistance of the blood vessels by causing vasodilation, which predisposes the animal to excessive heat loss and therefore hypothermia. Vasodilation and myocardial depression may also cause a fall in blood pressure that is roughly proportional to anesthetic depth. For this reason, IV fluid support is recommended in hypovolemic or hypotensive patients.
- Halothane causes some depression of respiration, and respiratory rate and tidal volume usually fall if anesthesia is prolonged. Respiratory arrest may occur at high concentrations. Halothane and all other inhalation anesthetics readily cross the placenta and may depress respiration in the newborn.
- Halothane is moderately lipid soluble. A portion of the administered dose is retained in body fat stores and subsequently metabolized in the liver. Halothane and its metabolites have been associated with hepatotoxicity and liver necrosis in human patients. There is no clear evidence at present that hepatotoxicity occurs with halothane use in veterinary patients; however, the use of alternative inhalation agents is probably advisable for patients with liver disease.
- Halothane may increase cerebral blood flow, which may lead to increased intracranial pressure in patients with head trauma or brain tumors.
- Halothane produces adequate muscle relaxation but only slight analgesia. The use of postoperative analgesics is advisable with this agent. Halothane and nitrous oxide are sometimes used in combination to achieve better analgesia.
- Halothane use is associated with malignant hyperthermia, a rare but often fatal disorder of thermoregulation. Affected animals show increased temperature, muscle rigidity, and cardiac arrhythmias, and may die. Treatment consists of removal from halothane, cooling, and administration of oxygen and specific drugs such as dantrolene.

Isoflurane
Physical and chemical properties

Isoflurane, a halogenated ether, is chemically similar to sevoflurane and methoxyflurane. The margin of safety of this agent is apparently greater than that of halothane or methoxyflurane, which has led to its wide acceptance in veterinary anesthesia despite its slightly greater cost. Isoflurane is approved for use only in dogs and horses, although it has gained widespread use in other species.

The chief physical and chemical properties of isoflurane are as follows:
- The vapor pressure of isoflurane is very close to that of halothane. Because of its volatile nature, isoflurane is normally used in a precision vaporizer. Some halothane vaporizers have been adapted successfully for isoflurane administration, although this practice is discouraged by manufacturers.
- The blood:gas solubility coefficient of isoflurane is extremely low. This, combined with the relatively low tissue solubility of this agent, results in extremely rapid induction and recovery. Isoflurane is better suited to mask or chamber induction than are slower-acting agents such as methoxyflurane or halothane. Unfortunately, some animals appear to be irritated by isoflurane vapors and

resist mask induction. Recovery from anesthesia is also rapid, and the anesthetist must refrain from turning off the anesthetic machine vaporizer until the end of surgery because return of consciousness may occur as rapidly as 1 to 2 minutes after isoflurane administration is discontinued. The low solubility coefficient of isoflurane also allows the anesthetist to change the patient's depth of anesthesia rapidly during the course of anesthesia. An animal that appears too deep or too light usually responds rapidly (within 1 or 2 minutes) after adjustment of the anesthetic level.

- The MAC of isoflurane is higher than that of halothane and thus it is less potent. Anesthesia is maintained in most patients at a concentration of 1.5% to 2.5% isoflurane in oxygen.
- The rubber solubility of isoflurane is low, and there is little absorption of this anesthetic by rubber-containing components.
- Isoflurane is stable at room temperature, and no preservative is necessary. This is an advantage because there is no preservative residue to accumulate in isoflurane vaporizers. (These vaporizers, however, still require periodic maintenance and calibration).

Pharmacologic effects

Of the volatile anesthetics commonly used in veterinary anesthesia, isoflurane is considered to have the fewest adverse effects on the heart.

- When used at normal anesthetic levels, isoflurane maintains cardiac performance close to that of preanesthetic levels. It causes only a small decrease in cardiac output, with little or no depression of myocardial cells and little effect on heart rate. Isoflurane does not sensitize the myocardium to the effects of epinephrine to the same extent as halothane does and is therefore not as arrhythmogenic. Because of its minimal effect on the heart, isoflurane is considered to be the inhalation agent of choice for patients with cardiac disease. As with halothane, however, vasodilation and decreased blood pressure may be observed, particularly at deeper levels of anesthesia.
- Isoflurane depresses respiration. The effect of isoflurane on respiration is more pronounced than that of halothane. The alveolar concentration that can cause apnea is as little as 3% in some dogs.
- Isoflurane does not increase cerebral blood flow as much as halothane and is considered a better anesthetic for animals with head trauma or brain tumors.
- Nearly all of the isoflurane administered to a patient is exhaled quickly once the vaporizer is turned off. Isoflurane has low fat solubility; consequently, there is little retention of isoflurane in body fat stores, little hepatic metabolism, and very little renal excretion of metabolites. For this reason isoflurane is well suited to animals with liver or kidney disease. Isoflurane is also a good anesthetic for use in neonatal and geriatric animals, in which hepatic metabo-lism and renal excretion mechanisms may be less efficient than in the healthy adult animal.
- Isoflurane induces adequate good muscle relaxation.
- Isoflurane has little or no analgesic effect in the postanesthetic period. The use of postoperative analgesics is advisable because this lack of analgesic effect, combined with the rapid recoveries experienced with this agent, may lead to pain and excitement during recovery.

Sevoflurane

Sevoflurane (Ultane, SevoFlo) is gaining popularity as an anesthetic agent, particularly for horses. Chemically, it is a halogenated ether closely related to isoflurane and shares many of the same characteristics. Sevoflurane is labeled for use in dogs but has been used in many other species.

Physical and chemical properties

The chemical and physical properties of sevoflurane include the following:
- The vapor pressure of sevoflurane is lower than isoflurane, and a precision vaporizer intended for use with sevoflurane is required. The vaporizer should be designed to deliver up to 8% sevoflurane.
- The solubility coefficient is very low, allowing even more rapid induction and recovery than isoflurane. Observed time to intubation has been reported as 5 to 7 minutes after mask induction (compared with 6 to 8 minutes for isoflurane). Mask induction with sevoflurane is typically associated with less struggling than isoflurane induction. Because of these characteristics, sevoflurane is the agent best suited to mask and chamber inductions and is also a good agent for cesarean sections. The rapid and quiet recoveries seen with sevoflurane use in horses has made this agent popular in equine anesthesia, despite its relatively high cost (currently, approximately 10 times that of isoflurane).
- The MAC is greater than isoflurane. Sevoflurane is therefore a less potent agent than isoflurane and higher concentrations are required to induce and maintain anesthesia. A concentration of 6% to 8% is required for mask induction (compared with 3% to 5% for isoflurane), and 2.5% to 4% is the normal maintenance range (compared with isoflurane, 1.5% to 2.5%).
- Sevoflurane reacts with the potassium hydroxide (KOH) or sodium hydroxide (NaOH) in soda lime to produce a chemical (Compound A) that can cause renal tubular damage in rats. This effect is most pronounced in closed circle systems, in low flow systems, and at high sevoflurane concentrations. Renal damage has not been reported in dogs or cats anesthetized with sevoflurane, and the potential for nephrotoxicity appears to be low in these species.

Pharmacologic effects

- Sevoflurane has a greater effect on the heart than isoflurane does, although less than halothane. Cardiac output is depressed at high concentrations. Vasodilation is also seen, and blood pressure may be reduced. Hypotension has been cited as the most common undesirable side effect of sevoflurane anesthesia (Branson et al, 2001). Sevoflurane does not sensitize the heart to the arrhythmogenic effect of epinephrine.
- Sevoflurane may depress respiration slightly more than isoflurane. Apnea (lasting at least 30 seconds) and tachypnea have both been reported.
- There is minimal biotransformation in the liver, and most of this agent is excreted by the lungs.
- Sevoflurane does not significantly increase cerebral blood flow and can be used for anesthesia of patients with head trauma or brain tumors.
- Sevoflurane induces adequate muscle relaxation.
- Paddling, excitement, and muscle fasciculations have been reported, primarily during the recovery period.

- Sevoflurane has no analgesic effect. Because of the rapid recoveries seen with this agent, an analgesic agent must be administered before the patient wakes up after a painful operation.

Methoxyflurane

Although it is difficult to obtain in some countries because of limited production, methoxyflurane is a useful anesthetic agent in small animal patients.

Physical and chemical properties

- The vapor pressure of methoxyflurane is significantly lower than that of halothane or isoflurane, and as a result methoxyflurane may be safely used in a nonprecision vaporizer. Because an anesthetic machine with a nonprecision vaporizer is considerably less expensive than one with a precision vaporizer, the initial equipment costs are less for methoxyflurane anesthesia than they are for other inhalation agents.
- The solubility coefficient of methoxyflurane is considerably higher than that of halothane or isoflurane, as is the lipid solubility. These two factors combine to produce slow induction and recovery rates in animals anesthetized with methoxyflurane. Because of the slow induction rates, it is not generally advocated that this agent be used for mask induction or chamber induction because stage II of general anesthesia (excitement stage) may be prolonged.
- The MAC of methoxyflurane is considerably lower than that of the other volatile inhalation anesthetics. It is the most potent inhalation anesthetic in common use.
- Methoxyflurane has considerable solubility in rubber or plastics and readily dissolves in reservoir bags, hoses, and endotracheal tubes. This may lead to deterioration of these products unless they are rinsed out immediately after use. The solubility of methoxyflurane in rubber or plastic anesthetic machine parts may also result in considerable release of methoxyflurane gas into the anesthetic circuit even after the vaporizer has been turned off.
- As with halothane, methoxyflurane requires the addition of a preservative to extend its shelf life. The accumulation of preservative may interfere with vaporizer function; however, cleaning and maintenance procedures for nonprecision vaporizers are much easier than those for precision vaporizers.

Pharmacologic effects

Methoxyflurane has a good margin of safety in both the dog and cat.

- Methoxyflurane causes less sensitization of the myocardium to the arrhythmogenic effects of catecholamines than does halothane.
- Methoxyflurane is the most potent respiratory depressant of all the inhalation anesthetics. It decreases both the respiratory rate and tidal volume, and it is important to monitor anesthetized animals to ensure adequate ventilation. However, the anesthetist should avoid continuous bagging of a patient under methoxyflurane anesthesia unless the vaporizer setting is reduced. Failure to reduce the setting may lead to excessive anesthetic being delivered to the patient (because the concentration of anesthetic increases as oxygen is forced through a nonprecision vaporizer by the bagging procedure).

- Because of its high lipid solubility, methoxyflurane is retained in body fat stores so that more than half of the anesthetic delivered to the animal is eventually metabolized and excreted by the liver and kidney. Fluoride ions and other potentially toxic metabolites are produced as a result of hepatic metabolism, and the presence within the kidney of these toxic metabolites may lead to renal damage, particularly if flunixin (Banamine), tetracyclines, or other potentially nephrotoxic drugs are administered concurrently. This effect has been well documented in human anesthesia, although its occurrence in veterinary anesthesia appears to be limited to dehydrated animals with preexisting renal damage. Urine-concentrating ability may be impaired for up to 3 days after methoxyflurane use, even in healthy patients. From the standpoint of operating room personnel, the persistence of methoxyflurane within body fat raises some concern about long-term health effects (see Chapter 5).
- Methoxyflurane causes marked skeletal muscle relaxation and may have some analgesic effect (because some of the drug remains in the tissues even after recovery). This allows surgery to proceed at relatively light planes of anesthesia, minimizing cardiovascular depression. The analgesic effect of this agent and the relatively slow recovery rate also ensure that recovery from methoxyflurane anesthesia is generally smooth, and patient distress seldom occurs.

Other Halogenated Agents
Enflurane

Enflurane, a volatile gaseous anesthetic used in human medicine, has not found wide acceptance in veterinary anesthesia. Induction and recovery are relatively rapid and smooth, with minimal effects on heart rate and minimal sensitization of the myocardium to catecholamines. However, enflurane causes profound depression of respiration, and spontaneous ventilation of the patient is poor under this anesthetic. Analgesia and muscle relaxation are poor, especially at concentrations over 3.5%. In the dog, enflurane also induces significant muscle hyperactivity, and seizure-like muscle spasms may result.

Desflurane

Desflurane is a recently introduced volatile anesthetic agent that is occasionally used in veterinary medicine. Desflurane has a chemical structure similar to isoflurane and, like isoflurane, undergoes very little metabolism in the body. Desflurane has the lowest solubility coefficient of the volatile anesthetics used in veterinary anesthesia and is known for "single breath" inductions in humans.

The vapor pressure of desflurane is extremely high, and this agent requires a special vaporizer for its use. The high cost of desflurane vaporizers is a significant factor limiting the use of this agent in veterinary medicine.

Other properties of desflurane include the following:
- As with isoflurane, desflurane vapors are irritating to breathe.
- The MAC varies considerably between individuals but is much greater than isoflurane, indicating that desflurane is a less potent agent. Because of the variability of the MAC between individuals, patient depth should be very closely monitored to determine if depth is appropriate.
- Desflurane does not sensitize the myocardium to epinephrine.

- Desflurane is reported to cause transient increases in heart rate and blood pressure in humans. This phenomenon (called *sympathetic storm*) has not been reported in dogs.
- Desflurane causes dose-related respiratory depression.
- Desflurane may cause the production of carbon monoxide when passed through dry carbon dioxide absorbent.

Nitrous Oxide
Physical and pharmacologic properties

Nitrous oxide (N_2O) is an odorless gas that can be used as an adjunct to anesthesia with other inhalation agents. It should not be used as the sole anesthetic agent in domestic animals. Unlike other inhalation anesthetics, nitrous oxide is available in compressed gas tanks and does not require a vaporizer. It is mixed with oxygen in the anesthetic machine before being delivered to the patient.

The property that limits the use of nitrous oxide in veterinary anesthesia is its lack of potency (that is, a high MAC) in domestic species. The MAC of nitrous oxide in humans is approximately 100%, whereas the MAC in the dog and horse is close to 200% and in the cat is approximately 250%. As these figures demonstrate, it is impossible to achieve a surgical plane of anesthesia in a healthy dog or cat with nitrous oxide alone.

Other properties of nitrous oxide can be summarized as follows:
- The use of nitrous oxide with another inhalation anesthetic (such as halothane) usually allows the anesthetist to lower the concentration of the other agent being administered. Nitrous oxide reduces the MAC (and therefore the vaporizer setting) of other anesthetics by 20% to 30%. This reduces the risk of adverse effects on the cardiovascular, pulmonary, and other systems and allows faster recoveries. Nitrous oxide also has been shown to speed the uptake of other anesthetic gases into the bloodstream by the second gas effect when used at high concentrations (50% to 70% of the total gas flow). This effect allows more rapid induction.
- Nitrous oxide has an extremely low solubility coefficient and is associated with rapid induction and recovery rates. It is therefore a helpful addition to slow-acting agents such as methoxyflurane. It does little to enhance induction with rapid-acting agents such as isoflurane.
- Nitrous oxide has little effect on the cardiovascular, respiratory, hepatic, or urinary systems and is considered to have a wide margin of safety. Nitrous oxide offers good analgesia but is not a good muscle relaxant.

Despite these advantages, the use of nitrous oxide in veterinary anesthesia has declined in recent years. One reason is the increased cost of N_2O anesthesia, compared with anesthesia with an inhalation agent alone. Another reason is the increased use of isoflurane and sevoflurane, which provide rapid induction and recovery even without the concurrent use of nitrous oxide.

Special precautions

The use of nitrous oxide is associated with several potential problems, including the following:

Fire hazard. Nitrous oxide is not flammable, but like oxygen it supports combustion.

Risk of hypoxia. The use of nitrous oxide in an anesthetic machine limits the amount of oxygen that is delivered to the patient to the extent that nitrous oxide replaces oxygen in the circuit. Because the minimal amount of nitrous oxide necessary to achieve analgesic effects is 50% (and values of 60% to 66% are recommended), the use of this agent decreases the amount of oxygen delivered to the patient by 50% to 66%. When anesthetizing a small patient (cat or small dog), the anesthetist should ensure that at least 30 ml/kg/min of oxygen is delivered to the patient and that the oxygen content of the inspired gases is at least 33%. This can be achieved by ensuring that the nitrous oxide flow (in liters per minute) is no more than twice the oxygen flow and that oxygen flow rates less than 500 ml/min are avoided.

The patient breathing nitrous oxide is at increased risk of hypoxia and should be monitored closely for cyanosis and cardiac arrhythmias. Sao_2 and Pao_2 values are helpful, if available. Because of the risk of hypoxia, animals with preexisting lung disease are poor candidates for N_2O anesthesia. For all patients, care should also be taken when adjusting the flowmeter of the anesthetic machine to avoid confusing oxygen controls with those for nitrous oxide.

Diffusion into air pockets. Because of its low solubility coefficient, nitrous oxide is able to diffuse into trapped air pockets within the body. This diffusion may result in an increase in the amount of gas within an organ and consequent distension of the organ containing trapped gas. For this reason, the use of nitrous oxide is contraindicated in animals with intestinal obstruction, gastric torsion, pneumothorax, or diaphragmatic hernia. As there is normally a large amount of gas in the equine gut, nitrous oxide may cause undesirable dilation of the intestines in this species.

Use in closed anesthesia systems. Nitrous oxide should never be used in a closed anesthetic circuit (that is, one with low oxygen flow rates, see Chapter 4) unless the anesthetist uses an oxygen monitor to determine oxygen levels in the inspired gas. Because oxygen is removed from a closed system by the animal's metabolism, the level of nitrous oxide in the circuit may increase to dangerous levels, resulting in hypoxia.

Diffusion hypoxia. During recovery from anesthesia, nitrous oxide will readily exit from the body via the respiratory system. Because of the rapid outpouring of nitrous oxide into the lungs, a state of diffusion hypoxia may occur. In this condition, oxygen molecules normally found in the alveoli are displaced by the large numbers of nitrous oxide molecules exiting from the body. Diffusion hypoxia can be prevented by keeping the animal on high oxygen flow rates for at least 5 minutes after the nitrous oxide has been turned off and ensuring that the animal is frequently bagged with pure oxygen.

Waste anesthetic gas hazards. Exposure of operating room personnel to waste nitrous oxide has been linked to several health disorders (see Chapter 5).

AGENTS USED IN THE POSTANESTHETIC PERIOD

Two classes of drugs, reversing agents and analeptics, are available to hasten recovery after anesthesia. An *analeptic agent* is a drug that causes general CNS stimulation. The most commonly used analeptic agent is doxapram. A *reversing agent* is a drug that negates the effect of a specific anesthetic or preanesthetic agent (usually by competing with the anesthetic for specific receptor sites) and speeds up recovery. Several reversing agents are discussed in Chapter 1.

Although useful, these drugs should not be substituted for careful anesthetic technique. The anesthetist should rely primarily on precise control of anesthetic depth to ensure rapid and smooth patient recovery. However, the use of reversing agents and analeptics in selected patients may be of value.

Doxapram

Doxapram (Dopram) is a respiratory stimulant and analeptic agent. When given intravenously, doxapram will increase respiratory rate and depth and may accelerate arousal from barbiturate or inhalation anesthesia. The required dose is much greater for patients that have undergone injectable anesthesia than it is for patients recovering from inhalation anesthesia.

Doxapram is also useful for stimulating respiration in newborn puppies and kittens delivered by cesarean section: two or three drops placed under the tongue may greatly increase respiration rate and depth.

Although doxapram has a wide margin of safety, it may cause tachycardia and arrhythmias in some patients and should be used with caution in animals with cardiac disease. Doxapram must be used only in the presence of adequate oxygen levels in the brain, otherwise CNS damage may result. Doxapram must not be used in patients with a history of seizures because the drug will lower the seizure threshold.

KEY POINTS

1. Injectable anesthetics are eliminated by redistribution, liver metabolism, and renal excretion. Inhalation anesthetics are eliminated primarily by exhalation from the lungs. Some inhalation anesthetics also undergo liver metabolism and renal excretion.
2. Both injectable and inhalation anesthetics have a wide margin of safety; however, most agents have depressant effects on the cardiovascular, respiratory, and thermoregulatory systems.
3. Injectable anesthetics include barbiturates, cyclohexamines, neuroleptanalgesic agents, propofol, and etomidate.
4. Several classes of barbiturates are available for veterinary anesthesia, including intermediate-acting barbiturates such as pentobarbital, short-acting barbiturates such as thiopental, and ultrashort-acting barbiturates such as methohexital. These classes differ in their lipid solubility, duration of effect, and distribution within the body.
5. Barbiturates are commonly used as induction agents and are normally administered by titration to achieve the minimum effective dose.
6. Barbiturates may cause respiratory depression and respiratory acidosis. Other adverse effects include tissue necrosis (when injected perivascularly), cardiac arrhythmias, and excitement during anesthetic induction and/or recovery.
7. Barbiturates show unusual potency in patients that are acidotic, hypoproteinemic, or hypotensive. They may cause prolonged sleeping times in sighthounds.
8. Pentobarbital can be given intravenously or intramuscularly to achieve anesthesia, but this drug is seldom used in dogs or cats because its use is associated with poor muscle relaxation, lack of analgesia, respiratory depression, and prolonged recoveries.

9. Thiopental has a rapid onset of action and short duration and is a commonly used induction agent in dogs and cats. Transient apnea may be seen during induction. Methohexital is an alternative agent for use in sighthounds.

10. Cyclohexamine agents such as ketamine and tiletamine produce a state of dissociative anesthesia characterized by exaggerated reflex responses, central nervous system (CNS) excitement, apneustic respiration, tachycardia, and increased muscle tone. These agents may be given by intramuscular injection in cats or intravenous injection in cats or dogs. Concurrent use of a tranquilizer (such as diazepam, zolazepam, acepromazine, xylazine, or medetomidine) is recommended to promote muscle relaxation and to prevent excitement during recovery.

11. Neuroleptanalgesia is a profound hypnotic state produced by the administration of an opioid and a tranquilizing agent. These agents provide relatively safe induction in debilitated patients.

12. Propofol and etomidate are recently introduced induction agents that can be given by repeat injection to maintain anesthesia.

13. The inhalation agents in common use are isoflurane, halothane, and sevoflurane. Each of these agents is administered by means of an anesthetic machine and either a mask or an endotracheal tube. These agents enter the body by absorption through the alveolus, at a rate that depends on the solubility coefficient of the agent.

14. Anesthetic agents vary in their solubility coefficient, vapor pressure, and minimum alveolar concentration (MAC). These properties affect the speed of induction and recovery, the type of vaporizer that should be used, and the vaporizer setting that is required for anesthesia.

15. All inhalation anesthetics may cause respiratory depression and decrease cardiac output and blood pressure. In addition, halothane may potentiate cardiac arrhythmias. Of the commonly used agents, isoflurane and sevoflurane are considered to have the greatest margin of safety and the shortest induction and recovery times.

16. Isoflurane and sevoflurane are eliminated almost entirely through respiration. Halothane and methoxyflurane undergo some hepatic metabolism and renal excretion as well as respiratory elimination.

17. Nitrous oxide has few cardiovascular or respiratory side effects and is a useful adjunct to other agents. It is too weak to be used as a sole anesthetic agent in animals. The anesthetist must be aware of the risk of hypoxia associated with this agent, particularly in the period immediately after discontinuation of the agent.

18. Reversing agents and analeptics may be given after anesthesia to hasten anesthetic recovery. Doxapram is a nonspecific respiratory stimulant that may accelerate arousal from barbiturate or inhalation anesthesia.

REVIEW QUESTIONS

1. Etomidate is particularly well suited for induction of dogs with which of the following problems?
   a. Severe cardiac disease
   b. Renal failure
   c. Orthopedic disease
   d. Pediatric (younger than 4 weeks)

2. Injectable drugs that are highly fat soluble are likely to be taken up by the brain more quickly than drugs that are not fat soluble.
   True   False

3. Which of the following is an example of a dissociative anesthetic?
   a. Thiopental sodium
   b. Pentobarbital sodium
   c. Ketamine hydrochloride
   d. Propofol

4. One of the disadvantages of the drug methohexital is that animals that are anesthetized with it often may demonstrate excitement during recovery.
   True   False

5. Metabolism and elimination of ketamine hydrochloride are the same in the dog as they are in the cat.
   True   False

6. Compared with methoxyflurane, halothane is considered to have a:
   a. Higher vapor pressure
   b. Similar vapor pressure
   c. Lower vapor pressure

7. Halothane may sensitize the heart to catecholamines.
   True   False

8. Halothane is moderately soluble in rubber, which may result in release of this gas from anesthetic equipment.
   True   False

9. An anesthetic agent that has a low solubility coefficient will result in

   _____ induction and recovery time.
   a. Slow
   b. Moderate
   c. Fast

10. Which of the following has the lowest solubility coefficient?
    a. Halothane
    b. Isoflurane
    c. Methoxyflurane
    d. Sevoflurane

11. As a rough guideline, to safely maintain a surgical plane of anesthesia, the
    vaporizer should be set at _____ × MAC.
    a. 0.5
    b. 1
    c. 1.5
    d. 2
    e. 2.5
12. Isoflurane is a more potent cardiac depressant than halothane.
    True   False
13. Propofol sometimes causes transient apnea. To avoid this, the anesthetist should:
    a. Give by infusion only
    b. Premedicate with opioids
    c. Administer IV only
    d. Titrate this drug in several boluses
14. To be considered effective, nitrous oxide should be used at a minimum
    concentration of:
    a. 3%
    b. 30% to 40%
    c. 50% to 60%
    d. More than 80%
    e. None of the above ranges are correct
15. One problem frequently associated with recovery from tiletamine-zolazepam
    in dogs is:
    a. Excitement
    b. Bradycardia
    c. Hypotension
    d. Laryngospasm

For the following questions, more than one answer may be correct.

16. Effects of halothane on the body include:
    a. Vasodilation
    b. Nystagmus
    c. Sensitization of myocardium to catecholamines
    d. Depression of myocardial cells
    e. Respiratory depression
17. Effects that barbiturates may have on the body include:
    a. Reduction of respiratory rate
    b. Tachycardia
    c. Cardiac arrhythmias
    d. Decreased blood pressure
18. The concentration of barbiturate entering the brain is affected by a variety of
    factors such as:
    a. Perfusion of the brain
    b. Lipid solubility of the drug
    c. Plasma protein levels
    d. Blood pH of the animal

19. Effects that are commonly seen after administration of a cyclohexamine drug include:
    a. Increased blood pressure
    b. Increased heart rate
    c. Increased CSF pressure
    d. Increased intraocular pressure
20. Effects that isoflurane may have on the body include:
    a. Hepatic toxicity
    b. Accumulation in body fat stores
    c. Depression of respiration
    d. Seizures during recovery
21. MAC will vary with:
    a. Temperature of the patient
    b. Age of the patient
    c. Concurrent use of other drugs
    d. Anesthetic agent
22. Factors that may affect the speed of the induction process with a volatile gaseous anesthetic include:
    a. Solubility coefficient of the agent
    b. Vaporizer setting
    c. MAC of the agent
    d. Concurrent use of atropine
23. Nitrous oxide may be included as part of an anesthetic protocol because it:
    a. May provide a second gas effect
    b. Will reduce the amount of volatile anesthetic needed
    c. Has minimal depressant effects on the respiratory or cardiovascular centers
    d. Can replace oxygen in the anesthetic circuit
24. When pentobarbital sodium is used as an anesthetic, which of the following may be noted:
    a. Relatively slow onset of action
    b. Respiratory depression
    c. Poor analgesia
    d. Slow recovery
    e. Easily reversed
25. Which of the following drugs may be safely and effectively given IM or IV in a cat?
    a. Thiopental sodium
    b. Telazol
    c. Ketamine hydrochloride
    d. Methohexital sodium

ANSWERS FOR CHAPTER 3

1. a	2. True	3. c	4. True	5. False
6. a	7. True	8. True	9. c	10. d
11. c	12. False	13. d	14. c	15. a
16. a, c, d, e	17. a, c, d	18. a, b, c, d	19. a, b, c, d	20. c
21. a, b, c, d	22. a, b	23. a, b, c	24. a, b, c, d	25. b, c

Selected Readings

Branson KR et al: A multisite case report on the clinical use of sevoflurane in dogs, *J Am Anim Hosp Assoc* 37(5):420-432, 2001.

Clarke KW: Desflurane and sevoflurane, *Vet Clin North Am Small Anim Pract* 29(3): 793-810, 1999.

Haskins SC: Opinions in small animal anesthesia, *Vet Clin North Am Small Anim Pract* 22(2):326-469, 1992.

Mama K: New drugs in feline anesthesia, *Compendium Small Animal* 20(2):125-138, 1998.

Muir WW III, Hubbell JAE, Skarda RT, et al: *Handbook of veterinary anesthesia,* ed 3, St Louis, 2000, Mosby.

Pablo LS, Bailey JE: Etomidate and telazol, *Vet Clin North Am Small Anim Pract* 29(3): 779-792, 1999.

Paddleford RR: *Manual of small animal anesthesia,* New York, 1988, Churchill Livingstone.

Short CE, Bufalaria A: Propofol anesthesia, *Vet Clin North Am Small Anim Pract* 29(3):747-778, 1999.

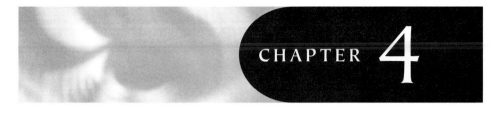

CHAPTER 4

Anesthetic Equipment

PERFORMANCE OBJECTIVES

After completion of this chapter, the reader will be able to:
- Define the terms *fresh gas, bagging, VOC, VIC, closed system, open system,* and *line pressure.*
- Identify equipment that is used for the induction and maintenance of general anesthesia in the dog or cat.
- Differentiate among the various types of endotracheal tubes and list the advantages and disadvantages of each.
- List the advantages and disadvantages of cuffed versus noncuffed tubes.
- Describe the function of each component of an anesthetic machine.
- Trace the flow of oxygen through an anesthetic machine and patient breathing circuit for a circle system and Bain apparatus.
- State the differences between a rebreathing and a nonrebreathing system with regard to equipment, airflow pattern, and indications for use.
- Understand the advantages and disadvantages of both rebreathing and nonrebreathing systems.
- Differentiate between a precision and nonprecision vaporizer and recognize the advantages and disadvantages of each.
- Understand the importance of flow rates as they relate to anesthetic concentration within the breathing circuit, type of circuit (closed versus open), safety for the patient, and waste gas production.
- Understand the advantages and disadvantages of low-flow anesthesia and how it differs from conventional anesthesia.
- Explain the procedure that should be followed to prepare an anesthetic machine for use.
- Describe the proper maintenance procedures for anesthetic machines and associated equipment.

Before the introduction of anesthetic machines, administration of anesthesia was a relatively hazardous undertaking. Anesthetic liquids such as ether or chloroform were poured onto a cloth that was then held over the patient's nose and mouth until the desired depth of anesthesia was achieved. Alternatively, the patient was sometimes required to inhale vapors rising from a jar of liquid anesthetic. The development of modern anesthetic equipment allowed the administration of precise amounts of anesthetic under controlled conditions, greatly increasing the safety and convenience of inhalation anesthesia.

This chapter describes the function and use of anesthetic equipment and the maintenance procedures that are likely to be the responsibility of the veterinary technician in practice. Useful equipment for routine intravenous (IV) induction and inhalation anesthesia are listed in Appendix C. Of the many types of equipment used for anesthesia, only endotracheal tubes, the anesthetic machine, and the breathing circuit are discussed in this chapter.

ENDOTRACHEAL TUBES

Endotracheal tubes are used to deliver anesthetic gas from the breathing circuit to the patient's lungs. Many types of endotracheal tubes are available for veterinary anesthesia. Endotracheal tubes have a slanted (beveled) end that is passed through the mouth or nose and into the trachea (Fig. 4-1). This end is referred to as the *patient-end* of the tube. The other end of the endotracheal tube protrudes from the mouth or nose, is connected to the breathing circuit of the anesthetic machine, and is referred to as the *machine-* or *circuit-end* of the tube.

Tubes used in small animal practice are usually made of red rubber, vinyl plastic, silicone rubber, or polyvinyl chloride. Red rubber endotracheal tubes are relatively inexpensive and common in veterinary practice. The technician should be aware of some potential problems associated with their use, including the following:

- Rubber tubes may absorb disinfectant solutions, causing the outer surface of the tube to become dry and cracked after prolonged use. If residual disinfectant contacts the patient's oropharynx or trachea, irritation may result.

Murphy eye

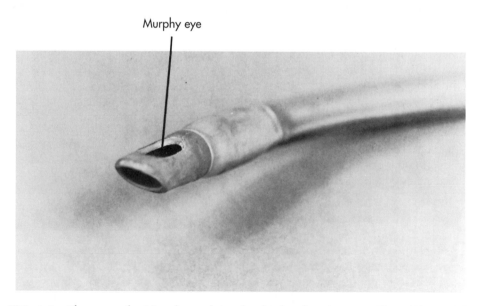

FIG. 4-1   Close-up of a Murphy endotracheal tube showing eye. (*From Warren RG: Small animal anesthesia, St Louis, 1983, Mosby.*)

- Rubber tubes are extremely flexible, and kinking or collapse of the tube is a potential hazard, particularly for small tubes. Specialized rubber tubes, called *spiral* or *anode tubes,* contain a coil of metal or nylon embedded in the rubber. These tubes are flexible but resist kinking or collapse from external pressure. This is particularly useful for procedures that require flexion of the head and neck.

Tubes made of transparent vinyl plastic are also used in veterinary anesthesia. These tubes are less porous than rubber and resist cracking. However, they are less flexible than rubber and tend to become stiff with age.

Silicone rubber tubes, although expensive, are well suited to veterinary anesthesia. They are smooth, flexible, and less irritating to tissues than either rubber or vinyl plastic tubes. Polyvinyl chloride tubes are also flexible and easily conform to the curve of the airway.

Whether manufactured from rubber, silicone rubber, polyvinyl chloride, or vinyl plastic, endotracheal tubes are available in several shapes and sizes. The two types of tubes most commonly used in veterinary practice are the Murphy tube and the Magill tube. Both have a beveled (slanted) patient-end, but they differ in that the Murphy tube has an eye near the bevel, whereas the Magill tube does not (see Fig. 4-1). The eye helps prevent complete obstruction of the tube if the bevel is plugged by mucus or by the tracheal wall.

Unfortunately, several different systems of size classification have been used in the past, which has led to some confusion when selecting tubes (Table 4-1). The classification used most commonly is based on the internal diameter (ID) of the tube as expressed in millimeters. The ID of each tube is written on its surface (Fig. 4-2). Endotracheal tubes ranging from 5 to 18 mm ID are suitable for use in dogs (Table 4-2). The endotracheal tubes used most commonly in cats are those with IDs of 3, 3.5, 4, and 4.5 mm. Very small animals may be more easily intubated with a special type of tube called a *Cole endotracheal tube* (Fig. 4-3).

TABLE 4-1		
A Comparison of Three Systems Used to Classify Endotracheal Tubes		
MAGILL SCALE	FRENCH SCALE	INTERNAL DIAMETER SCALE (mm)
00	13	4
0	16	5
	18	
1	20	
2	22	6
3	24	7
4	26	8
5	28	
6		9
7	30	10
8	32	11
9	34	12
10	36	

Modified from Warren RG: *Small animal anesthesia,* St Louis, 1989, Mosby.

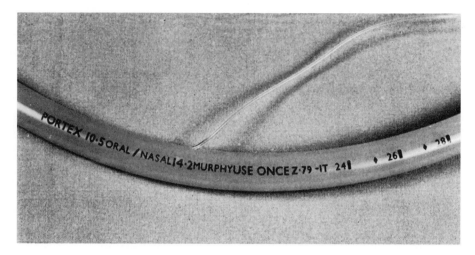

FIG. 4-2   Detail of endotracheal tube with internal diameter of 10.5 mm. (*From Warren RG: Small animal anesthesia, St Louis, 1983, Mosby.*)

Tubes may be labeled *oral* or *nasal* according to their intended use in humans; however, endotracheal tubes are almost always passed orally in small animals to avoid damage to the sensitive nasal turbinates (the scroll-shaped passages within the nose).

Endotracheal tubes may be obtained with or without cuffs. The cuff is a balloonlike inflatable structure located near the beveled end of the tube. When this cuff is inflated with air, it provides a seal between the tube and the trachea. Air is injected into the cuff by a small tube connected to it. A pilot balloon on the small tube indicates if the cuff is inflated.

The use of cuffed tubes offers the following three advantages over tubes without cuffs:

1. The inflated cuff helps prevent leakage of waste gas around the tube and therefore reduces operating room pollution.
2. Use of cuffed tubes reduces the risk of aspiration of blood, saliva, vomitus, and other material into the lungs.
3. Animals intubated with cuffed tubes are prevented from breathing room air, which may otherwise enter the breathing passages by flowing around the outside of the tube. Animals breathing significant amounts of room air are difficult to maintain at adequate anesthetic depth because room air dilutes the anesthetic vapor.

Despite these advantages, cuffed tubes should be used with caution, especially in small patients. The cuff of the tube may exert significant pressure on the tracheal mucosa and cause local necrosis, particularly after prolonged use. A special type of cuff, called a *high-volume, low-pressure cuff* is designed to gently conform to the contour of the tracheal wall, reducing (but not eliminating) the risk of tracheal trauma. Uncuffed tubes may be preferred to cuffed tubes in very small patients and in patients at significant risk of tracheal damage. Alternatively, a cuffed tube can be used with the cuff not inflated.

TABLE 4-2

Guide for Selection of Veterinary Endotracheal Tubes According to Body Weight and Species

SIZE	INTERNAL DIAMETER (mm)
CATS	
2 kg	3
4	4
6	4.5
DOGS	
2 kg	4-5
4	6
7	6-7
9	7-8
12	8
14-18	9-11
18-20	12-14
20-25	14-16
25-30	16
40	16-18
HORSES	
Foals	9-14
Small ponies	14-16
Adult thoroughbred	26-30
Adult draft horse	30-36
LIVESTOCK	
Calves (3 months)	9-12
Calves (6 months)	14-18
Yearlings	22
Mature cows	26
Large bulls	30
Sheep and goats	7-9
Pig (25 kg)	6
Pig (50 kg)	9
Large sows or boars	10-14

Modified from Warren RG: *Small animal anesthesia,* St Louis, 1989, Mosby.

The use of endotracheal tubes is outlined in detail in Chapter 2; however, the following additional points should be noted:

- Endotracheal tubes should have a slippery surface to avoid trauma to the trachea. Some materials are naturally slippery, whereas others require lubrication with water or commercial lubricant.
- When correctly used, endotracheal tubes reduce mechanical dead space (see Chapter 2). For this to be achieved, the endotracheal tube should be no longer than the distance between the mouth and the tip of the shoulder or thoracic inlet. If the tube protrudes more than 2 cm beyond the nose, it is too long and should be cut shorter or replaced. Ideally, the endotracheal tube should only extend two thirds down the neck, to reduce the risk of intubating one bronchus.

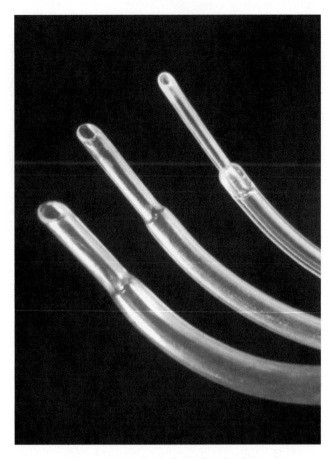

FIG. 4-3   Cole endotracheal tubes.

- Special considerations apply when endotracheal tubes are used in conjunction with laser surgery. Lasers create intense heat, and in a high-oxygen environment such as the trachea there is a risk of fire and the endotracheal tube may ignite. The anesthetist may use special fire-resistant laser tubes or adapt regular tubes by wrapping them with metal tape. It may also be advisable to pack the area where lasers are to be used with saline-soaked sponges and fill the cuff of the endotracheal tube with water instead of air.

ANESTHETIC MACHINES AND BREATHING CIRCUITS

The anesthetic machine and breathing circuit (Fig. 4-4) are designed to deliver a volatile gaseous anesthetic (usually halothane, isoflurane, or sevoflurane) to and from a patient by means of a circuit of corrugated tubing. The anesthetic is contained within a carrier gas, which is either oxygen (O_2) alone or oxygen in combination with nitrous oxide (N_2O). To achieve this result, the anesthetic machine and breathing circuit must perform several important functions, including the following:
- Oxygen must be delivered (with or without nitrous oxide) at a controlled flow rate.

- A designated concentration of liquid anesthetic (usually isoflurane, halothane, or sevoflurane) must be vaporized, mixed with oxygen (and nitrous oxide, if used), and delivered to the patient.
- Exhaled gases must be moved away from the patient and either disposed through a scavenging system or recirculated to the patient. If the exhaled gases are recirculated, the machine must remove carbon dioxide (CO_2) before returning the gases to the patient.

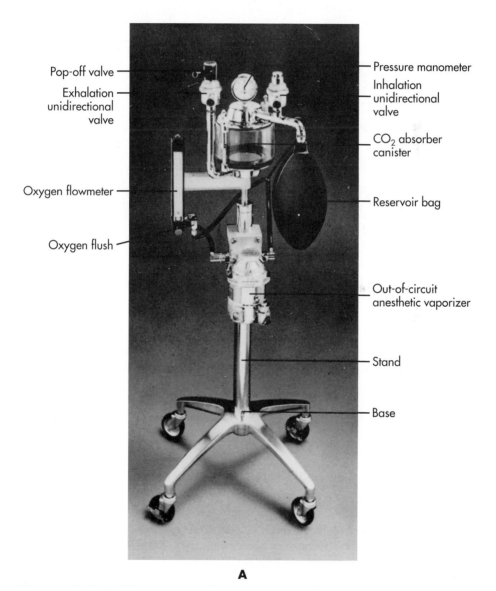

A

FIG. 4-4   A, Basic inhalation anesthesia machine with an out-of-circuit precision vaporizer.   *Continued*

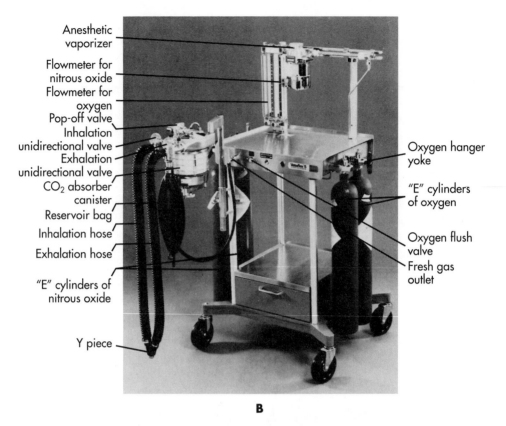

Anesthetic vaporizer

Flowmeter for nitrous oxide

Flowmeter for oxygen

Pop-off valve

Inhalation unidirectional valve

Exhalation unidirectional valve

CO₂ absorber canister

Reservoir bag

Inhalation hose

Exhalation hose

"E" cylinders of nitrous oxide

Y piece

Oxygen hanger yoke

"E" cylinders of oxygen

Oxygen flush valve

Fresh gas outlet

B

FIG. 4-4, cont'd B, Two-gas inhalation anesthesia machine with out-of-circuit precision vaporizer for methoxyflurane.

Anesthetic machines are used not only for inhalation anesthesia but also as a means of delivering oxygen to patients that are critically ill. In these situations, the machine is used with the vaporizer (that is, the anesthetic source) turned off, and the hoses deliver oxygen to an endotracheal tube or to a mask held over the patient's face.

Different models of anesthetic machines vary in cost, from $5000 for a basic model to more than $100,000 for an advanced machine with built-in monitors and multiple vaporizers.

COMPONENTS OF THE ANESTHESIA DELIVERY SYSTEM

The components of the anesthesia delivery system and the way in which an anesthetic machine works can best be understood by following the path of oxygen starting with the oxygen tank, passing through the machine to the patient, and returning again to the machine. For the sake of clarity, one type of anesthetic setup (that is, the circle system using a precision vaporizer) is described. This system is illustrated schematically in Fig. 4-5. It has three parts: a compressed gas supply (consisting of compressed gas cylinders or tanks, tank pressure gauges, and a pressure-reducing valve), the anesthetic machine (consisting of a flowmeter and vaporizer), and the

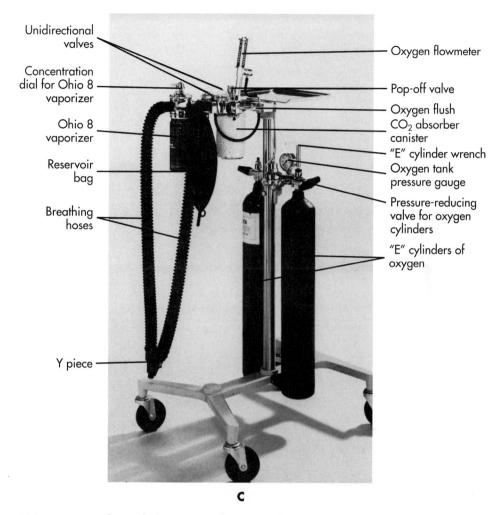

Unidirectional valves

Concentration dial for Ohio 8 vaporizer

Ohio 8 vaporizer

Reservoir bag

Breathing hoses

Y piece

Oxygen flowmeter

Pop-off valve

Oxygen flush

CO_2 absorber canister

"E" cylinder wrench

Oxygen tank pressure gauge

Pressure-reducing valve for oxygen cylinders

"E" cylinders of oxygen

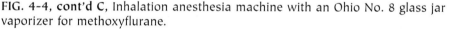

C

FIG. 4-4, **cont'd C,** Inhalation anesthesia machine with an Ohio No. 8 glass jar vaporizer for methoxyflurane.

breathing circuit (consisting of unidirectional valves, hoses and a reservoir bag, pop-off valve, carbon dioxide absorber, oxygen flush valve, pressure manometer, and negative pressure relief valve).

Compressed Gas Supply

Oxygen is necessary to sustain life and must be continuously supplied to every patient throughout anesthesia. In the healthy awake patient breathing room air (21% oxygen), the concentration of oxygen in the alveolus is 13%, in arterial blood 12%, in capillary blood at tissue level 5%, and in the tissues only 2%.

Although these levels are adequate for normal function in the awake patient, anesthetized patients may not achieve them and easily become hypoxic. This is because the anesthetized patient has a reduced tidal volume compared with the

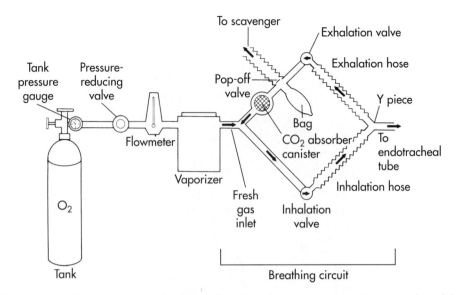

FIG. 4-5 Schematic of anesthetic machine (circle system, vaporizer out of circle). (Redrawn from Hartsfield SN: Machines and breathing systems for administration of inhalation anesthetics. *In Short CE, editor:* Principles and practice of veterinary anesthesia, *Baltimore, 1987, Williams & Wilkins.*)

awake animal, and the amount of air taken in with each breath is therefore smaller. It is therefore desirable to increase the amount of oxygen available to the patient, to at least 30% of the inspired air. Anesthetic machines are designed to provide up to 100% oxygen. If nitrous oxide is used, the amount of oxygen provided should be no less than 33% (that is, the oxygen flow rate must be at least one third of the total flow rate).

Oxygen flow from the machine to the patient not only meets the metabolic requirements of the animal but also passes through the vaporizer and carries vaporized anesthetic to the patient. Anesthetic machines are designed so that no anesthetic can be delivered to the patient unless oxygen is present to act as a carrier gas.

Gas cylinders

Oxygen used for anesthesia is provided as a compressed gas contained in metal cylinders. The gas is held under pressure in the cylinder so that a large amount of gas may be stored in a relatively small container. These cylinders may be small, in which case they are usually attached to the anesthetic machine (E cylinders, illustrated in Fig. 4-4, *B* and *C*). Large cylinders, which stand separately from the machine (Fig. 4-6), are also available. The capacities of several types of cylinders are given in Table 4-3. Cylinders normally remain the property of the company that supplies the oxygen. Empty cylinders are periodically picked up, and full cylinders are delivered by company personnel.

Oxygen starts to flow into the machine when the outlet valve on the top of the gas cylinder is opened in a counterclockwise direction (that is, to the left). When the flow is started, the outlet valve should be turned slowly until it is fully open.

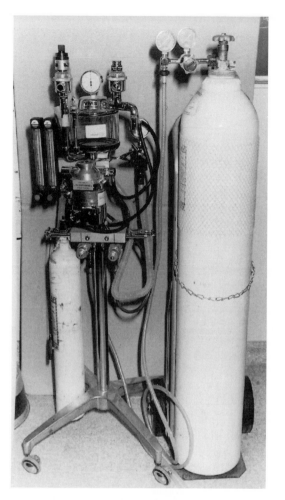

FIG. 4-6   Large cylinder connected to anesthetic machine.

	TABLE 4-3			

Capacity of Compressed Gas Cylinders

CYLINDER DIMENSIONS	EMPTY WEIGHT (kg)	CAPACITY (LITERS OF OXYGEN)	CAPACITY (LITERS OF NITROUS OXIDE)
E Cylinder			
4.25 inches OD × 26 inches	5.9	659	1590
G Cylinder			
8.5 inches OD × 51 inches	50	5331	13,836
H Cylinder			
9.25 inches OD × 51 inches	59	5570-7500	15,899

Modified from Warren RG: *Small animal anesthesia*, St Louis, 1989, Mosby.
OD, Outside diameter.

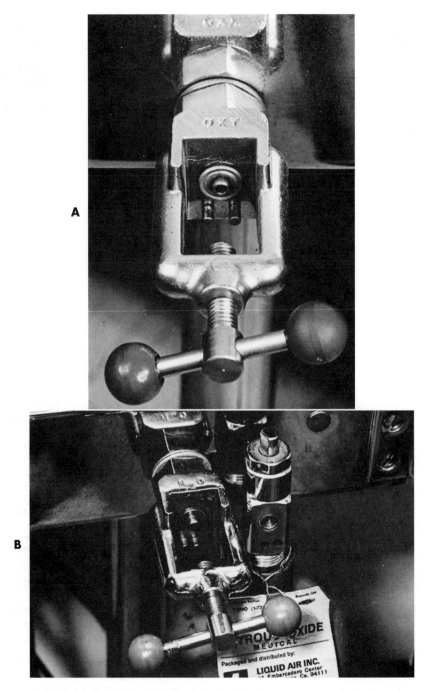

FIG. 4-7   Yokes, showing pin indexing. **A,** Pins for oxygen tank. **B,** Pins for nitrous oxide tank. (*From Warren RG:* Small animal anesthesia, *St Louis, 1983, Mosby.*)

The flow is discontinued when the valve is turned completely clockwise (that is, to the right). The mnemonic "left loose, right tight" has been used by several generations of anesthesia students as an aid in remembering these facts.

Some anesthetic machines are designed to provide not only oxygen but also nitrous oxide gas. Like oxygen, nitrous oxide is contained in a compressed gas cylinder. This may be a large freestanding tank or a smaller tank attached to the machine. Some machines have a device that discontinues nitrous oxide administration to the patient if the oxygen flow is cut off. This mechanism prevents inadvertent asphyxiation of the patient, which could occur if the patient breathed nitrous oxide in the absence of oxygen.

Gas cylinders that are part of the anesthetic machine are attached to it by a yoke (Fig. 4-7), whereas freestanding cylinders are connected to the machine by gas lines. Gas lines may take the form of flexible hose, or gas may be carried in pipes mounted within a wall. Often, gas lines are the primary source of oxygen and nitrous oxide, and cylinders are used as a backup supply or in locations where piped-in gas is unavailable.

Anesthetic machines are designed so that it is difficult or impossible to attach the wrong type of gas cylinder to the machine connections. The yokes for each gas are equipped with a pin index system so that an oxygen cylinder, for example, cannot be put on a nitrous oxide yoke (see Fig. 4-7). In addition, cylinders and gas lines are color-coded to prevent inadvertent use of an incorrect gas. Cylinder color codes vary by country. In the United States and Canada, nitrous oxide cylinders are blue, and oxygen cylinders are green (United States) or white (Canada) (Table 4-4).

Cylinders are designed to store large quantities of gas under pressure. The volume (in liters) of oxygen present in any E cylinder can be calculated by multiplying the pressure (in pounds per square inch [psi]) by 0.3. For a full E cylinder of oxygen, the pressure is approximately 2200 psi (15,000 kilopascals [kPa]) indicating that 660 L of oxygen gas (that is, 0.3 × 2200 psi) is contained in the tank. A reading of 1100 psi (7500 kPa) indicates the tank is approximately half full and therefore contains approximately 330 L of oxygen. The volume of the oxygen in the tank indicates to the anesthetist how much longer the tank can be used. For example, if the anesthetist selects an oxygen flow rate of 1 L/min, a full E tank containing 660 L of

TABLE 4-4					
Characteristics of Compressed Gas Cylinders					
GAS	FORMULA	COLOR	FULL TANK PRESSURE PSI AND kPa @21° C	PRESSURE (PSI AND kPa) AT WHICH TANK SHOULD BE CHANGED	STATE WITHIN CYLINDER
Oxygen	O_2	White or green	2200-2650 psi 15,000- 18,000 kPa	100-200 psi 680-1360 kPa	Gas
Nitrous oxide	N_2O	Blue	760 psi 5170 kPa	500 psi 3400 kPa	Liquid/Gas

Modified from Warren RG: *Small animal anesthesia*, St Louis, 1989, Mosby.

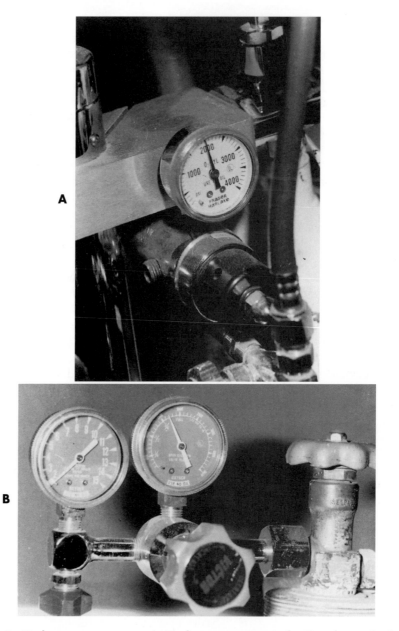

FIG. 4-8   Tank pressure gauges. A, Tank pressure gauge for E tank attached to anesthetic machine. B, Line pressure gauge (*left*) and tank pressure gauge (*right*) for large freestanding oxygen tank.

oxygen will last approximately 11 hours (that is, 660 minutes), and a half-full tank will last approximately 5½ hours (that is, 330 minutes). The volume in litres for the larger H cylinder can be calculated by multiplying the pressure (psi) by 1.7.

Tank pressure gauge

The pressure of oxygen being delivered by any given tank is indicated by a pressure gauge attached to the cylinder (Fig. 4-8, *A* and *B*). The tank pressure gauge will read zero when the tank is empty. It also reads zero when the tank is turned off and the remaining gas in the line has been evacuated (that is, "bled off"). When the tank valve is opened, the gauge reading rises to indicate the pressure of gas remaining in the tank.

During use, oxygen is gradually released from the tank and the pressure within the tank falls, as indicated by the reading on the tank pressure gauge (which usually sits directly above or immediately adjacent to the tank, see Fig. 4-8, *A*). The anesthetist may notice a considerable drop in indicated pressure during a lengthy anesthesia. The anesthetist must, of course, periodically monitor the oxygen tank pressure gauge during each procedure and change the tank when the valve indicates that the tank is close to empty. Because of the gradual way in which oxygen tank pressure falls, the anesthetist can rely on the gauge to roughly indicate the amount of oxygen remaining. Usually it is unnecessary to change oxygen tanks until the pressure drops below 100 to 200 psi (680 to 1360 kPa), indicating only 30 to 60 L of oxygen remaining in the tank. Tanks should be changed between procedures (not during) if possible.

Nitrous oxide is also stored in compressed air tanks (normally blue) although at considerably less pressure than oxygen. The normal pressure for a full nitrous oxide tank is 760 psi (5170 kPa). Unlike oxygen, nitrous oxide is present in both the liquid and gas states within the pressurized tank. The pressure gauge reads only the pressure of the gas within the tank and not that of the liquid. As the gas leaves the tank, more liquid evaporates and enters the gas state. As a result, the pressure of the gas within the tank will not change until all of the liquid has evaporated. The anesthetist therefore should not expect the nitrous oxide tank gauge reading to change—even after several hours of anesthesia—unless the tank is close to empty. It follows that the pressure gauge reading on a nitrous oxide tank will not tell the anesthetist how full the tank is. This information can only be determined by weighing the tank before use. An E cylinder of nitrous oxide weighs approximately 8 kg (18 lb) when full and about 5.9 kg (13 lb) when empty. The full and empty weights are normally stamped on the outside of each cylinder.

Because weighing the cylinder is seldom an option, the question arises: how does the anesthetist know when to change the nitrous oxide tank? Although the pressure gauge reads full (760 psi), the anesthetist does not know the exact amount of nitrous oxide present in the tank (unless a full tank was just started). The gauge reading does not change until the liquid nitrous oxide is exhausted and the tank is nearly empty (5 to 10 minutes left, depending on the flow rate) and a tank change is required. Nitrous oxide tanks therefore should be changed as soon as the tank pressure gauge starts to drop below 500 psi (3400 kPa).

Pressure-reducing valve

As a gas moves from a high-pressure tank into the anesthetic machine, the pressure is reduced by a pressure-reducing valve, also called a *pressure regulator*. The use of a pressure-reducing valve allows a constant flow of gas into the machine regardless of the pressure changes within the tank and provides a safe operating pressure for the machine. Oxygen leaving a tank at a pressure of up to 2200 psi (15,000 kPa) must be reduced to a constant pressure of 40 to 50 psi (340 kPa) before entering the anesthetic machine. Oxygen provided through gas lines is also delivered at a pressure of 50 psi. For small tanks and gas lines, the line pressure is preset at 50 psi, and there is only one gauge, which reads the tank pressure (see Fig. 4-8, *A*). In the case of large tanks, there may be two gauges, one showing the pressure in the gas cylinder and one showing the line pressure entering the machine (which should be adjusted to 40 to 50 psi*) (see Fig. 4-8, *B*).

Anesthetic Machine

Oxygen and nitrous oxide from the compressed gas supply lines enter the anesthetic machine through a low-pressure hose (see Figs. 4-4 and 4-5). The function of the anesthetic machine is to mix oxygen with the desired amount of anesthetic and deliver this mixture (called *fresh gas*) to the breathing circuit.

Flowmeter

Oxygen and nitrous oxide entering the anesthetic machine first pass through a flowmeter. The flowmeter allows the anesthetist to set the gas flow rate, which is the amount of oxygen that travels through the machine to be delivered to the patient. Flow rates are expressed in liters of gas per minute (L/min). If a machine is set up to use both nitrous oxide and oxygen, there must be separate flowmeters so that the flow rates of the two gases can be monitored and adjusted separately. To prevent the controls for oxygen and nitrous oxide from being confused, they are touch coded and profile coded (feel and look different), may be color coded (green or white for oxygen, blue for nitrous oxide), and are labeled according to the gas they regulate. Some machines provide two flowmeters for oxygen: one for flow rates greater than 1 L/min and one to accurately adjust flow rates less than 1 L/min.

Each flowmeter consists of a dial attached to a glass cylinder of graduated diameter. Within the cylinder is a rotor or ball that indicates the gas flow rate (of either oxygen or nitrous oxide) on a scale that measures liters of gas per minute. Each gas enters the bottom of its respective flowmeter and exits at the top. When the dial is turned, a valve within the flowmeter opens and gas enters the cylinder. The ball or rotor rises, indicating the amount of gas flow. The anesthetist controls the gas flow by adjusting the valve. For flowmeters that have a ball indicator, the center of the ball should be read to determine the flow rate. In the case of a rotor indicator, the reading should be taken at the top of the rotor.

It is the flowmeter, rather than the tank pressure gauge, that indicates the amount of oxygen or nitrous oxide being delivered to the patient. When the anesthetist opens the oxygen tank, the tank pressure gauge will indicate the pressure of gas being released from the tank and the line pressure gauge (if present) indicates the pressure of the oxygen leaving the pressure reducing valve and entering the machine.

---

*If a ventilator is in use (see Chapter 7), it may be necessary to increase the pressure to 60 to 65 psi to provide sufficient driving pressure for the ventilator.

However, this does not necessarily mean that the patient receives any oxygen. Oxygen flow through the machine is turned on or shut off by the flowmeter. If it is set at zero flow, the patient does not receive any oxygen.

The flowmeters allow the anesthetist to accurately control the relative amounts of oxygen and nitrous oxide received by the animal. If the nitrous oxide flowmeter is set to deliver 2 L/min of nitrous oxide to the patient and the oxygen flowmeter is adjusted to deliver 1 L/min of oxygen to the patient, the resulting mixture will be a 2:1 ratio of nitrous oxide to oxygen. (This represents approximately 67% nitrous oxide and 33% oxygen.) Some machines automatically set the O_2 and N_2O proportions, and an adjustment of the flow rate of one gas will automatically change the flow rate of the other.

When using nitrous oxide, the anesthetist should ensure that the nitrous oxide/oxygen ratio never exceeds 2:1, or the patient will receive insufficient oxygen and asphyxiation may result. It is also imperative that a minimum of 10 to 15 ml/kg/min of oxygen flow be delivered throughout anesthesia to any patient receiving a mixture of nitrous oxide and oxygen (30 ml/kg/min for small patients). Flow rates lower than 500 ml/min should be avoided.

As oxygen or nitrous oxide passes through the flowmeter, the gas pressure is further reduced, from 50 psi (340 kPa) to 15 psi (100 kPa). This pressure is only slightly above atmospheric pressure and is the optimum pressure for passage of gas to the patient.

Vaporizer

Oxygen gas exits at the top of the oxygen flowmeter and continues through the low-pressure system to the vaporizer (see Figs. 4-4 and 4-5.) The function of the vaporizer is to convert a liquid anesthetic such as halothane, isoflurane, or sevoflurane to a vapor state and to add controlled amounts of the vaporized anesthetic to the carrier gases (O_2 and N_2O) flowing through the machine. The vaporized anesthetic can only be released from the vaporizer by dialing a flow of carrier gas, which moves the anesthetic from the vaporizer into the breathing circuit of the anesthetic machine. No anesthetic is delivered to the patient if the flowmeters read zero because there is no flow of carrier gases into the vaporizer. Anesthetic vaporizers are further discussed in a separate section on pp. 187-196. After passing through the vaporizer, the oxygen (and nitrous oxide, if used) carrying the vaporized anesthetic continues to the fresh gas inlet. The breathing circuit is constructed so that this mixture of gases, commonly known as *fresh gas,* does not return to the vaporizer.

Breathing Circuit

The breathing circuit is the system that carries anesthetic and oxygen from the vaporizer to the patient and conveys expired gases away from the patient. The breathing circuit may be incorporated into the anesthetic machine (as in the circle system) or it may be a separate unit, such as a Bain circuit. In the commonly used circle rebreathing system, the breathing circuit contains the unidirectional (or one-way) valves, reservoir bag, pop-off (or pressure relief) valve, carbon dioxide canister, oxygen flush valve, negative pressure relief valve, and pressure manometer.

Once fresh gas enters the anesthetic circuit, there are a variety of flow paths, depending on the type of machine used (Fig. 4-9). Most commonly, fresh gas enters the circle system just upstream from the inspiratory unidirectional valve and downstream from the carbon dioxide absorber.

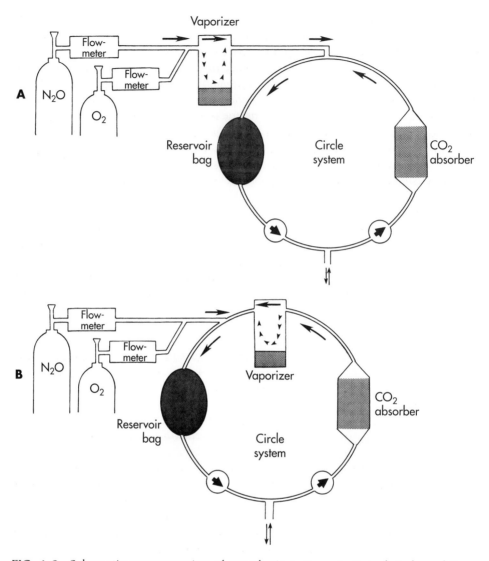

FIG. 4-9 Schematic representation of anesthetic system. A, Out of circle and B, in circle. (*From Warren RG: Small animal anesthesia, St Louis, 1983, Mosby.*)

Unidirectional valves

Fresh gas flowing through the breathing circuit passes through a one-way valve, called the *inhalation unidirectional valve* or *inhalation flutter valve* (see Figs. 4-4 and 4-5). The inhalation unidirectional valve allows gases to flow in only one direction (toward the patient). The valve may be a rigid disk that opens and "flutters" as gas flows past it, or it may be a flap.

When the patient inhales, the inhalation flutter valve opens, allowing the oxygen and anesthetic to enter the hoses. The gases travel through the inspiratory hose to the Y piece and are directed into the endotracheal tube or mask. Upon reaching the patient's lungs, oxygen and anesthetic molecules are absorbed and enter the blood-stream. At the same time, carbon dioxide and anesthetic molecules are released from the bloodstream, enter the alveoli, and are exhaled on the next breath.

Exhaled gases leave the patient and travel through another hose to reenter the breathing circuit. At the point at which the exhalation hose attaches to the machine, there is another unidirectional valve, commonly called the *exhalation* or *expiratory unidirectional valve,* or *exhalation flutter valve* (see Figs. 4-4 and 4-5). As with the inhalation valve, this valve controls the direction of gas flow and only allows gases to flow one way through the breathing circuit (in this case, away from the patient). This prevents expired gases from returning to the patient without first passing through the absorber canister, where carbon dioxide is removed.

Reservoir bag

Between breaths, fresh gas enters and fills the circuit between the expiratory valve and the carbon dioxide absorber, inflating a black rubber bag called the *reservoir bag* or *rebreathing bag* (see Figs. 4-4 and 4-5.) This bag is gradually filled as gases enter the circuit or the patient exhales, and is deflated when the patient inhales. The bag therefore expands and contracts continuously, reflecting the patient's respirations.

The reservoir bag serves a number of functions, including the following:

- The bag stores gas. It is easier for a patient to breathe from a reservoir bag than to rely solely on a continuous flow of air through a piece of tubing.
- Movement of the bag with the animal's respirations indicates to the anesthetist that the endotracheal tube is within the trachea and not the esophagus and therefore is a useful check on the location of the endotracheal tube.
- The bag allows the anesthetist to observe the animal's respirations. Both the respiratory rate and the size of each breath are indicated by the movement of the bag. Inadequate movement of the bag may indicate that the patient is breathing room air rather than gas from the machine. Often this occurs because the endotracheal tube is too small or because the cuff is inadequately inflated and air is passing around the tube. Alternatively, minimal movement of the reservoir bag may indicate that the patient's tidal volume is small, alerting the anesthetist to possible respiratory problems.
- The reservoir bag allows the anesthetist to deliver oxygen (with or without anesthetic) to the patient by means of "bagging." In this procedure the reser-voir bag is gently squeezed, forcing oxygen and anesthetic into the patient's lungs and causing the patient's chest to rise slightly. It is advisable to "bag" an anesthetized patient every 5 to 20 minutes to gently inflate the lungs with fresh oxygen and anesthetic. Use of this technique to manually ventilate the patient's lungs is further described in Chapter 7.

There are three reasons why bagging may be beneficial to the anesthetized patient:

1. Bagging helps to reverse a condition called *atelectasis,* in which the alveoli in certain sections of the lungs are collapsed and not useful for oxygen and anesthetic transfer to the patient. Bagging the patient helps reinflate the collapsed alveoli.
2. Anesthetized patients have a decreased ability to breathe, and the volume of gas inhaled with each breath may be as little as 50% of normal. By bagging the animal, the anesthetist flushes the airways and alveoli with fresh gas,

removing air that has increased carbon dioxide (CO_2) content and reduced anesthetic and oxygen content.

3. Bagging may be a lifesaving procedure if the patient is not breathing (a condition called *respiratory arrest*). Bagging allows the anesthetist to assist or control ventilation by delivering oxygen directly to the lungs and is an effective means of artificial respiration.

The reservoir bag should have a minimum volume of 60 ml/kg of patient weight. Bags are available in various sizes, from 500 ml (for very small patients) to 30 L (intended for use in horses). The most common sizes used for small animal anesthesia are 1-, 2-, and 3-L bags. If the rebreathing bag is too small, the reservoir may not be large enough for the animal to breathe easily. Also, a bag that is too small may become overinflated very rapidly, allowing pressure to build up in the patient's airways and alveoli. On the other hand, if the bag is too large it is difficult to monitor the patient's breathing because there is little movement with inspiration or expiration. Use of a large bag also makes it more difficult to assess the amount of gas being delivered to an animal when bagging a patient.

The anesthetist should ensure that the reservoir bag is properly inflated during anesthesia. The optimum size is approximately three fourths full. If the fresh gas flow is in excess of the patient's demand for oxygen and anesthetic (as is most often the case), the bag will tend toward being full. If the pressure builds in the system, the excess gas will be vented through the pop-off valve (see the next section), provided this is left open. The reservoir bag should not be allowed to overfill under pressure (assuming the appearance of an inflated beach ball), because this will increase pressure in the breathing circuit (called *back pressure*) and make it difficult for the animal to exhale. There is also some risk that the excessive pressure may rupture alveoli in the patient's lungs. The most common cause of an overfilled reservoir bag is failure to open the pop-off valve adequately.

On the other hand, the bag should not be allowed to empty completely when the animal inhales, because this defeats its purpose, which is to act as a reservoir. Complete emptying of the bag indicates that the gas flow is inadequate, that the bag is too small, or that the pop-off valve is open too much.

Pop-off valve (pressure relief valve)

Almost all anesthetic machine circuits contain a pressure relief valve, also called a *pop-off valve, exhaust valve, adjusting pressure limiting (APL) valve,* or *overflow valve* (see Figs. 4-4 and 4-5.) This valve is similar to a tap in that it can be turned fully open, partly open, or closed off entirely, allowing varying amounts of gas to exit from the system.

The main purpose of the pop-off valve is to allow excess gas (including oxygen, nitrous oxide, nitrogen, inhalation anesthetic, and carbon dioxide) to exit from the anesthetic circuit and enter the scavenging system. By venting excess gas, the pop-off valve prevents the buildup of excessive pressure or volume of gases within the circuit. If allowed to occur, this excess pressure would eventually reach the animal's lungs, causing the alveoli to distend and possibly rupture. The pop-off valve is normally kept open when the patient is breathing spontaneously, unless a low-flow technique is used (see Procedure 4-1). The anesthetist should adjust the pop-off valve periodically during the anesthetic procedure to maintain optimum gas volume within the circuit (as indicated by the distension of the reservoir bag, see previous section). If the animal is to be bagged the pop-off valve is closed, because otherwise the gases will escape through the scavenger when pressure is put on the reservoir bag, rather than going to the patient. However, a closed pop-off valve may allow pressure to build up in the circuit, and therefore the pop-off valve should be periodically opened to allow venting of excess gas.

It should be evident that the gas flow rate (determined by the flowmeter setting), the size of the rebreathing bag, and the position of the pop-off valve (open or closed) are related. Normally, the anesthetist selects a flow rate and adjusts the pop-off valve so that the reservoir bag is optimally inflated.

Carbon dioxide absorber

Any gases that do not exit from the system through the pop-off valve are directed to the carbon dioxide absorber canister before being returned to the patient (see Figs. 4-4 and 4-5.) Gas may enter the canister through the bottom or the top, depending on the design. The canister contains an absorbing chemical, either soda lime, which is a mixture of calcium hydroxide ($Ca[OH]_2$), sodium hydroxide ($NaOH$), and potassium hydroxide (KOH), or barium hydroxide lime. In soda lime, the main absorbing ingredient is $Ca(OH)_2$, which removes carbon dioxide from the gases that percolate through the canister. The chemical reaction that takes place within a canister containing soda lime is as follows:

$$2\ CO_2 + Ca(OH)_2 + 2\ NaOH \rightarrow Na_2CO_3 + CaCO_3 + 2H_2O + heat$$

The heat released by this reaction is sufficient to raise the temperature of the carbon dioxide absorber canister, and it may become warm during use. The water produced by this reaction is captured in a trap that lies immediately below the absorbing granules.

Soda lime and barium hydroxide lime granules do not last indefinitely: after several hours of use, the granules become exhausted and will no longer absorb carbon dioxide molecules. The use of depleted granules is not advised because this may result in the delivery of excessive amounts of carbon dioxide to the patient, leading to hypercapnia. There are several ways in which the anesthetist may become aware of granules that are exhausted and must be replaced, including the following:

- Fresh granules, containing mainly $Ca(OH)_2$, can be chipped or crumbled with finger pressure, whereas granules saturated with carbon dioxide (containing mainly calcium carbonate [$CaCO_3$]) become hard and brittle. This test can be used to determine the saturation of the granules before or after the anesthetic procedure.
- The color of the granules may indicate their degree of saturation. Absorber granules contain a pH indicator that causes the granules to change color when they are saturated with carbon dioxide. This color change will vary with the type of indicator used: some granules become whiter in appearance when exhausted, whereas other granules are normally white or pink and turn blue when exhausted. The color reaction is time limited, and granules that have changed color (indicating saturation with carbon dioxide) may return to the original color after a few hours although they are still saturated with carbon dioxide. Thus it is important that the anesthetist remove granules that have

changed color as soon as possible after using an anesthetic machine. Granules should be discarded when one third to one half have changed color.

Oxygen flush valve

Many anesthetic machines have a valve marked "oxygen flush." This valve, if depressed, allows oxygen to bypass the flowmeter and vaporizer and enter the machine between the unidirectional valves, often at the carbon dioxide absorber. Pure oxygen is thereby delivered directly to the breathing circuit at a flow rate of 35 to 75 L/min. This feature is particularly useful when delivering oxygen to a critically ill patient, and it also can be used to rapidly fill a depleted reservoir bag. The oxygen flush is also useful at the end of the anesthetic period, such as when it allows the anesthetist to add pure oxygen to the system, thereby diluting the residual anesthetic being exhaled by the animal. *The oxygen flush should not be used with certain nonrebreathing systems (such as the Bain system) because a high flow rate of oxygen into this type of circuit can seriously damage an animal's lungs.*

Pressure manometer

Many machines have a pressure manometer (also called a *pressure gauge,* not to be confused with the tank pressure gauge) often situated on top of the carbon dioxide absorber canister (Fig. 4-10). This gauge measures the pressure of the gases within the breathing system (expressed in centimeters of water [cm H_2O] or in millimeters of mercury [mm Hg]). This pressure, in turn, reflects the pressure of the gas in the animal's airway and lungs. Pressures over 15 cm H_2O (11 mm Hg) indicate a buildup of air within the machine, usually because the pop-off valve is not sufficiently open or because the oxygen flow rate is too high.

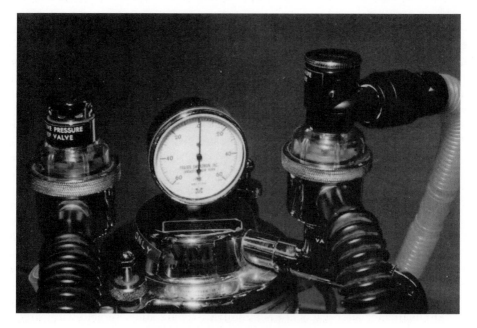

FIG. 4-10   Pressure manometer.

The pressure manometer is a useful aid when bagging an animal because it indicates the approximate pressure being exerted on the animal's lungs when the anesthetist squeezes the reservoir bag. In the case of cats and dogs with healthy lungs, the pressure should not exceed 15 to 20 cm H_2O (11 to 15 mm Hg) during bagging. For horses with normal lungs the pressure should not exceed 25 cm H_2O. Higher pressure may be needed in an animal with pulmonary dysfunction, such as a dog with gastric dilation/volvulus or a colicky, bloated horse. In the case of the dog with gastric dilation/volvulus, pressures of 30 to 35 cm may be needed to deliver a reasonable tidal breath, and in bloated horses pressures up to 50 to 55 cm may be necessary.

Negative pressure relief valve

Some machines have an additional valve called the *negative pressure relief valve*. This valve is designed to open and admit room air to the circuit if, for some reason, a negative pressure (partial vacuum) is detected in the circuit. This may happen when an active scavenging system is attached to the circuit, particularly if excessive suction is present.

Negative pressure may also develop in the circuit if the oxygen flow rate is too low or if the tank runs out of oxygen. With room air added to the circuit, the negative pressure relief valve ensures that the patient always receives some oxygen. It is preferable that the patient breathe room air (21% oxygen) rather than none at all, as would otherwise be the case if the tank ran out of oxygen.

VAPORIZERS

Of all the components of the anesthetic machine, the vaporizer is the most complicated and often the most expensive to purchase and service. The function of the vaporizer is to add anesthetic to the carrier gases (that is, either oxygen alone or oxygen plus nitrous oxide) that flow to the patient. Most vaporizers are designed for use with a specific agent, which is purchased in liquid form and put into the vaporizer before use. When oxygen passes through the vaporizer, a portion of the vaporized anesthetic is picked up by oxygen and the mixture is conveyed to the patient as a gas.

Almost all vaporizers have an indicator window at their base that allows the technician to inspect the amount of liquid anesthetic remaining in the vaporizer. This should be checked before the machine is used, and the vaporizer should be refilled if the level indicates that over half of the anesthetic has evaporated. Some anesthetics (halothane, methoxyflurane) contain a preservative that eventually accumulates within the vaporizer, causing a yellow discoloration of the liquid. Servicing or vaporizer flushing is recommended if this discoloration is apparent because vaporizer function may be impaired by high levels of preservative.

Some vaporizers are designed such that they are subject to leakage if the anesthetic machine is tipped over or shaken vigorously. Under these circumstances, liquid anesthetic enters bypass channels of the vaporizer and a potentially lethal dose of anesthetic may be delivered to the next patient. If an anesthetic machine is tipped or shaken, the anesthetic leak can be remedied by running oxygen through the machine (with the vaporizer dial turned off) for 15 minutes. Emptying anesthetic machine vaporizers before transport is the best way to avoid this problem.

TABLE 4-5		
Comparison of Precision and Nonprecision Vaporizers		
PARAMETERS	PRECISION VAPORIZER	NONPRECISION VAPORIZER
Temperature compensation	Output not affected by temperature in most models	Output affected by temperature
Flow compensation	Output not affected over a wide range of flow rates	Output affected by flow rate
Back pressure compensation	Changes in back pressure do not affect output	Changes in back pressure affect output
Maintenance requirements	Requires periodic factory recalibration and cleaning	Minimal; can be done by hospital staff
Cost	High	Minimal
Anesthetics commonly used	Isoflurane sevoflurane, halothane (that is, those with high vapor pressure)	Methoxyflurane (that is, those with low vapor pressure); isoflurane and halothane with low-flow techniques
Control over anesthetic concentration	Precise; given as a percentage	Not precise; given as a control lever setting (1-10)
Position relative to anesthetic circuit	Out of circle (VOC)	In circle (VIC)

Anesthetic machines may be equipped with either a precision or nonprecision vaporizer. The characteristics of these two types of vaporizers are summarized in Table 4-5.

Precision Vaporizers

A precision vaporizer is designed to deliver an exact concentration of anesthetic as selected by the anesthetist. The dial of a precision vaporizer (Fig. 4-11) is graduated in percent concentration (for example, 1%, 2%). For most patients, a concentration of 1.5 times the minimum alveolar concentration (MAC) value of that anesthetic will result in a moderate depth of anesthesia. For example, the MAC of isoflurane in the dog is 1.2%. A concentration of approximately 2% isoflurane therefore can be expected to maintain surgical anesthesia in most dogs. Halothane has a slightly lower MAC (0.87%), and a vaporizer setting between 1% and 1.5% is often adequate to maintain anesthesia. Sevoflurane has a high MAC (approximately 2.3), and the maintenance level can be expected to be close to 3.5%. This is only a rough guideline, and the anesthetist must, of course, monitor each animal's response to the anesthetic to determine the optimum setting for that individual.

Precision vaporizers are expensive, but they offer the advantage of closely controlling the delivery of anesthetic. This is of particular importance if the anesthetic used has a high vapor pressure (as is the case for sevoflurane, halothane, and isoflurane). Anesthetics with a high vapor pressure readily vaporize and may reach concentrations of 30% or greater within the anesthetic circuit if the amount of vapor being delivered to the breathing circuit is not controlled. Because the maximum safe con-

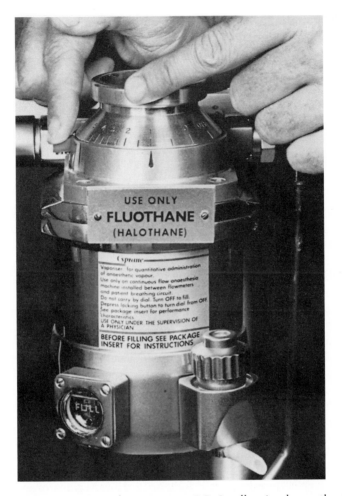

FIG. 4-11   Precision vaporizer. (*From Warren RG:* Small animal anesthesia, *St Louis, 1983, Mosby.*)

centration for isoflurane and halothane is less than 5% and most patients are satisfactorily maintained at 1% to 2%, uncontrolled delivery of anesthetic vapor will result in excessively high levels that could be dangerous for the patient. It is therefore customary to use halothane, isoflurane, and sevoflurane in a precision vaporizer, affording the anesthetist more exact control of the anesthetic concentration in the circuit. (Information on the use of halothane or isoflurane in a nonprecision vaporizer is given in the section on low-flow anesthesia.)

Not all anesthetics require this degree of control. For example, methoxyflurane has a low vapor pressure (that is, it does not vaporize readily) and will only produce a maximum of 4% concentration in the carrier gases. For an anesthetic with a high blood:gas solubility and slow onset of action, this anesthetic level is relatively safe for most patients, so a nonprecision vaporizer is adequate for methoxyflurane delivery.

A variety of precision anesthetic vaporizers are available. Examples include the Tec series (3 through 6), Ohmeda, and Drager models. Each vaporizer is designed for use with an anesthetic of a particular vapor pressure; therefore vaporizers are labeled for use with one anesthetic only. There is one exception to this rule: halothane and isoflurane have similar vapor pressures and may be used interchangeably in some vaporizers, although this practice is not recommended by vaporizer manufacturers.

Most vaporizers have keyed filler systems that help prevent inadvertent introduction of the wrong anesthetic into the vaporizer. If the wrong anesthetic is accidentally put into a vaporizer (for example, halothane into a methoxyflurane vaporizer), the vaporizer must be drained and flushed with oxygen (1 L/min) until it is dry. Gas exiting the vaporizer should be scavenged.

Nonprecision Vaporizers

Not all machines are equipped with precision vaporizers. Nonprecision vaporizers are available that are much simpler in design and much less expensive than precision vaporizers. They are acceptable for use with anesthetics that have a low vapor pressure (for example, methoxyflurane) and, under certain circumstances, may also be used with anesthetics that have a high vapor pressure (for example, isoflurane and halothane).

One example of a nonprecision vaporizer is the Ohio No. 8 vaporizer, which consists of a glass jar containing a wick. The wick absorbs anesthetic contained in the jar and increases the surface area available for vaporization, thus increasing saturation of the carrier gas with anesthetic. In a nonprecision vaporizer, the concentration of the anesthetic delivered to the patient is unknown because the vaporizer dial settings are unrelated to specific amounts of vapor delivered from the vaporizer. It therefore cannot be given as a percentage and is indicated only by a control lever setting (Fig. 4-12). The anesthetist varies the amount of anesthetic delivered to the patient by opening or closing the control valve, basing this decision on the patient's depth of anesthesia. This type of control is adequate for methoxyflurane, which has a low vapor pressure and will only achieve a maximum of 4% concentration even if the vaporizer is fully open. However, many anesthetists have traditionally thought that this control is inadequate for more volatile anesthetics such as halothane or isoflurane, which can achieve very high concentrations in such a system and lead to a rapid increase in patient depth. However, a nonprecision vaporizer such as the Stephens Universal Vaporizer can be safely used with isoflurane or halothane because it has been purposely made inefficient by removal of the wick, allowing halothane or isoflurane to be delivered at a concentration suitable for anesthesia (see Procedure 4-1, p. 201). The two advantages of this system are as follows:

1. It can be used with low flow rates and is therefore economical.
2. The initial cost is somewhat less than that of a precision vaporizer.

Use of isoflurane or halothane in this type of vaporizer is discussed in Procedure 4-1.

VOC versus VIC

The anesthetist may occasionally find an anesthetic machine referred to as *VOC* or *VIC*. The letters VOC are an abbreviation for *vaporizer out of circuit* and indicate that the vaporizer is not placed within the breathing circuit itself (see Fig. 4-9, *A*).

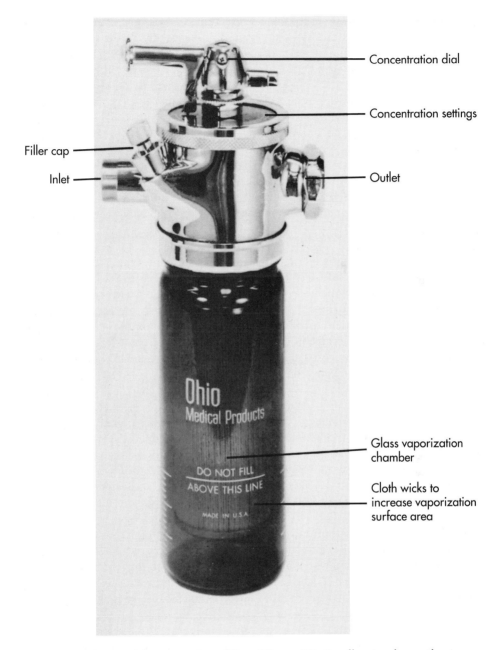

Concentration dial

Concentration settings

Filler cap

Inlet

Outlet

Glass vaporization chamber

Cloth wicks to increase vaporization surface area

Ohio
Medical Products

DO NOT FILL
ABOVE THIS LINE

MADE IN U.S.A.

FIG. 4-12 Nonprecision vaporizer. (*From Warren RG:* Small animal anesthesia, *St Louis, 1983, Mosby.*)

The "circuit" referred to includes the unidirectional valves, hoses, carbon dioxide absorber canister, pop-off valve, and reservoir bag as described earlier in this chapter. The letters VIC indicate a *vaporizer in circuit* (see Fig. 4-9, *B*). In this type of machine (for example, the Ohio No. 8 or Stephens vaporizer) the carrier gases enter the circuit directly from the flowmeter. The vaporizer (which is nonprecision in this case) is part of the circuit, and exhaled gases reenter the vaporizer each time they flow through the circuit.

It is reasonable to ask at this point why precision vaporizers are found out of circuit and nonprecision vaporizers are found in circuit. The position of a vaporizer in circuit or out of circuit is governed by the resistance it offers to the flow of gases. Nonprecision vaporizers offer little resistance to gas flow and do not impede the flow of gases around the breathing circuit. Precision vaporizers, however, offer a high resistance to gas flow and must be placed out of the breathing circuit.

Factors That Influence Vaporizer Function

When an anesthetic machine is used, it is easy to assume that the concentration of anesthetic delivered depends only on the vaporizer setting. However, the concentration delivered may be affected by other factors, including temperature, carrier gas flow rate, and back pressure.* Newer precision vaporizers are compensated for all three factors and can deliver the concentration indicated on their dials with little error or variation. However, technicians working with older precision vaporizers or nonprecision vaporizers such as the Ohio 8 or Stephens vaporizer should realize that these do not automatically compensate for factors.

Temperature

Volatile anesthetics, like all liquids, vaporize more readily at a high temperature than at a low temperature. If a vaporizer is not constructed to compensate for temperature changes, the amount of anesthetic vaporized will vary with changes in room temperature. If a noncompensated vaporizer is used in a cold room, the amount of anesthetic vaporized may be considerably less than that indicated on the dial. Conversely, in a warm room, the amount vaporized may be greater than the reading on the dial.

Temperature compensation is also important because at high oxygen flow rates, the passage of oxygen will cause the temperature of the liquid anesthetic to fall. Unless the vaporizer has built-in compensation for this effect, this leads to decreased vaporization and a decreased concentration of anesthetic being delivered to the patient. The result is that at high flow rates, a noncompensated vaporizer may deliver less anesthetic than the amount indicated by the dial.

Most precision vaporizers are temperature compensated to prevent variation of anesthetic output. Older models that are not temperature compensated provide a thermometer and temperature adjustment scale that allow the anesthetist to adjust the vaporizer setting to account for temperature changes within the vaporizer.

---

*Other reasons why the concentration of anesthetic may not be the same as that indicated by the vaporizer include uptake or release of anesthetic by rubber machine components and dilution of fresh gas by the patient's expired gases at the start and end of anesthesia.

Carrier gas flow rate

Just as temperature influences the rate of vaporization of a volatile anesthetic, the amount of gas that flows over the liquid anesthetic (the carrier gas flow rate) will also affect it. In a vaporizer that is not flow compensated, the concentration of anesthetic that is delivered at an oxygen flow rate of 3 L/min may differ from that released at a flow rate of 500 ml/min. Most modern precision vaporizers are designed to compensate for this variation and will vaporize the amount of anesthetic indicated on the vaporizer dial throughout a wide range of clinically useful flow rates. Older halothane vaporizers such as the Tek 2 series are not flow compensated, however, and come equipped with a chart that estimates the vaporizer output for a given dial setting over a range of flow rates.

For any precision vaporizer, flow compensation is not unlimited. Flows that are very high (that is, in excess of 10 L/min) or very low (that is, below 500 ml/min) may affect the vaporizer output even in a flow compensated precision vaporizer. The vaporizer setting does not accurately reflect the concentration of anesthetic released at these extreme flow rates.

Another complication, seen even with precision vaporizers, is that the amount of anesthetic received by the animal is affected by the carrier gas flow rate to the breathing circuit. High flows that approach the patient's minute ventilation (the total amount of gas a patient breathes in a minute) will bring the circuit concentration close to the dialed setting and thus the concentration the patient receives will be close to the dialed concentration. Lower flows result in less fresh anesthetic gas being delivered to the circuit and more rebreathing of the patient's expired gases that have lower concentrations of anesthetic because anesthetic has been taken up by the animal. This lowers the anesthetic concentration within the circuit. For example, if a 20-kg dog is connected to an anesthetic machine with a flow rate of 300 ml/kg/min (in this case, 6 L/min) and a vaporizer setting of 2%, the actual concentration of anesthetic being breathed by the animal is close to 2%. If the flow is reduced to 100 ml/kg/min (in this case, 2 L/min), then to 50 ml/kg/min (1 L/min), and finally to 10 ml/kg/min (200 ml/min), the percent concentration of anesthetic being inspired may drop to 1.8%, 1.2%, and 0.8%, respectively. In each case the vaporizer is delivering a 2% concentration to the circuit, but at the lower fresh gas flows less anesthetic is delivered to the circuit while the patient's expired gases increasingly dilute the anesthetic in the circuit. This is why precision vaporizer settings must be increased if low oxygen flow rates are used (see Procedure 4-1).

Back pressure

A vaporizer that is not back pressure compensated will release additional anesthetic if gas from the circuit passes through it under pressure. This may occur, for example, when the animal is bagged. Most precision vaporizers are designed to compensate for back pressure effects so that bagging does not affect the amount of anesthetic released by these vaporizers.* However, nonprecision vaporizers do not compensate for this effect.

---

*Despite back pressure compensation, an increased amount of anesthetic may be delivered to a patient that is bagged continuously. This occurs because the volume of gas entering the lungs in a ventilated animal is greater than that breathed by the anesthetized patient on its own. It is therefore important to reduce the setting for both precision and nonprecision vaporizers when continuously bagging a patient, particularly if patient depth seems excessive.

Nonprecision vaporizer function

Nonprecision vaporizers do not compensate for changes in temperature, carrier gas flow rates, or back pressure. This has several serious implications that must be understood by the anesthetist using this type of vaporizer.

- *Lack of temperature compensation.* At any given setting, the vaporizer will deliver a greater concentration of anesthetic in a warm room than in a cold room. The vaporizers also do not compensate for the drop in temperature that accompanies vaporization at high flow rates.
- *Lack of flow compensation.* The amount of anesthetic delivered to the patient will increase if the patient's ventilation increases or the flow rate is increased. Increased ventilation results in increased flow of gas through the vaporizer and thus will deliver more anesthetic to the patient. Eventually the high flow rates will cause the temperature of the anesthetic in the vaporizer to fall, and the concentration of anesthetic may decrease. The variation of anesthetic output with flow rate is much less in a flow-compensated precision vaporizer, in which anesthetic output will not vary despite changes in respiratory rate or depth or changes in oxygen flow rate.
- *Lack of back pressure compensation.* Because nonprecision vaporizers are not back pressure compensated, a buildup of pressure within the circuit (as may occur when the patient is bagged or a ventilator is used) may result in increased concentration of anesthetic being delivered to the patient and may result in excessive anesthetic depth. Controlled ventilation therefore is difficult with nonprecision vaporizers. The anesthetist must ensure that the vaporizer setting is greatly reduced (or the vaporizer is turned off) when bagging the animal or when delivering intermittent positive pressure ventilation by means of a ventilator. In contrast, when a precision out-of-circuit vaporizer is used, it is not normally necessary to turn the vaporizer off when bagging the patient because of the back-pressure compensation of these vaporizers.
- *Monitoring.* The use of a nonprecision vaporizer with a volatile anesthetic such as isoflurane offers less precise control over anesthetic depth than does a standard precision vaporizer. Close monitoring of the patient is essential, particularly during the first 5 minutes of anesthesia, when patient depth increases rapidly.
- *Use with nonrebreathing systems.* Nonprecision vaporizers are difficult to adapt to nonrebreathing systems such as the Bain circuit.

OPERATION OF THE ANESTHETIC MACHINE

The anesthetist operating any anesthetic machine has a number of options regarding its use. The most important decision is the type of breathing system to be used. There are three systems in common use: total rebreathing (closed), partial rebreathing (semiclosed), and nonrebreathing (open). The choice of system to be used is important because it will determine the following:

- Whether the gases that have been exhaled will be recirculated back to the patient ("rebreathed").
- Oxygen and nitrous oxide flow rates
- Position of the pop-off valve (closed or open)
- Type of equipment used (for example, whether a Bain system will be required)

Rebreathing Systems

In the system described thus far in this chapter (a circle system with a VOC precision vaporizer), the gases exhaled by the patient travel through the expiratory hose and the expiratory unidirectional valve and enter the carbon dioxide canister. They are then directed into the reservoir bag and back toward the patient through the inhalation unidirectional valve. These exhaled gases include oxygen, anesthetic vapor, carbon dioxide (removed by the CO_2 absorber), nitrogen, water vapor, and nitrous oxide (if used). At this point, fresh oxygen and anesthetic vapor enter the circuit from the vaporizer and mix with the patient's exhaled gases. The flow of gas through the anesthetic machine therefore is circular (reservoir bag, inhalation unidirectional valve, inspiration hose, animal, expiration hose, exhalation unidirectional valve, carbon dioxide canister, back to the inhalation unidirectional valve). The machine adapts to the patient's ventilation patterns and maintains a constant flow of gas to the patient through the use of a reservoir bag, pop-off valve, and negative pressure relief valve.

This type of system allows recirculation of exhaled gases to the patient and therefore is called a *rebreathing system*. It is also sometimes referred to as a *circle system*. The patient rebreathes its own exhaled gases, from which carbon dioxide has been removed and a certain amount of fresh oxygen and anesthetic are continuously added.

Rebreathing systems are further subdivided into total rebreathing systems (also called *closed systems*) in which all of the gases exhaled by the patient remain in the circuit, and partial rebreathing systems (also called *semiclosed systems*), in which some gases exhaled by the patient remain in the circuit, and some exit through the pop-off valve into the scavenger.

The main difference between these systems lies in the amount of oxygen and nitrous oxide that is delivered to the patient, called the *flow rate*. In a closed, total rebreathing system, the oxygen flow rate is relatively low, providing only the oxygen necessary to meet the patient's metabolic requirements. A total rebreathing system recirculates all of the exhaled gases (with the exception of carbon dioxide, which is removed by the absorber), and only a small amount of fresh oxygen and anesthetic are added to the system. The amount of oxygen used by the patient is closely matched by the amount of oxygen entering the circuit from the vaporizer. In this type of system, it may be necessary to turn the pop-off valve almost to the closed position to prevent gases from escaping, particularly if the suction from the scavenger is strong.

In the semiclosed, partial rebreathing system, the flow rate of fresh oxygen, nitrous oxide, and anesthetic entering the system must be considerably higher than that for the closed, total rebreathing system. The pop-off valve is left partly open, allowing some exhaled gases to escape. Although some of the exhaled gases are recirculated to the patient, much of the exhaled gases exit by means of the scavenger. The exiting gases are replaced by fresh oxygen and anesthetic entering the circuit.

Nonrebreathing Systems

The total and partial rebreathing systems just discussed are well suited to many patients. However, in some circumstance the anesthetist may prefer to use a different type of anesthetic setup, called a *nonrebreathing system*. In a nonrebreathing system, little or no exhaled gases are returned to the patient; instead they are evacuated by a scavenger connected to a pop-off valve or exit port. If no gases are returned to the patient, the system is described as open; if some gases return, the system is described as semiopen. The characteristics of rebreathing and nonrebreathing systems are compared in Table 4-6.

As with the rebreathing system, the nonrebreathing system can best be understood by following the path of an oxygen molecule from the tank, to the patient, and finally to the scavenger. Just as in a rebreathing system, oxygen (and nitrous oxide gas, if used) flows from the tank, through a flowmeter and into the vaporizer. At this point, however, gases exiting the vaporizer go directly into a hose for delivery to the patient, bypassing the inhalation flutter valve. Exhaled gases pass through another hose and may enter a reservoir bag, but they do not enter a carbon dioxide canister. The gas is then released into a scavenger through a pop-off valve, pressure relief valve, or other mechanism. Because most of the gases exit through the scavenger and are not returned to the patient, the system is accurately described as nonrebreathing.

TABLE 4-6

Comparison of Rebreathing and Nonrebreathing Systems

PARAMETERS	NONREBREATHING (OPEN OR SEMIOPEN)	REBREATHING (SEMICLOSED OR CLOSED SYSTEM)
CO_2 absorption	Not required	Must have CO_2 absorber canister
Changes in depth of anesthesia	Quickly	Slowly
Flow rates	High flow rates: must equal or exceed the respiratory minute volume	Low-flow rates: only to meet the metabolic oxygen requirement
Cost of operation	High because of the amount of oxygen and anesthetic used	Low, because less oxygen and anesthetic used
Amount of waste gas produced	High	Minimal
Pop-off valve position	Full open, or no pop-off	Closed (total rebreathing) or partly open (partial rebreathing)
Heat and moisture conservation (from exhaled gases)	Poor	Good
Vaporizer position	No circle, or VOC	VOC or VIC
Size of animal	Any size: limited only by the total gas flow that is delivered. Generally recommended for animal under 7 kg.	Only for animals over 7 kg (if pediatric hoses used, can be used for animals 3-7 kg also)

It is evident that several components that are used in a circle system are not required in a nonrebreathing system. These include the carbon dioxide canister and the unidirectional valves.

Although most anesthetic machines are designed to be used as a rebreathing or partial rebreathing system, a conventional anesthetic machine (with a CO_2 absorber canister and unidirectional valves) can be converted to a nonrebreathing system. This is achieved with a high oxygen flow rate (200 to 300 ml/kg/min) or flow rates that match or exceed the patient's minute ventilation. This effectively flushes most of the exhaled gases through the pop-off valve. Alternatively, the anesthetic machine may be easily converted to a nonrebreathing system through the use of attachments such as the Bain system (The Kendall Company, Boston, Massachusetts) (Figs. 4-13 and 4-14), the Ayres T piece, the Mapleson A system (Magill), the Kuhn circuit, the Norman mask elbow, an anesthetic chamber, or similar equipment. Each of these attachments delivers the fresh gas from the vaporizer to the animal and conducts the expired gases to a scavenger. Most systems have a fresh gas inlet, reservoir bag, tubing, scavenger outlet, and endotracheal tube connection but differ as to where the fresh gas enters the circuit, the position of the reservoir bag, and the location of the exhalation port.

Because the Bain system is a commonly used nonrebreathing attachment, it will be discussed in more detail here. Readers are referred to more detailed reference texts or equipment manufacturers for information on other systems.

The Bain system consists of inner tubing (which conducts fresh gas to the patient and corresponds to the inspiratory hose of a rebreathing system) surrounded by larger, corrugated tubing (which conducts gas away from the patient and corresponds

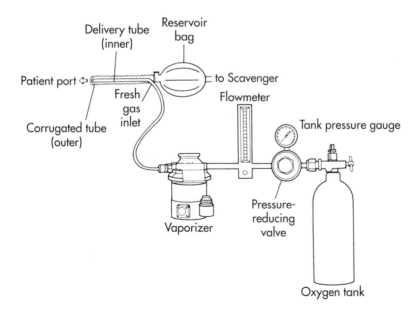

FIG. 4-13 Components of an anesthesia delivery system with a Bain circuit. (Redrawn from Hodgson DS: The case for nonrebreathing circuits for very small animals. *In Haskins SC:* Vet Clin North Am Small Anim Pract 22(2):326-469, 1992.)

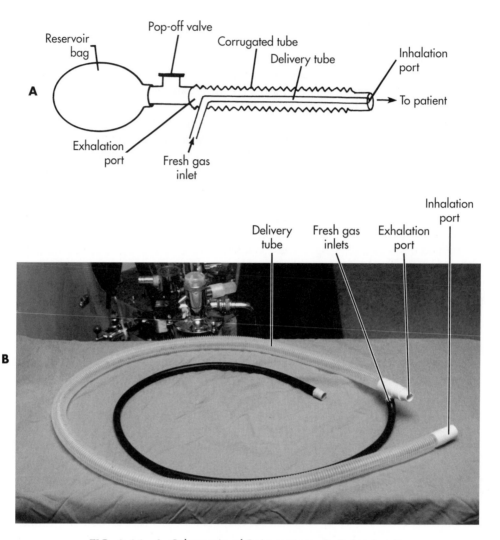

FIG. 4-14 A, Schematic of Bain system. B, Bain circuit.

to the expiratory hose in a rebreathing system). The arrangement of the tubing into an inner and outer hose (called a *coaxial system*) makes the setup less cumbersome and allows the incoming gases to be warmed slightly by the exhaled gases that surround them, before reaching the patient. When a Bain circuit is used or cleaned, care must be taken to ensure that the inner tubing does not detach from the rest of the apparatus, or gas will not be delivered to the next patient.

Gas from the outer, exhalation tubing enters a reservoir bag before exiting the system. In an open system with minimal rebreathing, the bag is not strictly necessary but facilitates monitoring of respirations and permits manual ventilation if necessary. Some Bain circuits are not equipped with an overflow valve or pop-off valve, and it may be necessary to cut the tail of the reservoir bag to allow the escape of waste gases. In this case, the tail of the reservoir bag should be connected to the scavenging system to allow proper disposal of the waste gas. It may be necessary to partially clamp the outlet of the reservoir bag with a paper clip or screw clamp to act as a pop-off valve and allow the anesthetist to control the rate at which the reservoir bag empties. Alternatively, a Bain mount is available that allows the use of an uncut bag. This mount features a pop-off valve, which allows easy scavenging and bagging.

When a nonrebreathing system such as the Bain is the used, the oxygen flow rate is normally high (usually at least 130 ml/kg/min), and a large proportion of the exhaled gases enters the scavenger. Some rebreathing of gas can occur if a reservoir bag is present, particularly during peak inspiration, if the respiratory rate is rapid, or the length of the Bain circuit is shorter than it should be for the size of the patient. The amount of rebreathing depends on the oxygen flow rate and therefore can be controlled by the anesthetist. If the anesthetist selects a high oxygen flow rate (for example, 2 L/min for a 5-kg cat), there is little return of exhaled gases to the patient. The system is therefore truly nonrebreathing, and the reservoir bag outlet is kept fully open. At lower flow rates (for example, 500 ml of oxygen per minute for a 5-kg cat), significant rebreathing of exhaled gases may occur even with a Bain circuit, and the setup would be more properly classified as a partial rebreathing system rather than a nonrebreathing system. Because the Bain system does not remove carbon dioxide from exhaled gases, low flow rates should be avoided because they may cause the patient to inhale excessive amounts of carbon dioxide gas.

Choice of Rebreathing versus Nonrebreathing System

The decision of whether to use a rebreathing system (such as the conventional anesthetic machine setup) or a nonrebreathing system (such as the Bain) is made on the basis of the following factors:

- *Patient size.* Nonrebreathing systems offer little resistance to respiration, which is a significant advantage for very small patients. If a rebreathing system is used, the unidirectional valves, carbon dioxide canister, and pop-off valve increase the resistance to air movement within the system. Small patients may have difficulty inhaling with enough force to draw air from such a circuit into their lungs.* For this reason, anesthetists prefer nonrebreathing systems for patients weighing less than 7 kg (15 lb). If the circle system has pediatric hoses and unidirectional valves are of the newer designs (lightweight, nonsticky), a circle system can be used on patients as small as 2 kg. Patients smaller than 2 kg should be on a nonrebreathing circuit.
- *Convenience.* Nonrebreathing circuits such as the Bain are generally lighter than the Y piece and hose assembly of a rebreathing circuit and therefore cause less drag on the endotracheal tube.
- *Cost.* Total rebreathing (closed) systems are more economical than nonrebreathing (open) systems because gas flows are relatively low and less anesthetic and

---

*The size of the endotracheal tube has a greater effect on resistance than does the type of circuit used. The use of an endotracheal tube that is too small results in far greater resistance to air passage than that offered by the remainder of the anesthetic circuit, even in a rebreathing setup.

oxygen are used. Partial rebreathing (semiclosed) systems are not as economical as total rebreathing systems but require much less oxygen and anesthetic (on a per kilogram basis) than nonrebreathing systems such as the Bain. For this reason, rebreathing systems (either total or partial rebreathing) are commonly used in large patients, which would require prohibitively large amounts of anesthetic and oxygen in a nonrebreathing system.

- *Control.* The speed at which the anesthetist can change anesthetic depth depends in part on the type of system used. A rebreathing system has a relatively slow turnover of gases because the flow rate of fresh oxygen and anesthetic into the system is low compared to the volume of the circuit (see Box 4-1). A nonrebreathing system allows a much faster turnover of gases because flow rates of fresh gas are higher relative to the volume of the circuit and the fresh gas is often delivered close to the circuit's connection to the endotracheal tube. This means that changes made in the (precision) vaporizer setting will result in rapid changes in anesthetic concentration within a nonrebreathing system, and the percentage of anesthetic breathed by the patient is very close to that indicated by the dial. However, changes in anesthetic concentration within a rebreathing system require a longer time, and the concentration of anesthetic inhaled by the patient may not be the same as that indicated on the dial for several minutes after the dial setting is changed.*

- *Conservation of heat and moisture.* Fresh gas entering a breathing system from the vaporizer is relatively cool and dry, compared with the patient's exhaled gases. Inspired fresh anesthetic gases have a relative humidity close to 0% and a temperature of approximately 16° C, whereas exhaled gases have a relative humidity of almost 100% and a temperature close to 25° C. Rebreathing systems automatically warm and humidify fresh gas that enters the circuit as it mixes with the patient's expired gases. In nonrebreathing systems, the warmed and humidified gases exhaled by the patient exit through the scavenger, and the patient breathes only the cool, dry fresh gas. Nonrebreathing systems are therefore associated with significant heat and water loss from the patient. In addition, the dry anesthetic gases may impair ciliary function and dry the airways.

- *Production of waste gas.* Total rebreathing systems release little waste anesthetic gas because oxygen flow rates are low and exhaled gases are recirculated rather than vented through the pop-off valve.

The use of total rebreathing systems is outlined in Procedure 4-1.

Carrier Gas Flow Rates

For each anesthetic procedure, the anesthetist is faced with the problem of deciding how much flow (or volume) of carrier gas is required. Usually the carrier gas is oxygen alone, but if both oxygen and nitrous oxide are used, flow rate determinations must consider the total flow of gas as well as the individual flow rates of each gas. Thus it may be decided that for a particular patient and machine setup, a total

---

*The type of volatile anesthetic used will also determine how quickly anesthetic depth can be changed, regardless of oxygen flow rates or the type of circuit used. (See discussion on blood:gas solubility coefficients in Chapter 3.)

PROCEDURE 4-1   Procedure for Operation of a Total Rebreathing System

If a total rebreathing (closed) system is used, the anesthetist should take the following active steps to ensure patient safety:

- Check the machine for leaks before use. If leaks are present, oxygen may escape from the circuit and room air may leak into and dilute the oxygen in the circuit. In a total rebreathing system the oxygen flow rate is low and any loss of oxygen or its dilution by room air may be detrimental. The pop-off valve is normally closed, or almost so to prevent oxygen escape.

- Induction is the most challenging period of anesthesia when low oxygen flows are used. The reservoir bag should be emptied and filled with oxygen 2 to 3 times during the first 15 minutes of anesthesia and every 30 minutes thereafter to help prevent patient hypoxia and to eliminate nitrogen (N_2) that is being exhaled by the patient (a process known as *denitrogenization*). Alternatively, the anesthetist may provide 5 to 10 minutes of high oxygen flow (200 ml/kg/min) at the start of anesthesia, until the patient reaches a surgical plane. The pop-off valve should be open when these flow rates are used. This flushes room air out of the system and replaces it with oxygen. Thereafter, much lower flow rates (7 to 15 ml/kg/min) can be used, and the pop-off valve should be closed. This amount of oxygen will meet the metabolic oxygen requirements of the anesthetized patient.

- Closely monitor the reservoir bag if a total rebreathing system is used. If the bag becomes smaller, then a leak is present in the system, the pop-off valve is open too much, or the flow rate of oxygen is inadequate. On the other hand, if the bag becomes distended, it indicates that fresh gas flow exceeds the patient's demand for oxygen and anesthetic (which can occur if the patient is too deep, too cold, or any other factor reduces patient demand for oxygen). In this case, after the patient has been checked and it is certain the patient is not having problems, either the oxygen flow rate should be reduced or the pop-off valve should be opened. It is wise to leave the pop-off valve slightly open during low-flow anesthesia, in case pressure in the circuit rises and excess gas must be vented.

- It may be difficult to change the patient's depth quickly. If a rapid change in anesthetic depth is required, the vaporizer setting should be changed and the breathing system converted to a partial rebreathing system by increasing the oxygen flow rate and opening the pop-off valve. If low oxygen flow rates are maintained, changes in the vaporizer setting may not affect the concentration of anesthetic in the circuit for several minutes.

- If a precision vaporizer is used for low-flow, closed circuit anesthesia, the setting required during the maintenance period will often be well above the setting normally used to maintain surgical anesthesia with a semiclosed or open system. In a total rebreathing system with an out of circuit vaporizer, the vaporizer concentration required may be 1% to 2% higher than that used for a partial rebreathing system (at least until a state of equilibrium is reached, such that concentrations in the brain and blood are equal to the concentration of anesthetic in the circuit). In a closed system this may take a considerable period of time to occur, due to the low gas flow rate, see Box 4-1.

- In contrast, if an in-circuit nonprecision vaporizer is used for low-flow, closed circuit anesthesia, the required vaporizer setting will usually be lower than that

---

PROCEDURE 4-1   **Procedure for Operation of a Total Rebreathing System—cont'd**

used for a partial rebreathing system. When a vaporizer in circle is used, if the fresh gas flow is decreased to the circuit, the anesthetic concentration in the circuit will increase because the fresh gas flow is so low that it does not dilute the anesthetic circuit concentration. Fresh gas flow will dilute what is in the circuit as long as all other factors remain the same, such as patient ventilation and temperature.

- The low oxygen flow rates used in a total rebreathing system may be inadequate for accurate delivery of anesthetic by some vaporizers. Consult the vaporizer manual for minimum recommended flow rates and be aware that the anesthetic concentration indicated by the dial may be incorrect at lower flows. Total rebreathing systems should not be used at all with certain vaporizers, including the Fluothane Tek-2, Copper Kettle, and Vernitrol.
- Nonprecision vaporizers are sometimes used to deliver halothane or isoflurane in a closed, total rebreathing system. Ohio No. 8 vaporizers (nonprecision) can be used with halothane or isoflurane, but the wick should be removed and no more than 100 ml of anesthetic should be put into the vaporizer. For the first 2 minutes, a setting of 6 to "fully open" should be used, and thereafter a setting between 2 and 6 is usually adequate.
- If a Stephens vaporizer (nonprecision) is used to deliver halothane or isoflurane at low oxygen flow rates, the metal sleeve should be fully retracted and the anesthetic should only be filled to the anesthetic level line. A vaporizer setting of 4 is used for the first 2 minutes, and for the maintenance period a setting between "off" and 4 is usually adequate.
- Low flow rates are unsuitable for Bain or other nonrebreathing systems.

BOX 4-1 Time Constants

The concept of time constants helps explain why a change in vaporizer setting takes time to be reflected in the circuit (and in the patient) and also gives the anesthetist a rough idea as to how long he or she can expect for a change anesthetic concentration to occur. Consider a circuit that has a total volume of about 5 L (2 L for the reservoir bag, 1.5 L for the carbon dioxide absorber, and 1.5 L in the inspiratory and expiratory hoses). If the anesthetic is delivered in fresh gas to the circuit at a flow rate of 2 L/min, this yields one time constant of: total volume/fresh gas flow rate = 5 L/2 L/min = 2.5 minutes. It takes 5 time constants to effect a 95% change in circuit concentration. In this example, if the vaporizer dial setting is changed, it will take 12.5 minutes (2.5 minutes × 5) before the anesthetic concentration in the circuit reaches 95% of the new dial setting. In contrast, if the anesthetist is using a low-flow technique (for example, an oxygen flow rate of 200 ml or 0.2 L) with a circuit volume of 5 L, then 1 time constant is 5 L/0.2 L/min = 25 minutes. This amounts to a total time of 5 × 25 minutes = 125 minutes! This explains why there is such a time lag between making a vaporizer dial change and seeing an effect in the circuit if low flows are used. There are two ways to change the concentration more rapidly: turn up the fresh gas flow rate and shorten the time constant for the circuit being used, or make a big change in the vaporizer dial setting.

flow of 1 L/min is required. The 1 L may consist of pure oxygen or some combination of nitrous oxide and oxygen (for example, 600 ml/min of nitrous oxide and 400 ml/min of oxygen). If nitrous oxide is used, the nitrous oxide flow should be 1.5 to 2 times the oxygen flow rate.

The calculation of the flow rate to be used for each anesthetic procedure is based on several factors, including the period of anesthesia (that is, induction, maintenance, or recovery) and whether a rebreathing or nonrebreathing system is preferred. These factors are summarized in Box 4-2.

Flow rates during induction

It is customary to use higher flow rates during induction than during the maintenance period. This is particularly true if mask induction or chamber induction is used. Use of high flow rates in the induction period allows the anesthetist to saturate the anesthetic circuit with carrier gas and anesthetic and dilute the expired gases of the patient. Otherwise, expired nitrogen gas (N_2), which comprises almost 80% of the air in patient's lungs and bloodstream at the start of the anesthetic period, will enter the circuit and dilute out the anesthetic vapor and oxygen. If high flow rates are used, the nitrogen will be evacuated by the scavenger within a few minutes. The flow rate can be decreased once the patient reaches the desired plane of anesthesia.

- For mask induction it is generally agreed that a flow rate per minute should equal 30 times the tidal volume for cats and small dogs (somewhat less for larger

---

BOX 4-2 Recommended Flow Rates

INDUCTION
Chamber Induction
- 5 L/min

Face Mask Induction
- 300 ml/kg/min, or 1-3 L/min for animals under 10 kg, 3-5 L/min for animals over 10 kg

Intravenous Induction
- 200 ml/kg/min (500 ml to 5 L/min depending on patient size)

MAINTENANCE
Nonrebreathing Systems
- Bain: 130-200 ml/kg/min
- Other systems: 200-300 ml/kg/min

Rebreathing Systems
- Total rebreathing (closed) system: minimum of 15 ml/kg/min; use of N_2O is inadvisable at this flow rate.
- Partial rebreathing (semiclosed system): 25-50 ml/kg/min.
- Semiclosed system with minimal rebreathing: 150-200 ml/kg/min.

Flow rates in excess of 2 L/min should be avoided when using nonprecision vaporizers.

Many vaporizers deliver inaccurate amounts of anesthetic at flow rates less than 500 ml/min or greater than 10 L/min.

Nitrous oxide flow rate should be 1.5 to 2 times the oxygen flow rate.

dogs). Because the tidal volume of most animals is approximately 10 ml/kg/min, the recommended flow rate for small patients is approximately 300 ml/kg/min. For animals under 10 kg, 1 to 3 L is usually adequate, and 3 to 5 L/min is suggested for animals over 10 kg.

- A flow rate of 5 L/min is recommended for chamber induction.
- For animals induced with an injectable anesthetic and subsequently intubated and connected to an anesthetic machine, the minimum flow rate during the initial anesthetic period is the respiratory minute volume, which is the tidal volume (10 ml/kg) times the number of breaths per minute. A figure of 200 ml/kg/min is commonly used, which results in a flow rate between 500 ml and 5 L/min, depending on the size of the animal and the preference of a rebreathing (low oxygen flow) or nonrebreathing (high oxygen flow) system.

Flow rates in the maintenance period

Once the animal achieves a satisfactory level of anesthetic depth, the flow rate may be safely reduced to a maintenance level. This value depends on the type of system used (total rebreathing, partial rebreathing, or nonrebreathing).

Nonrebreathing systems require relatively high flow rates on a per kilogram basis because the removal of carbon dioxide from the circuit is dependent on fresh gas flow. Fresh gas must be continuously provided to ensure that there is minimal rebreathing of exhaled gases. The recommended flow rate for a Bain circuit is 130 to 200 ml/kg/min. For a 5-kg animal, this flow rate is 650 ml to 1 L/min of pure oxygen. If nitrous oxide is used, flow rates of 600 ml nitrous oxide and 400 ml of oxygen per minute (a ratio of 1.5:1) would be appropriate.

For other types of nonrebreathing circuits, flow rates of 200 to 300 ml/kg/minute are generally accepted.

Rebreathing systems require relatively low flow rates compared with nonrebreathing systems because carbon dioxide absorption is available and the expired gases are returned to the patient. Provided the carbon dioxide absorber canister is effective and there are no leaks in the system, the carrier gas and anesthetic can be recycled continuously and only a small amount of fresh gas is required. For a total rebreathing (closed) system, the oxygen flow must only equal the oxygen requirements of the animal. The minimum oxygen requirement for the anesthetized animal is 5 to 10 ml/kg/min, although a value of 15 ml/kg/min is usually recommended. (See Procedure 4-1.) The anesthetist should be aware that flow rates less than 500 ml/min will not allow some precision vaporizers and flowmeters to accurately deliver the dialed vaporizer concentration and oxygen flow.

Flow rates of 25 to 50 ml/kg/min are recommended for partial rebreathing systems.

Flow rates at the end of anesthesia

It is recommended that the flow rates be increased immediately after the vaporizer is turned off. During this time, anesthetic gas is exhaled by the patient and its elimination from the circuit will be hastened with slightly higher fresh gas flow rates (especially for a rebreathing circuit). A flow rate similar to that used during induction is recommended to evacuate this anesthetic and to allow the patient to breathe pure oxygen. The anesthetist should periodically remove expired gases from the circuit by opening the pop-off valve and evacuating the reservoir bag. The bag can be refilled using the oxygen flush control.

Summary

Within the aforementioned guidelines, there is considerable leeway for the anesthetist's own judgment in determining the flow rate for any particular procedure. (See Boxes 4-2 and 4-3 for a summary of currently recommended flow rates and examples of flow rate calculations.) In many cases, the ultimate decision may be based on economic factors: low gas flow rates are more economical than high flow rates because less oxygen, nitrous oxide, and anesthetic are used. If the patient is small, the flow rate, even with a nonrebreathing system, is likely to be less than 1.5 L/min, and the cost of anesthetic and oxygen is relatively minor. Economic considerations are more important when considering whether to use a total or partial rebreathing system for a larger animal. Partial rebreathing systems use higher flow rates and, for this reason, are considerably more expensive than total rebreathing systems.

Safety Concerns with a Total Rebreathing System

Although total rebreathing systems are more economical than partial rebreathing systems, there are serious safety concerns that must be addressed when a total rebreathing system is used:

- *Carbon dioxide accumulation.* If the carbon dioxide absorber in a closed system is not operating efficiently, exhaled carbon dioxide will build up within the circuit. This is less likely to happen in a semiclosed, partial rebreathing system, in which some CO_2 is vented to the scavenger.
- *Increased pressure in the anesthetic circuit.* In a total rebreathing system, the volume of gas in the system may increase as fresh gas enters the circuit, particularly if the fresh gas flow exceeds the patient's uptake of oxygen and anesthetic and if the pop-off valve is closed. As a result, excessive pressure may build up in the circuit, making it difficult for the animal to exhale. In a partial rebreathing system, the pop-off valve is partly to fully open and excessive gas is vented.
- *Oxygen depletion and nitrous oxide accumulation.* In any anesthetic machine setup, oxygen is gradually depleted as the patient breathes the circulating gas. This is normally compensated by fresh oxygen entering the circuit. In a total rebreathing system, the oxygen flow rate is low and the amount of fresh oxygen added to the circuit may not entirely compensate for this loss. This is particularly serious if nitrous oxide is used in addition to oxygen, because the relative amount of nitrous oxide in the circuit may increase as the amount of oxygen decreases. As a result, the patient may breathe dangerously high levels of nitrous oxide gas. This effect is less likely to occur in a partial rebreathing system, in which nitrous oxide escapes through the pop-off valve and oxygen flow rates are higher. The use of a minimum of 30 ml/kg/min of oxygen in the presence of nitrous oxide prevents N_2O buildup, but this flow rate is not possible in a total rebreathing system. Total rebreathing (closed) systems therefore are not recommended if nitrous oxide is part of the anesthetic protocol, unless an oxygen monitor is used to measure inspired oxygen.

These disadvantages must be balanced against the economic advantages of a low-flow system (that is, less oxygen and anesthetic used) and the fact that little or

BOX 4-3 *Examples of Flow Rates*

1. Given a 5-kg cat and an anesthetic machine with a precision vaporizer, what type of circuit and flow rate would normally be used? Calculate the flow rates for oxygen alone and for oxygen and nitrous oxide used together (maintenance).

   Answer: Because the cat weighs less than 7 kg, a Bain or other nonrebreathing system is preferred. The flow rate recommended for the Bain system is 130 to 200 ml/kg/min. Thus the anesthetist could select 200 ml × 5 kg = 1000 ml or 1 L of gas flow per minute. If nitrous oxide is used for this animal, a 2:1 ratio of N_2O/O_2 should be provided. For a 1-L total flow of gas, this is equal to:
   Oxygen: One third of 1 L/min = 333 ml/min
   Nitrous oxide: Two thirds of 1 L/min = 667 ml/min

   If nitrous oxide is used, the anesthetist must ensure that the animal receives adequate oxygen (30 ml/kg/min). For this cat, the minimum is 30 ml of oxygen per minute × 5 kg × 150 ml of oxygen per minute. (Therefore 333 ml is safe.)

2. Given a 25-kg dog and a precision vaporizer, what type of circuit and flow rate would be preferred during the maintenance period?

   Answer: For economic reasons, the type of circuit used would probably be a circle system. If a total rebreathing system is used, the minimum oxygen flow rate is 15 ml × 25 kg/min, which is 375 ml/min. (For some vaporizers, this flow rate is too low and should be increased to a minimum of 500 ml/min.) If, as is more common, a partial rebreathing system is used, the flow rate should be 25 to 50 ml/kg/min. For this animal, the flow rate would therefore be 625 ml to 1.25 L of oxygen per minute. If the anesthetist wishes to increase the flow rate to achieve a nonrebreathing system, the flow rate would be calculated as 150 to 200 ml/kg/min, which is 3.75 to 5 L/min in this patient.

   The oxygen flow rate therefore can be set at a minimum of 400 to 500 ml/min and at a maximum of 5 L/min (if the pop-off valve is completely open and the animal is not rebreathing any expired gases). Many anesthetists would choose a flow rate midway between these two extremes, approximately 1 to 1.5 L/min.

3. Given a 15-kg dog anesthetized with a nonprecision methoxyflurane system, what would be the recommended flow rate during the maintenance period if:
   a. A semiclosed, partial rebreathing system is used?
   b. Minimal rebreathing is desired?

   Answer: If the dog is on a semiclosed system, the flow rate should be 25 to 50 ml/kg/min. For this animal, the flow rate therefore would be 375 to 750 ml/min. If minimal rebreathing is desired, the anesthetist should use a flow rate of 200 ml/kg/min, which is 3 L/min. However, because the vaporizer in this example is not compensated for flow rate, it would be inadvisable to use a flow rate over 2 L/min.

no waste anesthetic gas is produced when flow rates are low. Procedures used in the operation of a total rebreathing system are listed in Procedure 4-1.

In many situations (for example, where continuous monitoring of the patient and the anesthetic machine is not possible) the anesthetist may prefer to use a partial rather than a total rebreathing setup for the safety reasons just outlined. The anesthetist may choose to err on the side of wasting some gas by using higher gas flow rates rather than risk accumulation of carbon dioxide and depletion of oxygen within the circuit. Conversion from a total rebreathing system to a partial rebreathing system can be easily achieved by keeping the pop-off valve at least partially open (except when bagging the patient) and by maintaining a higher oxygen flow rate.

CARE AND USE OF ANESTHETIC EQUIPMENT
Daily Setup

Before use each day, the anesthetic machine should be assembled and thoroughly checked for problems. Procedure 4-2 is a checklist to be followed when setting up anesthetic equipment.

Ongoing Maintenance

As with any piece of equipment, the anesthetic machine requires periodic maintenance to ensure proper performance. A routine maintenance checklist includes the components listed in Procedure 4-1.

PROCEDURE 4-2   Setting Up Anesthetic Equipment

1. Assemble all needed supplies.
2. Inflate the endotracheal tube cuffs and record the amount of air required.
3. Check the laryngoscope light.
4. Draw up and label the injectable preanesthetic and anesthetic agents.
5. Warm IV fluids to be used.
6. Rotate the vaporizer dial to ensure smooth function. Turn to "off."
7. Check the amount of anesthetic in the vaporizer and replenish as necessary. Ensure that the vaporizer and flowmeter are off before filling the vaporizer.
8. Check that the gas cylinders are correctly mounted in the yokes, then turn on the gas cylinders using a cylinder wrench or similar device. Tanks should be opened slowly and turned to full open position for use. The oxygen tank should be changed if the tank pressure gauge indicates a pressure less than 100 psi (680 kPa). A cutoff of 200 psi (1360 kPa) is advisable if a long anesthesia is planned or if high flow rates are to be used. A nitrous oxide tank should be changed if nitrous oxide pressure is less than 500 psi (3400 kPa).
9. With the oxygen tank open, check the flowmeter controls to ensure proper function.
10. Assemble the appropriate circuit (nonrebreathing circuit or hoses and Y piece) and connect to the machine. The gas flow should be mentally traced from the tank to the patient and back to the machine and scavenger to ensure that connections are correctly assembled.
11. Connect the pop-off valve to the scavenger and turn on the scavenger.
12. Attach the reservoir bag to the machine or nonrebreathing circuit.
13. Change the carbon dioxide absorber canister contents if necessary. This procedure is best done immediately after machine use, when color changes are most evident.
14. Test the machine for leaks (see Chapter 5).

Oxygen and nitrous oxide tanks

After use, the outlet valve of each tank should be closed by turning it clockwise (that is, to the right). Failure to turn off the gas valve will result in excessive pressure on the regulator and, in some cases, leakage of gas from the tank.

Oxygen pressure remaining in the machine after closure of the tank (line pressure) should be removed with the oxygen flush valve or by turning the flowmeter to a high rate of flow. Failure to evacuate line pressure may damage the tank pressure gauge and pressure-reducing valve.

Petroleum or petroleum distillate products (for example, grease and gasoline) should not be used on oxygen tanks or their connections. An explosion may occur when the tank is opened and these materials contact oxygen released from the tank. Silicon or Teflon-based lubricants are generally safe for use.

Flowmeter

The dial of each flowmeter should be returned to the off position (full clockwise) for storage. Failure to do so may result in a sudden rush of air into the flowmeter when the oxygen tank is opened, which may jam the float or ball at the top of the flowmeter tube. Care should be taken not to overtighten the flowmeter knob when turning the flowmeter off.

Flowmeter accuracy can be assessed easily by setting the flow at, for example, 2 L/min and ensuring that a 2-L bag connected to the machine fills in approximately 1 minute.

Vaporizer

Before an anesthetic procedure is initiated, it is a good idea to fill the vaporizer with anesthetic if the anesthetic level is half full or less, (unless the planned procedure is very short). A keyed filling device should be used for this purpose. Vaporizers should be turned off when the machine is not in use. The vaporizer should always be set to "off" before being filled with a liquid anesthetic.

Precision vaporizers designed for halothane or methoxyflurane should be emptied of anesthetic every 6 to 12 months to help remove the buildup of preservative within the vaporizer. Isoflurane is supplied without a preservative, and periodic emptying is not usually necessary.

Despite periodic emptying, a halothane precision vaporizer may eventually become clogged with preservative and other residue. When this occurs, the anesthetic levels produced by the vaporizer will not correlate with the percentage indicated by the dial, the dial movement may become sticky, and the anesthetic in the vaporizer may turn brown. The anesthetist may become aware of the problem when patients can no longer be maintained at a satisfactory anesthetic depth even at high vaporizer settings. Halothane precision vaporizers should be cleaned and recalibrated by the manufacturer or other qualified personnel every 2 to 3 years to prevent this problem. It may be necessary to remove the vaporizer from the anesthetic machine and send it away for servicing. Many companies provide a "loaner" replacement during the servicing period. Vaporizers for isoflurane or sevoflurane do not accumulate preservative residue, but cleaning, wick change, and recalibration is advisable every 2 to 3 years, depending on frequency of use.

Carbon dioxide absorber canister

Barium hydroxide lime or soda lime granules should be checked after each anesthetic procedure. Granules that change color or that cannot be crushed with finger pressure should be replaced. Because the granules contain corrosive chemicals (NaOH and KOH), they should not be handled with bare hands, and chemical-resistant gloves should be used for this purpose. Care should be taken to avoid inhalation of dust when the granules are removed or replenished. Use of a ventilation fan or breathing protection (a mask or respirator) may be necessary when pouring new granules into the canister.

When the granules are replaced, they should not be tightly packed. At least 1 cm (one half inch) of air space should be left between the granules and the top of the canister to allow unimpeded airflow out of the canister. Gentle shaking of the canister during and after filling helps prevent channels from forming in the granules, which could reduce the efficiency of the absorber. The canister should be periodically checked for worn gaskets and improper seals.

When replenishing soda lime or barium hydroxide lime granules, the technician must ensure that dust does not enter the tubing or hoses of the machine, because it may be inhaled by the patient and is corrosive to mucous membranes. Also, water may collect in the trap below the CO_2 canister and should be periodically removed.

Cleaning machine parts

Flutter valves require periodic removal and cleaning with a disinfectant to prevent a buildup of water vapor, mucus, dust from the soda lime or barium hydroxide lime, and other material. Access to the valves is obtained by unscrewing the plastic caps that lie over the valves. Valves that are not cleaned may become sticky and adhere to the machine housing, impeding airflow through the circuit. After cleaning these valves (or any part of the machine or circuit, for that matter), the anesthetist must make certain that they are working properly.

After each anesthetic procedure, removable machine parts (such as the hoses, Y piece, Bain circuit or other nonrebreathing system, and the reservoir bag) should be washed in a mild soapy solution and thoroughly rinsed with water. A surgical scrub brush or bottle brush is useful in cleaning equipment surfaces. After cleaning, the equipment should be air dried. Other machine parts (such as the compressed air tanks, pop-off valve, and CO_2 canister) should be wiped with a disinfectant solution on a weekly basis.

Disinfecting anesthetic equipment

Some anesthetic equipment components will require more thorough disinfection. This is particularly true of equipment that contacts the patient's airway or oral cavity, including the endotracheal tube, laryngoscope blade, esophageal stethoscope, and face mask. If the equipment is used on a patient harboring certain viruses or bacteria (including feline upper respiratory viruses, *Bordetella*, and other respiratory pathogens), infection may be transmitted to the next patient. Laryngoscope blades should be cleaned with alcohol or benzalkonium chloride and air dried to prevent disease transmission between patients. The batteries and bulb should be replaced as necessary.

Cleaning endotracheal tubes

Gauze, adhesive tape, and the adapter should be removed from endotracheal tubes before cleaning and disinfection. Unfortunately, there is no ideal agent for disinfection of endotracheal tubes. Chlorhexidine is relatively harmless to tissues but is not effective against all microorganisms and spores. Glutaraldehyde solutions (2%) are effective against many microorganisms but are stable for only 2 to 4 weeks and must be periodically replaced. Ethylene oxide is an effective sterilizing agent but requires special equipment for safe use. Both glutaraldehyde and ethylene oxide are potentially toxic and may cause severe tissue injury to hospital personnel and to the patient if the anesthetic equipment or supplies are not properly handled. Personnel who work with these chemicals must have special training in their safe use.

All items exposed to any chemical solution should be thoroughly rinsed with water after cleaning and dried before use. Some chemicals may be absorbed by rubber, and if they are not completely removed by rinsing, they may cause burns when in contact with the patient's airway or skin. Ethylene oxide is particularly well absorbed by materials being sterilized, and endotracheal tubes exposed to this substance or glutaraldehyde have been known to cause tracheal necrosis.

After prolonged use rubber items deteriorate and must be replaced. Autoclaving causes rubber surfaces to become brittle and crack. Prolonged exposure to disinfectants or rubber-soluble anesthetics (such as methoxyflurane) may also cause rubber surfaces to deteriorate. Endotracheal tubes, masks, and reservoir bags should be periodically checked for wear and discarded if necessary. Endotracheal tubes with leaking or nonfunctional cuffs should also be discarded.

KEY POINTS

1. Many different types and sizes of endotracheal tubes are available for use in veterinary patients.
2. The anesthetic machine delivers volatile gas anesthetic and carrier gases (oxygen with or without nitrous oxide) to the patient and moves exhaled gases away from the patient. If gases are recirculated, the machine removes carbon dioxide from them before returning them to the patient.
3. Anesthetic machines can be used as a source of oxygen in emergencies.
4. Compressed oxygen cylinders contain oxygen gas under high pressure (up to 2200 psi or 15,000 kPa). Various sizes of oxygen cylinders are available; these may be freestanding or attach to the anesthesia machine but are always color coded. Large cylinders contain more oxygen and function for a longer time than small cylinders. For all oxygen cylinders, tank pressure is gradually reduced as the cylinder empties. Oxygen cylinders should be changed when the pressure reaches 100 to 200 psi.
5. Nitrous oxide cylinders are blue and contain nitrous oxide gas and liquid at a pressure of up to 760 psi (5100 kPa). As the tank empties, tank pressure is maintained until most of the nitrous oxide is gone. Therefore tanks should be changed when the pressure starts to drop below 500 psi.
6. The pressure reducing valve allows a constant flow of gas to enter the machine and provides a safe operating pressure (50 psi) for the machine.

KEY POINTS—cont'd

7. For each type of carrier gas, the flow rate is set by its respective flowmeter. Flows are generally expressed in liters per minute. The flow rate indicates to the anesthetist how much gas is being delivered to the patient at any given time. When using nitrous oxide, the anesthetist should set a nitrous oxide/oxygen ratio of 2:1.

8. Liquid anesthetic is vaporized and added to the carrier gas in the vaporizer. The combination of anesthetic vapor, oxygen, and nitrous oxide (if present) is called *fresh gas*.

9. Vaporizers may be precision or nonprecision, based on their construction. Precision vaporizers are commonly used for anesthetics with high vapor pressures and provide compensation for variations in temperature, gas flow rate, and back pressure. Precision vaporizers are found outside of the anesthetic circuit (VOC), whereas nonprecision vaporizers are found inside the anesthetic circuit (VIC).

10. The reservoir bag (rebreathing bag) can be used to monitor the animal's ventilation and to deliver oxygen (with or without anesthetic) to the patient by a process called *bagging*.

11. Inhalation and exhalation unidirectional valves allow one-way flow of gas through the breathing circuit.

12. Waste gas exits the machine at the pop-off valve, which should be connected to a scavenger.

13. Carbon dioxide is removed from the circuit by an absorber canister containing granules. Most types of granules exhibit a color change when they have become saturated with CO_2 and require replacement.

14. The pressure manometer measures the pressure of gases within the anesthetic circuit.

15. Anesthetic circuits may be classified as rebreathing (either closed or semiclosed) or nonrebreathing. Rebreathing systems use lower oxygen flow rates but must provide for carbon dioxide absorption. Nonrebreathing systems, such as the Bain system, require relatively high flow rates and are commonly used in small patients.

16. Carrier gas flow rates vary with the period of anesthesia and type of anesthetic circuit used (that is, rebreathing or nonrebreathing). High flow rates are used during induction and recovery for all systems and also during the maintenance period of anesthesia if a nonrebreathing system is used.

17. Anesthetic equipment requires routine cleaning, inspection, and maintenance.

REVIEW QUESTIONS

1. When the oxygen tank is half full, the tank pressure gauge will read approximately:
   a. 1100 psi
   b. 2000 psi
   c. 500 psi
   d. 2200 psi
   e. None of the above

2. The pressure gauge of a nitrous oxide tank will read _____ psi when the tank is full.
   a. 2200
   b. 1100
   c. 900
   d. 500
   e. 760

3. When the nitrous oxide tank is half full, the pressure gauge will read

   _____ psi.
   a. 760
   b. 350
   c. 100
   d. 500

4. Nitrous oxide is present in the tank as a _____ .
   a. Liquid
   b. Gas
   c. Liquid and a gas

5. The amount of oxygen an animal is receiving is indicated by the:
   a. Oxygen tank pressure gauge
   b. Flowmeter
   c. Pressure manometer
   d. Vaporizer setting

6. Flowmeters that have a ball for reading the gauge should be read from the

   _____ of the ball.
   a. Top
   b. Bottom
   c. Middle

7. The most commonly recommended ratio for nitrous oxide and oxygen flow rates is :
   a. 50% oxygen and 50% nitrous oxide
   b. 80% oxygen and 20% nitrous oxide
   c. 23% oxygen and 77% nitrous oxide
   d. 77% oxygen and 23% nitrous oxide
   e. 33% oxygen and 67% nitrous oxide

8. The minimum size for the reservoir bag can be calculated as _____.
   a. 20 ml/kg
   b. 60 ml/kg
   c. 80 ml/kg
   d. 100 ml/kg

9. The flutter valves on an anesthetic machine help _____.
   a. Control the direction of movement of gases
   b. Maintain a full reservoir bag
   c. Remove carbon dioxide
   d. Vaporize the liquid anesthetic

10. The pop-off valve is part of the anesthetic machine and helps:
    a. Vaporize the liquid anesthetic
    b. Prevent excess gas pressure from building up within the breathing circuit
    c. Keep the oxygen flowing in one direction only
    d. Prevent waste gases from reentering the vaporizer

11. In small animal anesthesia, when the pressure manometer reading exceeds

    _____ cm of water pressure, it indicates there is a buildup of
    pressure within the circuit that could be dangerous.
    a. 5
    b. 10
    c. 15
    d. 20

12. Rebreathing systems are best reserved for animals over 7 kg.
    True   False

13. Rebreathing is determined primarily by the:
    a. Fresh gas flow
    b. Type of anesthetic
    c. Presence of a reservoir bag
    d. Open or shut pop-off valve

14. Nonrebreathing systems should have maintenance flow rates that are:
    a. Very high (130 ml/kg/min)
    b. Very low (10 ml/kg/min)
    c. Moderate (50 ml/kg/min)

15. The negative pressure relief valve is particularly useful when:
    a. Nitrous oxide is being used.
    b. There is no scavenging system.
    c. There is a failure of oxygen flow through the system.
    d. The carbon dioxide absorber is no longer functioning.

16. The tidal volume of an animal is considered to be _____ ml/kg of
    body weight.
    a. 5-10
    b. 10-15
    c. 15-20
    d. 20-25

For the following questions, more than one answer may be correct.

17. A reservoir bag that is not moving may indicate:
    a. The endotracheal tube is not in the trachea.
    b. The animal has a decreased tidal volume.
    c. There is a leak around the endotracheal tube.
    d. The vaporizer is empty.
18. The anesthetist will know when the granules in the carbon dioxide absorber have been depleted because the:
    a. Anesthetist will smell waste carbon dioxide
    b. Granules will be brittle
    c. Granules may change color
    d. Granules may be hard
19. An increase in the depth of anesthesia can be achieved quickly by:
    a. Having high oxygen flow rates
    b. Having high vaporizer settings
    c. Using a closed anesthetic system
    d. Bagging the animal with the precision vaporizer at a higher setting
20. The concentration of anesthetic delivered from a nonprecision vaporizer may depend on the:
    a. Temperature of the liquid anesthetic
    b. Flow of the carrier gas through the vaporizer
    c. Back pressure
    d. Type of anesthetic in the vaporizer
21. The advantages of a nonprecision vaporizer include:
    a. It is economical to buy
    b. It can be readily used with all anesthetics
    c. It is easy to clean and service
    d. It can be used out of circuit
22. Low-flow anesthesia means:
    a. Using oxygen flows of 25 to 50 ml/kg/min
    b. Using flows that only meet the metabolic requirements of the animal on oxygen
    c. Using flows that allow accurate measurement of halothane or isoflurane output
    d. Using flows that allow you to open the pop-off valve
23. The disadvantages of low-flow anesthesia include:
    a. Production of excess waste anesthetic gas
    b. It may allow carbon dioxide to accumulate in the circuit.
    c. It results in the use of more anesthetic in the maintenance period.
    d. It is difficult to use with nitrous oxide.
24. Using special techniques, nonprecision vaporizers can be used for:
    a. Low-flow anesthesia
    b. Delivery of nitrous oxide
    c. Elimination of carbon dioxide from the circuit
    d. Delivery of isoflurane

ANSWERS FOR CHAPTER 4

1. a	**2.** e	**3.** a	**4.** c	**5.** b
6. c	**7.** e	**8.** b	**9.** a	**10.** b
11. c	**12.** True	**13.** a	**14.** a	**15.** c
16. b	**17.** a, b, c	**18.** b, c, d	**19.** a, b, d	**20.** a, b, c, d
21. a, c	**22.** b	**23.** b, d	**24.** a, d	

Selected Readings

Bednarski RM, Gaynor JS, Muir WW III: Vaporizer in circle for delivery of isoflurane to dogs, *J Am Vet Med Assoc* 202(6):943-948, 1993.

Bednarski RM: Use of in-circle vaporizers to deliver isoflurane, *Compendium* 17:1377-1382, 1995.

Dyson DH: Influence of oxygen flows during anesthetic management, *Can Vet J* 32:752-754, 1991.

Hartsfield SM: Equipment for inhalation anesthesia, *Vet Clin North Am Small Anim Pract* 29(3):645-663, 1999.

Haskins SC: Opinions in small animal anesthesia, *Vet Clin North Am Small Anim Pract* 22(2):326-469, 1992.

Heavener JE, Flinders C, McMahon D, et al: *Technical manual of anesthesia*, New York, 1989, Raven Press.

Ludders JW, Stafford KL: Basic equipment for small animal anesthesia: use and maintenance, part II, *Compendium* 12(1):35-40, 1991.

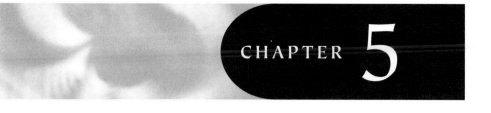

CHAPTER 5

Workplace Safety

PERFORMANCE OBJECTIVES

After completion of this chapter, the reader will be able to:
- Describe both the short-term and long-term effects of waste anesthetic gas on persons working in health care environments.
- Recognize ways in which the release of waste anesthetic gases may be minimized.
- Describe proper procedures for handling and transporting compressed gas cylinders.
- Outline the precautions necessary when handling potentially hazardous injectable agents.

V eterinary technicians may participate in the anesthetic management of several thousand animals during the course of their career. It is therefore essential that the technician be familiar with the human safety considerations involved in veterinary anesthesia. These can be divided into three categories: (1) hazards of waste anesthetic gas, (2) safety considerations for handling compressed gas cylinders, and (3) hazards associated with potent injectable agents.

This chapter outlines the precautions that the anesthetist can take to reduce, as much as possible, the health risks of working with anesthetic equipment, injectable drugs, and compressed gases.

HAZARDS OF WASTE ANESTHETIC GAS

Concerns have been raised regarding the possible adverse effects resulting from exposure of hospital personnel to waste anesthetic gas and vapors. The term *waste anesthetic gas* refers to nitrous oxide, halothane, isoflurane, and other volatile anesthetic vapors that are breathed out by the patient or that escape from the anesthetic machine. These vapors are breathed inadvertently by all personnel working in areas where animals are anesthetized or are recovering from inhalation anesthesia. Significant exposure to anesthetic vapors can also occur when emptying or filling anesthetic vaporizers. In addition, short-term exposure to high levels of anesthetic vapors can occur because of an accidental spill of liquid anesthetic.

Since the first study of waste anesthetic gas was published in 1967, many investigators have attempted to determine the toxicity of halothane, methoxyflurane, nitrous oxide, and other anesthetic agents to operating room personnel. Although some of the evidence is contradictory, it is suspected that exposure to high levels of waste anesthetic gas is associated with a higher than normal incidence of some health problems. The suspected health hazards can be divided into two categories: (1) short-term problems that occur during or immediately after exposure to these agents and (2) long-term problems that may become evident days, weeks, or years after exposure.

Short-Term Effects

The short-term problems associated with breathing waste gas appear to arise from a direct effect of anesthetic molecules on brain neurons. Persons working in environments with a high level of waste gas have reported symptoms such as fatigue, headache, drowsiness, nausea, depression, and irritability. Although these symptoms usually resolve spontaneously when the affected person leaves the area, the frequent occurrence of these symptoms may indicate that excessive levels of waste gas are present and that a potential for long-term toxicity exists.

Long-Term Effects

Long-term inhalation of air polluted with waste gas may be associated with serious health problems, including reproductive disorders, liver and kidney damage, bone marrow abnormalities, and chronic nervous system dysfunction. Evidence suggests that the risk of these disorders developing is not high in normal practice settings. The mechanism of long-term anesthetic gas toxicity is not fully understood but is thought to be the result of toxic metabolites produced by the breakdown of anesthetic gases within the liver and their subsequent excretion by the kidneys. These metabolites include inorganic fluoride or bromide ions, oxalic acid, and free radicals, all of which are known to have harmful effects on animal tissues.

It is widely accepted that anesthetic agents that are retained by the body and metabolized will have greater long-term toxicity than those that are quickly eliminated through the lungs. For this reason, isoflurane is thought to be the least toxic inhalation agent in common use (0.2% of the amount inhaled is retained and metabolized), followed by sevoflurane (3% is retained and metabolized). In contrast, approximately 20% of the halothane and 50% of the methoxyflurane administered to a patient are retained within the patient's body fat, to be metabolized in the liver and excreted through the kidneys. Although the patient may appear completely recovered from anesthesia induced by these agents, this appearance indicates only that the level of anesthetic in the brain is low. Significant amounts of anesthetic may linger in the liver, kidney, and body fat stores. Metabolites of halothane have been recovered from the urine of patients as long as 20 days after anesthesia. Human patients who inhale 50% nitrous oxide for 1 hour have been shown to have more than 100 parts per million (ppm) nitrous oxide in their expired breath for the next 3 hours. In the same way, the anesthetist who inhales waste anesthetic gas may retain the gas or its metabolites for a considerable period. For example, anesthetists may show traces of halothane in their breath 64 hours after administering this gas to a patient.

Although it is generally accepted that isoflurane is safer for staff than other halogenated anesthetics, safety concerns (including NIOSH recommendations and OSHA regulations), apply to all anesthetics.*

---

*OSHA, the United States Occupational Safety and Health Administration, is the government body that enforces safety and health regulations in the workplace. NIOSH, the National Institute for Occupational Safety and Health, conducts research into the prevention of work-related illness and injury and publishes recommendations on safety procedures.

Effects on reproduction

There is some evidence that high concentrations of waste anesthetic gas can adversely affect the reproductive system. In a comprehensive survey of nurse and physician anesthetists, the American Society of Anesthesiologists found that the risk of spontaneous abortion in this group was 1.3 to 2 times that of the normal population. Another study showed that the frequency of spontaneous abortion among working hospital anesthetists (18.2%) was higher than that observed among nonworking anesthetists (13.7%) and a control group (14.7%). The same study showed that 12% of the working anesthetists interviewed were infertile, compared with 6% of the control group.

Exposure to anesthetic gases also has been linked to an increase in congenital abnormalities in the children of pregnant operating room personnel. One study reported a 16% incidence of congenital abnormalities in children of practicing nurse-anesthetists, compared with a 6% incidence in a control group. Other studies have failed to show a statistically significant correlation between waste gas exposure and an increased incidence of congenital abnormalities.

Interpreting or comparing the results obtained by these and other studies is difficult because there are wide variations in the types of anesthetics used, in the amounts of waste gas exposure, and in the availability of control measures (such as scavengers). In most cases, operating room personnel were exposed to several agents simultaneously, and it is difficult to determine which agent or combination of agents was responsible for the adverse effects. It appears, however, that nitrous oxide is a potential reproductive hazard, because rats exposed to high levels of nitrous oxide had abnormalities in sperm morphology, reduced ovulation, fetal resorption, and abnormal fetal development.

A recent report (Hoerauf, 1999) suggests that exposure to even trace levels of waste anesthetic gas could cause genetic damage, as indicated by an increased incidence of sister chromatid exchanges. However, the study group was small, and other recent studies have so far failed to confirm these findings.

Oncogenic effects

Given that waste anesthetic gases may exert their adverse reproductive effects by altering DNA, investigators have attempted to determine whether these agents have the potential to cause other DNA-related changes, such as neoplasia. Several studies undertaken in the 1970s appeared to suggest that operating room personnel have an increased incidence of some types of cancer. These studies, however, have been criticized for inappropriate data collection and statistical analysis, and it is now generally thought that none of the commonly used anesthetic agents is carcinogenic at the levels found in veterinary hospitals.

Effects on the liver

In several studies researchers have investigated the incidence of liver disorders in personnel exposed to waste anesthetic gas. Halothane, in particular, is recognized as being potentially hepatotoxic. Metabolism of halothane in certain rare anesthetized individuals produces toxic by-products that may result in massive hepatic necrosis, termed *halothane hepatitis*.

The possible adverse effects of waste anesthetic gas on the liver were suggested by a study showing that the risk of liver disease in hospital operating room personnel is 1.5 times that of the general population. However, it is difficult to say with certainty whether the increased incidence of liver disease is associated with exposure to waste anesthetic gas or the result of other occupational hazards, such as viral hepatitis.

Effects on the kidney

It is well established that methoxyflurane has the potential to cause renal toxicity in human beings anesthetized with this agent, but the risk to operating room personnel has been more difficult to assess. Studies have indicated that there is a 1.2- to 1.4-fold increase in renal disease in female operating room personnel and a 1.2- to 1.7-fold increase in renal disease in female dental assistants compared with the general population. It has not been determined whether this increase is the result of the effect of methoxyflurane, nitrous oxide, other anesthetic agents, or other occupational factors working alone or in combination.

Neurologic effects

Because the mechanism of action of anesthetic agents involves their effect on neurons, various studies have investigated the effect of waste anesthetic gas on the central nervous system. It has been suggested that exposure to high levels of anesthetics produces a decline in performance of motor skills and short-term memory. However, the threshold at which they begin to affect performance has not been established.

Some studies have indicated that exposure to even low concentrations of anesthetic gas mixtures (for example, nitrous oxide 500 ppm and halothane 15 ppm) results in decreased cognitive and motor skills. Chronic exposure to nitrous oxide has been associated with increased risk of neurologic disease: a study of female dental assistants exposed to high levels of nitrous oxide showed them to have a 1.7- to 2.8-fold increase in the incidence of neurologic disease compared with the normal population. Dentists and dental assistants exposed to high levels of waste nitrous oxide reported muscle weakness, tingling sensations, and numbness.

Hematologic effects

In one study, exposure to high levels of waste nitrous oxide has been associated with bone marrow abnormalities in dentists who administer this gas.

Assessment of Risk

Despite the alarming list of potential health hazards, the average veterinary technician working in a veterinary clinic is not necessarily at high risk. It is difficult to determine a clear-cut assessment of risk for several reasons, including the following:

- Caution must be used in interpreting the epidemiologic evidence provided by these studies. The evidence produced by various studies (or within one study) is sometimes contradictory. For example, some studies have failed to show any association between the incidence of spontaneous abortion or congenital abnormalities and a history of exposure to waste gas, whereas other studies suggest the opposite.
- Although many epidemiologic studies indicate an increased incidence of health problems in persons working in an environment where exposure to waste gas

occurs, it does not necessarily follow that the anesthetic gases themselves are the causative agents. Other chemicals or other factors present in the operating room or dentist's office may contribute to increased incidence of health disorders.

- Many of the early studies have been faulted for low response rates, lack of verification of reported outcomes, and the possibility of bias. Some commentators have observed that the increased risks observed are small and could be due to uncontrolled variables.
- Most studies of the adverse effects of waste anesthetic gases do not measure the level of waste gas present in the working environment. Epidemiologic studies do not give information about the use of scavengers and procedures that reduce waste gas pollution. Without this information, interpretation of the studies is difficult.

The American Society of Anesthesiologists Task Force on Trace Anesthetic Gases (1999) suggests that although adverse health effects are associated with chronic exposure to high levels of waste anesthetic gas, studies have failed to demonstrate an association between trace levels of waste anesthetic gas (such as are found in scavenged hospitals) and adverse effects to hospital employees. The Task Force concluded that even at the maximum allowable dose of isoflurane, halothane, or nitrous oxide, there was no evidence of significant damage to the gonads, liver, kidney, or other organs, even in long-term studies. There are no data to suggest that waste anesthetic gases are a danger to hospital employees (including pregnant women) working in a scavenged environment.

Most authorities and regulatory agencies agree that exposure to high levels of waste anesthetic gas should be avoided and that controls should be introduced to reduce exposure. After reviewing the available literature, NIOSH recommended that the concentration of halothane, methoxyflurane, or isoflurane not exceed 2 ppm when used alone and not exceed 0.5 ppm when used with nitrous oxide. (The concentration at which the odor of halothane can be detected by the average person is 33 ppm or more, which is much higher than the maximum recommended level.) It is also suggested the nitrous oxide concentration not exceed 25 ppm. These levels were chosen because they were thought to be the lowest levels realistically achievable given current technology. The British Government Health Service Advisory Committee (1991) recommends a maximum of 100 ppm nitrous oxide, 50 ppm isoflurane, and 10 ppm halothane (maximum average reading over an 8-hour period).

Surveys of human and veterinary hospitals reveal a wide variation in the levels of waste anesthetic gas present in different locations within the clinic (Tables 5-1 and 5-2). The halothane concentration in the air of unscavenged surgery suites in human hospitals has been reported to be as high as 85 ppm, and concentrations of nitrous oxide have been measured as high as 7000 ppm. Veterinary hospitals using scavengers usually have isoflurane or halothane levels between 1 and 20 ppm and nitrous oxide levels between 50 and 200 ppm. As expected, air samples taken from surgery suites, surgical preparation rooms, and anesthetic recovery rooms are more likely to contain waste gas than samples taken elsewhere in the clinic. During the anesthetic period itself, the level of waste gas is highest immediately adjacent to the anesthetic machine, but the actual level varies with the duration of anesthesia, the flow rate of the carrier gas, the type of anesthetic system used (rebreathing or non-rebreathing), and most important, the use of an effective scavenging system.

TABLE 5-1	

Waste Anesthetic Gas (Halothane) Concentrations in Various Locations Within the Veterinary Hospital (Semiclosed Circuit, 1 L/Minute Oxygen Flow)

SAMPLING SITE	LEVEL OF CONTAMINATION (ppm)
PERSONNEL BREATHING ZONE	
With scavenging	1.45
No scavenging	2.00
Nose and mouth of patient just removed from anesthetic chamber	10.00
Air around unscavenged anesthetic chamber nose and mouth of anesthetized patient	10.00
Intubated, cuff inflated	3.25
Intubated, cuff not inflated	6.10
Air outside recovery cage door	1.07
Nose of patient in recovery cage	5.43

Modified from Short CE, Harvey RC: Anesthetic waste gases in veterinary medicine, *Cornell Vet* 73(4):363-374, 1983.

Reducing Exposure to Waste Anesthetic Gas

Given the potential health hazards associated with exposure to waste anesthetic gas, it is in the technician's best interest to minimize exposure as much as possible. The American College of Veterinary Anesthesiologists recommends that any veterinary facility using inhalant anesthetics should institute and maintain a control program for waste anesthetic gases, given the possibility that trace gases may adversely affect human health.

If proper equipment, techniques, and procedures are used, it is possible to reduce waste gas exposure to a level well below the NIOSH standards. This can be achieved through several means, including using a gas scavenging system, testing equipment for leaks, and using techniques and procedures that minimize exposure to waste gas.

TABLE 5-2	

Sources of Anesthetic Gas Contamination

TECHNIQUE OR SITUATION	LEVEL OF CONTAMINATION (ppm)
Room air when filling vaporizer	10
Reservoir bag emptied into room air	2.5- >10
Room air after spill of agent	10
Hands of personnel filling vaporizer	2.5- >10
Hands after washing	0
Clothing of personnel filling vaporizer	5.0-8.75
Residues in unwashed rubber components	1.8- >10

Modified from Short CE, Harvey RC: Anesthetic waste gases in veterinary medicine, *Cornell Vet* 73(4):363-374, 1983.

Use of a scavenging system

The installation and use of an effective gas scavenging system are the most important steps in reducing waste gas exposure. A 1982 survey of veterinary hospitals showed that scavenging reduces waste halothane concentrations by 64% to 94%. A scavenger consists of tubing attached to the anesthetic machine pop-off valve (or in the case of a nonrebreathing system, to the outlet port or tail of the reservoir bag). The function of a scavenger is to collect waste gas from the machine and conduct it to a disposal point outside the building.

From the regulatory perspective, OSHA's Hazard Chemical Standard (1910.1200) requires the employer to install adequate engineering controls to ensure that occupational exposure to any chemical never exceeds the permissible exposure limit. This is difficult or impossible to achieve in a veterinary clinic unless a waste anesthetic gas scavenger or activated charcoal canister is used. Scavenging should be used in every room where inhaled anesthetic gases are administered. Scavenging should include the exhaust not only from the anesthetic machine but also from ancillary equipment such as ventilators, anesthetic chambers, and capnometers.

Ideally, scavenging systems should be professionally installed when the veterinary clinic is built. However, it is not difficult to assemble and install an effective scavenging system in an established veterinary hospital. Scavenger parts may be purchased or can be readily assembled with simple materials. The hose or tubing of the scavenger may be constructed from plastic tubing, polyvinyl chloride (PVC) pipe, or other gas-impermeable material. Most modern anesthetic machines have fittings that allow easy connection to a scavenging system. Older machines can be retrofitted with adapters that can be connected to a scavenger hose. The international standard for scavenger system attachments for anesthetic machines is 30 mm.

Scavenging systems may be passive or active (Figs. 5-1 and 5-2). An active system uses suction created by a vacuum pump or fan to draw gas into the scavenger, whereas a passive system uses the positive pressure of the gas in the anesthetic machine to push gas into the scavenger. Although both active and passive scavenging systems appear to be effective when correctly assembled and operated, the most efficient system appears to be an active one with a dedicated vacuum pump. However, active scavenging systems are more costly than passive systems, they require more maintenance, and the operator must remember to turn on the system each day.

The most commonly used type of passive system discharges waste gas to the outdoors through a hole in the wall. This system is best suited for rooms adjacent to the exterior of the building and is ineffective for interior rooms where the distance to the outlet is more than 20 feet (7 m).

Another type of passive system can be set up by placing the end of the transfer hose adjacent to the room ventilation exhaust or nonrecirculating air conditioning system. This is acceptable provided the air is not recirculated within the building and the transfer hose is no more than 10 feet in length. Because anesthetic vapors are heavier than room air, the transfer hose should travel a downward course toward the exhaust. The waste gas must be discharged outdoors: passive systems that simply vent gases to the floor level are ineffective.

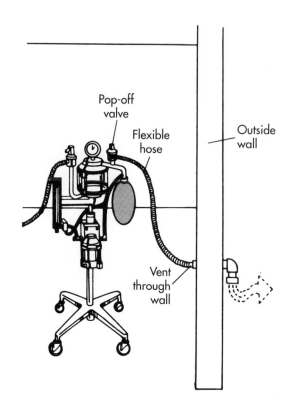

FIG. 5-1   Passive scavenging system.

Once the waste gas is collected by an active or passive system, it must be expelled outside of the building, away from doors, windows, and air intakes. Waste gas collected in the tubing should be totally confined within the scavenger hose from the pop-off valve to the point of discharge and must not be recirculated into the building air. Scavenger hoses that end discharge gas on the floor of the surgery room or into an attic or a basement, or that conduct the waste gas into a recirculating central vacuum system or recirculating ventilation exhaust, merely contaminate all building rooms with the waste gas.

Normally, use of a scavenging system with an anesthetic machine does not alter the operation of the machine. The anesthetist should, however, be aware of two potential difficulties that can occur when a scavenging system is present:

1. When an active scavenging system is used, the anesthetist should prevent the negative pressure (vacuum) from the scavenger from being excessively applied to the breathing circuit. If this is allowed to occur, the reservoir bag will collapse. Many machines are equipped with a negative pressure relief valve, adjacent to the pop-off valve, which opens automatically if negative pressure is detected in the circuit. The open valve admits room air to the circuit, thereby ensuring that a vacuum does not develop. When a machine that is not equipped with a negative pressure relief valve is used, the anesthetist should ensure that the reservoir bag is at least partially inflated with air or oxygen at all times.

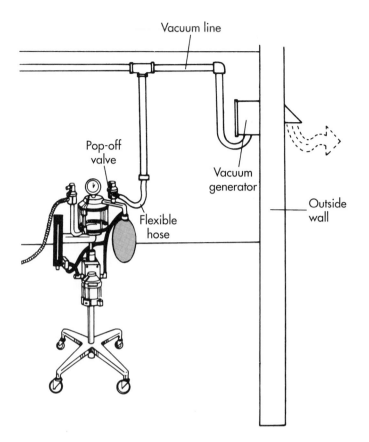

FIG. 5-2   Active scavenging system.

2. If either a passive or active scavenging system is in use, the anesthetist must
   be aware that an obstruction may occur and block waste gas entry into the
   system. If this happens, gas will accumulate within the anesthetic circuit. This
   situation is analogous to operating a machine with a closed pop-off valve and
   may result in excessive pressure developing within the circuit and the patient's
   lungs. To avoid this, many machines have scavenger interfaces that are equipped
   with a positive pressure relief valve that opens automatically if excessive
   pressure builds up within the circuit.

Regardless of whether an active or passive system is used, the anesthetist must
be able to connect an anesthetic machine or anesthetic chamber to a scavenger in
every room in which the machines are used. It is sometimes impractical to use a
scavenger when it is in a specialized room such as the x-ray room or when a mobile
anesthetic machine is used. In these situations, either anesthesia can be maintained
with an injectable agent, or an anesthetic machine with an activated charcoal cartridge
can be used (for example, f/air canister, A.M. Bickford, Inc.). These cartridges can
effectively absorb anesthetic vapors. To be effective, however, these cartridges must
be replaced after 12 hours of use or after a weight gain of 50 g. Additional
drawbacks of these units are their inability to absorb nitrous oxide and their relative
inefficiency at flow rates greater than 2 L/min.

For additional protection, masks with activated charcoal filters can be worn by personnel who are at special risk (such as pregnant workers). Like the activated charcoal canister for anesthetic machines, these are not effective in filtering out nitrous oxide vapors; however, organic vapor cartridges effectively absorb isoflurane, sevoflurane, halothane, and other anesthetic gases and vapors. Masks with cartridges designed for particulate matter do not absorb anesthetic vapors and should not be used.

Equipment leak testing

Although the installation of a scavenging device is the most important step in reducing anesthetic gas pollution, there are many other procedures and techniques that significantly reduce the anesthetist's risk of exposure. One of these is leak testing of anesthetic machines. Gas leaks from anesthetic machines are a significant source of operating room pollution and are not reduced by a scavenging system. Leakage may occur from any part of the machine in which nitrous oxide or gas anesthetic is present. The most common problems that can result in waste gas leakage are the following:

- The connections for nitrous oxide gas lines are not tightly secured.
- Rings, washers, and other seals joining nitrous oxide gas tanks to the machine hanger yokes are missing, worn, or out of position.
- The covering over a unidirectional valve is not tightly closed.
- The carbon dioxide absorber canister is not securely sealed. Leaks are often caused by improper positioning of the canister or by the presence of absorber granules on the seals around the canister.
- The connection between the pop-off valve and scavenger is not airtight.
- Breathing hoses, the reservoir bag, or the endotracheal tube have holes or are not securely connected to the machine.
- The vaporizer cap was not replaced after the vaporizer was last filled.

The anesthetist should routinely perform leak tests to determine the presence and location of waste gas leaks. The following are two types of tests:

1. *High-pressure tests,* which check for leaks in the nitrous oxide or oxygen supply. High-pressure leaks arise between gas tanks and the flowmeter, where the pressure is 50 pounds per square inch (psi) or greater.
2. *Low-pressure tests,* which check for anesthetic gases that escape from the anesthetic machine itself. The pressure of gas within the machine is approximately 15 psi. Low-pressure leaks may arise in any part of the anesthetic machine or breathing circuit that does not fit together tightly or that develops a hole.

High-pressure system tests

One test of the high-pressure system is to turn the nitrous oxide tank on and place a 1:1 solution of water and dishwashing liquid on all tank connections and joints. Each location is then observed for bubble formation, which indicates a leak.

Another useful high-pressure test is conducted by first turning on the nitrous oxide cylinder, noting the reading on the tank pressure gauge, and then turning the cylinder off. Throughout this procedure the flowmeter is set to zero, maintaining the pressure in the system (that is, line pressure is not evacuated). The tank pressure gauge should be checked again in 1 hour. If the pressure gauge reading is unchanged or has decreased by no more than 50 lb/in^2, the high-pressure system is leak free.

If the pressure is at or near zero, there is a leak somewhere between the cylinder and the flowmeter, and nitrous oxide is escaping into the room air. The most likely location of the leak is at the connection of the cylinder to the machine yoke.

It is also possible to check for high-pressure leaks of oxygen by following the same procedure as that outlined for the nitrous oxide. Although the escape of small amounts of oxygen poses little or no risk of health problems to the anesthetic machine operator, it may lead to premature emptying of the oxygen tank.

Low-pressure system tests: circle systems

Low-pressure leaks in circle systems are best detected by securing all connections, closing the pop-off valve, and placing a hand or stopper over the Y piece, thus closing off all avenues of gas escape from the machine. The oxygen tank is turned on and the flowmeter is adjusted to supply a flow rate of at least 2 L/min, and the reservoir bag is allowed to gradually fill with oxygen. The anesthetist should be able to squeeze the inflated bag with gentle pressure without causing escape of air from the bag. Because the only exits from the system (the pop-off valve and the Y piece) are closed, any escape of air indicates that a leak is present. Alternatively, the anesthetist can close the pop-off valve, occlude the Y piece, and pressurize the system to 30 to 40 cm of water, using the flowmeter. When the oxygen flowmeter is turned off, the pressure should be maintained for 10 seconds. When the system is pressured to 30 to 40 cm of water, the quantity of leakage can be measured by determining the flow rate of oxygen necessary to maintain a constant pressure in the system. The leak rate should be less than 200 ml/min. (This leak rate is determined by turning the flowmeter to the lowest level that maintains pressure.)

Low-pressure system tests: nonrebreathing systems

Nonrebreathing systems such as the Bain apparatus can also be checked for leaks. The external hose of the Bain circuit can be checked by attaching the apparatus to the inspiratory hose, occluding the patient port, and closing the pop-off valve. Oxygen is introduced into the system until the reservoir bag fills. When the pressure gauge reads 20 cm H_2O, the flowmeter is turned off, and the pressure is observed for the next 20 seconds. A significant decrease in pressure indicates that a leak is present. For a test of the internal hose, the fresh gas hose from the anesthesia machine is attached to the Bain circuit, the oxygen flow is set at 2 L/min, and the outlet port of the internal hose is occluded with the rubber end of a 3-ml syringe or with a finger, while the flowmeter is observed. If there is no leak, the bobbin in the oxygen flowmeter should drop to zero, indicating adequate back pressure.

For both nonrebreathing and rebreathing systems, the location of leaks may be determined by listening for the hiss of escaping air or by using a detergent solution as previously described.

High-pressure leak testing should be performed at least weekly if nitrous oxide is in use. Low-pressure leak testing should be done every time the machine is assembled. If leaks that cannot be resolved by the technician are detected, a manufacturer's representative or other qualified person should service the machine. Frequent, routine servicing of the anesthetic machine and breathing circuit by qualified personnel is helpful in detecting equipment problems that can lead to leaks but is not an adequate substitute for daily leak testing of the machine by the anesthetist.

Anesthetic techniques and procedures

The anesthetist, by his or her choice of anesthetic techniques, has considerable control over the amount of waste gas released into the room air. One survey of human hospitals found faulty work practices accounted for 94% to 99% of waste anesthetic gas released in scavenged operating rooms.

The steps in Procedure 5-1 are recommended to minimize waste gas release.

PROCEDURE 5-1   **Minimizing Waste Gas Release**

1. Use caution when inducing an animal in an anesthetic chamber. Anesthetic chambers were the greatest source of anesthetic pollution noted in a 1983 survey of veterinary facilities. Not only are large amounts of waste gas released when the chamber is opened, but also the fur of the patient is contaminated with anesthetic vapor. If a chamber is used, a scavenging system should be connected to it. Anesthetic chambers should have two inlet holes, to which the breathing hoses from the anesthetic machine can be attached after the Y piece is removed. In this way, the waste gases are evacuated through the machine and regular scavenger. Alternatively, the hose from a Bain system can be attached to one inlet, and the scavenger system can be directly attached to the other inlet. Either way, the chamber should be closed immediately after the patient is removed, and the oxygen flow should be continued for several minutes to purge waste gas into the scavenger, rather than releasing waste gas into the room air. Anesthetic chambers should be tightly sealed to avoid leakage and used only in a well-ventilated area. Chambers should be washed with soap and water after each use to remove residual anesthetic and contaminants from the animal.

2. Avoid using masks to maintain anesthesia. Significant amounts of anesthetic gas may escape from around the diaphragm of the mask and enter the room air. If the situation dictates the use of a mask, it should be fitted tightly over the animal's face. Face masks are available in a variety of sizes and should be chosen to fit the patient snugly but comfortably. When a mask is used, the sequence of events is the same as for an endotracheal tube: turn the oxygen on, place the mask on the patient, then turn the vaporizer on. This order should be reversed when ending the procedure.

3. Use cuffed endotracheal tubes when possible. Endotracheal tubes significantly reduce the escape of waste gas into room air, as compared with masks. To be effective, however, the tube must be of adequate size, and the cuff must be inflated and in good repair. Before use, inflate cuffs with air to check for leaks. After intubation of the patient, check the fit of the endotracheal tube within the trachea by closing the pop-off valve and gently squeezing the reservoir bag. (To prevent overinflation of the patient's lungs, ensure that the circuit pressure displayed on the manometer does not exceed 20 cm of water when applying pressure to the bag to check the cuff.) The cuff should not leak up to an airway pressure of 20 cm H_2O but should leak above 20 cm H_2O. Leakage at pressures over 20 cm is necessary to reduce the risk of barotrauma in case the pop-off valve is closed and accidentally forgotten.

4. When using a rebreathing system, ensure that the reservoir bag inflates and deflates synchronously with the patient's respirations (in other words, inflates on expiration and deflates on inspiration, with the volume of movement approximately equal to the animal's tidal volume). If this does not occur, one should suspect either an air leakage around the endotracheal tube or esophageal intubation. Significant release of waste gas can occur in either case. (It is also likely that the patient will wake up because a significant amount of room air enters the lungs in either case.)

5. The use of closed rebreathing systems may help minimize waste gas pollution. Anesthesia with open systems and high gas flows (that is, greater than 3 L/min) is associated with greater release of waste gas, particularly if effective scavenging is unavailable.

6. When working with small animals, do not turn the vaporizer or flowmeters on until the anesthetic machine is connected to the endotracheal tube and the cuff is inflated. The practice of filling the machine and reservoir bag with anesthetic gas before connecting the machine to a dog or cat should be discouraged. This practice is acceptable when working with large animals, and in this case the Y piece should be occluded with a rubber plug. When it is time to attach the circuit to the intubated patient, the connection should be made quickly. Once the anesthetic procedure is under way, avoid disconnecting the patient from the breathing circuit unnecessarily. If the patient is to be disconnected from the machine, the vaporizer setting and flowmeters should be turned to zero.

7. Do not release the contents of the reservoir bag into the room air. If it is necessary to empty the reservoir bag, leave it attached to the machine and evacuate the contents into the scavenger.

8. After the vaporizer is shut off, maintain the connection between the animal and the machine, having the animal breathe pure oxygen at 2 to 3 times the maintenance flow rate for several minutes. Periodically flush the system with oxygen by emptying the rebreathing bag through the pop-off valve. If possible, leave the patient attached to the machine until extubation occurs. This allows expired anesthetic to enter the scavenging system rather than the room air.

9. Ensure that all rooms in which anesthetic gases are released (for example, surgical prep room, operating room, recovery room, and radiography room) have adequate ventilation that provides at least 15 air changes per hour. A properly designed ventilation system helps eliminate residual waste gases not collected by the scavenging system (for example, those that arise from leaks or improper work practices).

10. One study found that concentrations of halothane and nitrous oxide were higher in recovery areas than in scavenged operating rooms. For the reduction of waste gas levels, it is usually necessary to have an exhaust fan or nonrecirculating ventilation system operating in the room where patients are recovering from anesthesia. Whenever possible, avoid being closer than 3 feet from the nose of an animal recovering from anesthesia.

11. Have anesthetic machines serviced at least annually by a qualified service technician to ensure minimal leakage through machine components. A log of evaluation and maintenance procedures and leakage testing should be maintained for each anesthetic machine, ventilator, and vaporizer.

Continued

PROCEDURE 5-1   **Minimizing Waste Gas Release—cont'd**

12. Inspect equipment often and perform necessary maintenance. The routine maintenance procedures for anesthetic machines are usually explained in the operations manual.

13. Hoses, reservoir bags, and endotracheal tubes that are cracked or worn should be discarded. Endotracheal tubes with nonfunctional or leaking cuffs should not be used.

14. After each procedure, wash hoses, reservoir bags, masks, endotracheal tubes, and all other rubber components of the anesthetic circuit with soap and water, flush well with water, and allow them to air dry. These components may absorb considerable amounts of anesthetic during use. Washing not only removes absorbed waste gas, but also reduces transfer of microorganisms between patients.

15. Emptying and filling vaporizers may release significant amounts of anesthetic vapor into the surrounding air. Anesthetics may also be spilled onto the technician's hands and clothing (see Table 5-2). Ideally, vaporizers should be filled at the end of the workday, as personnel are leaving the hospital. Use a filling device (a specialized attachment that transfers anesthetic directly into the vaporizer) rather than pouring from a bottle to replenish liquid anesthetic in the machine. Agent-specific keyed filler systems are preferred. If no filling device is available, use a bottle adapter with a spout to prevent spillage. Fill vaporizers in a well-ventilated area (ideally, outside of the building), and after filling a vaporizer, be sure that the filling port is properly closed. Use of an approved organic cartridge respirator (a device that fits over the mouth and nose and filters incoming air), vinyl or plastic gloves, a lab coat or plastic apron, and other protective equipment will also minimize exposure to anesthetic liquid or vapors. Hands should be washed immediately after filling a vaporizer because liquid anesthetics are readily absorbed through intact skin.

16. Vaporizers should be turned off when not in use.

17. If liquid anesthetic is spilled, high concentrations of anesthetic vapor will be present in the immediate area of the spill. Accidental spillage of even 1 ml of liquid anesthetic will produce up to 200 ml of gas vapor with a concentration of 1 million ppm. If a spill occurs, increase ventilation as much as possible during the cleanup by opening windows or using fans. Close doors to the rest of the building and turn off the central vacuum system to avoid spreading the fumes throughout the building. For anything other than a small spill, all personnel not involved in the cleanup should leave the area, and the remaining staff should wear approved protective clothing, vinyl or plastic (not latex or rubber) gloves, and organic cartridge respirators. Remove all contaminated articles, including lab coats. Pour absorbent material such as kitty litter on the spill so that the liquid is completely absorbed. Dispose of the litter in an airtight container outside the clinic. If the spill is large or if protective equipment is unavailable, all personnel should leave the building and the local fire department should be notified.

18. Cap empty anesthetic bottles before discarding them because residual anesthetic in the bottle may evaporate into the room air. For the same reason, store vaporizer-filling devices in a sealed plastic bag between uses.

Monitoring Waste Gas Levels

It is advisable to periodically monitor waste anesthetic gas levels to ensure that the NIOSH-recommended levels are not exceeded. If professional monitoring is required, an accredited industrial hygiene laboratory can be contacted for assistance. (Industrial hygienists are found in the yellow pages of the telephone directory under "occupational safety.") An occupational hygienist will usually visit the hospital to evaluate ventilation and scavenging techniques and to interview the anesthetist regarding procedures used to minimize waste gas release. Air samples should be collected from all areas in which anesthetics are used, and the level of waste gas in the collected air should be determined with an infrared spectrometer. The cost of such a visit ranges from $250 to $700.

Professional monitoring services are not always necessary. Clinic employees can inexpensively monitor waste gas levels using detector tubes or badges. Badges may detect only one chemical, such as halothane, isoflurane, or nitrous oxide or may be sensitive to all halogenated anesthetics. The badges (called *passive dosimeters*) are uncapped at the beginning of the exposure period, then worn by personnel in the surgical prep room, operating room, or recovery area, for a timed period when anesthetic gases are being used. Alternatively, the badge may be placed in a room for area monitoring. After exposure, the badge is recapped and returned to the supplier (usually an industrial health and safety supply house or a company specializing in OSHA compliance) for analysis. Results are given as a time-weighted average in parts per million. Cost, including analysis, is approximately $40 to $50 per badge.*

SAFE HANDLING OF COMPRESSED GASES
Fire Safety Precautions

There is a potential for fire in any room where oxygen or nitrous oxide is used. Oxygen and nitrous oxide are not flammable; however, both support combustion and cause fuels to burn more readily. It is recommended that no flames or sources of ignition (for example, matches, lighters, or Bunsen burners) be present in any room in which oxygen or nitrous oxide cylinders are stored or used. For obvious reasons, smoking also must be prohibited in all rooms in which oxygen is stored or used. Even static electricity can cause fires in areas in which oxygen and flammable materials are used together. (This is one of the reasons why ether, which is extremely flammable, is no longer used in anesthesia.)

Use and Storage of Compressed Gas Cylinders

Tanks of compressed gas can be viewed as a storehouse of tremendous amounts of energy, waiting for release. If gas is released too quickly, nearby personnel may be injured. Persons connecting compressed gas cylinders to an anesthetic machine or gas piping system should wear impact-resistant goggles to protect their eyes from jets of gas. If a cylinder leak occurs, never use your hand to try to stop the leak.

---

*Current suppliers include Lab Safety Supply (1-800-356-2501), Assay Technology (1-800-833-1258, and Vetamac (1-800-334-1583).

Gas may also be suddenly released when the tank is turned on. When turning on a compressed air tank that is connected to the anesthetic machine, use the appropriate wrench and turn the valve slowly to the full open position. Keep your head and face away from the valve outlet, pressure gauge, and pressure relief device.

If a cylinder is damaged, the sudden release of gas can have catastrophic consequences. If, for example, a cylinder is punctured or is knocked over and the regulator (the metal attachments at the top of the tank) or cylinder neck is broken off the tank, the force of the gas suddenly escaping from the tank may cause it to move like a rocket through a wall or roof. To prevent this occurrence, chain or belt large cylinders to a wall and always store them in an upright position. Valve caps should be used on all large cylinders that are not connected to gas lines to protect the valve from damage.

Gas cylinders should be stored away from emergency exits or areas with heavy traffic. If a cylinder must be moved to another location, a handcart should be used; do not drag or roll the cylinder.

Full tanks should be kept separate from empty tanks and also should be clearly labeled for quick identification. The use of tear-off labels helps eliminate confusion regarding the empty, in-use, or full status of a given compressed air cylinder. The current status of the tank is given on the outermost section of the label (Fig. 5-3). Cylinders should be used in the order that they are received (that is, first in, first out).

ACCIDENTAL EXPOSURE TO INJECTABLE AGENTS

All anesthetic agents are potentially toxic to personnel handling them. Skin exposure, eye splash, or oral ingestion of injectable drugs or inhalation agents may be hazardous (and in the case of oral ingestion, fatal).

The injectable drugs of most concern are the opioids used for the restraint and capture of wildlife, including etorphine (Immobilon, M99) and carfentanil (Wildnil). Etorphine has 10,000 times the potency of morphine and is absorbed readily through mucous membranes or broken skin. Exposure may also occur through accidental injection, eye splash, or oral ingestion.

Human exposure to even a minute amount of these agents by any route can cause rapid onset of unconsciousness, respiratory failure, and death. The following precautions should be taken:

- Never handle potent opioids such as etorphine unless you have been adequately trained in their safe use, potential adverse effects, and treatment in case of exposure.
- Never work alone when using potent opioids.
- Wear gloves. If exposure occurs, immediately wash skin and clothing with cold water.
- A reversal agent (diprenorphine, naloxone, naltrexon) must be drawn up ready for use. Note that up to three bottles (12 mg) of naloxone may be necessary to antagonize a single drop of these opioids.
- Dispose of needles and syringes in a closed container immediately after use. The syringes should be carefully taken apart, placed in a bucket, and rinsed with copious amounts of water.

Other injectable agents that may be hazardous include the cyclohexamines (ketamine, tiletamine), which have been reported to cause disorientation, excitement,

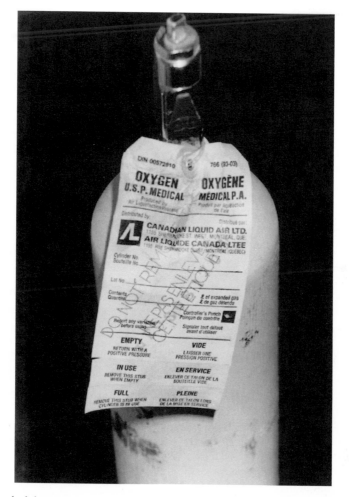

FIG. 5-3 Label for compressed gas tanks. Current status of tank is shown by printing at the bottom of the label. Label shown is from newly purchased tank and reads "FULL." When tank is connected to machine, lower portion of the label is removed so that remaining label reads "IN USE." When tank is empty, "IN USE" stub is removed, leaving the label that reads "EMPTY."

dizziness, and unconsciousness after an accidental eye splash. Human exposure to alpha-2 agonists (xylazine, detomidine, medetomidine) may cause profound sedation, hypotension, bradycardia, respiratory depression, and coma.

Safety precautions for prevention of exposure to any injectable agent include the use of personal protective equipment if there is a risk of spillage or eye splash, careful loading of syringes, and proper disposal of used needles and syringes. If accidental exposure occurs, the exposed person should receive prompt first aid (eye wash, flushing exposed skin with large amounts of water, respiratory support) and subsequent transport to a medical center.

1. Anesthesia presents several potential health risks to hospital personnel, including exposure to waste anesthetic gas and hazardous injectable agents and the handling of compressed gas cylinders.

2. Waste anesthetic gases and vapors are breathed by all personnel working in areas in which animals are anesthetized or are recovering from inhalation anesthesia. Filling or emptying vaporizers and the cleanup of accidental spills also may result in significant exposure.

3. Exposure to waste anesthetic gas is associated with short-term problems such as fatigue, headache, drowsiness, nausea, depression, and irritability.

4. Long-term exposure to waste anesthetic gases may be associated with reproductive disorders, liver and kidney damage, and nervous system dysfunction. The evidence of epidemiologic studies is sometimes contradictory and difficult to interpret. Most authorities recommend that exposure to high levels of waste anesthetic gas be avoided, particularly by pregnant women.

5. Anesthetics such as methoxyflurane and halothane, which undergo significant hepatic metabolism and renal excretion, are considered to be a greater hazard than anesthetics that are minimally eliminated by these routes (isoflurane, sevoflurane).

6. Waste anesthetic gases apparently do not have oncogenic (cancer-causing) effects.

7. The NIOSH recommendations for waste anesthetic gas concentrations limit exposure to 2 parts per million (ppm) or less for halothane, isoflurane, and methoxyflurane (0.5 ppm or less if nitrous oxide is concurrently used). Surveys of veterinary clinics show wide variations in waste gas levels, depending on the sampling site, scavenging system, and anesthetic techniques used.

8. Installation and use of an effective gas scavenging system greatly reduces waste gas exposure. Caution should be used to prevent the scavenger from applying negative pressure to the breathing circuit.

9. Equipment leak testing should be done on a daily basis to detect and allow correction of leakage from the anesthetic machine and compressed air cylinders. Tests should be done on both the high-pressure and low-pressure components of the machine.

10. Certain anesthetic techniques are associated with excessive release of waste gas. These include the use of anesthetic chambers, masks, and uncuffed endotracheal tubes. Procedures such as turning off the vaporizer before disconnecting the animal from the machine are helpful in reducing waste gas contamination of hospital air.

11. Vaporizers should be filled and emptied with care, using appropriate equipment and protective clothing.

12. Waste gas levels may be monitored by professional occupational hygienists or by the use of detector tubes or badges.

13. Compressed air cylinders should be transported, used, and stored with care. Special hazards include risk of fire in areas in which cylinders are stored and the risk of sudden release of pressurized gas from cylinders.

14. Potent injectable opioids such as etorphine have considerable potential to cause serious, even fatal reactions. Special training is necessary to safely handle these agents, and a narcotic reversing agent must be readily available in case of human exposure.

REVIEW QUESTIONS

1. Waste anesthetic gases are a potential hazard to personnel, but problems that arise are really only of a short-term nature.
   True   False
2. Long-term toxicity of inhalation anesthetics is thought to be caused by the release of toxic metabolites during the breakdown of these drugs.
   True   False
3. The anesthetic thought to be the least toxic to hospital personnel is:
   a. Isoflurane
   b. Halothane
   c. Methoxyflurane
   d. Nitrous oxide
4. In the United States, the National Institute for Occupational Safety and Health (NIOSH) recommends that the levels of waste anesthetic gases for anesthetics such as isoflurane, halothane, or methoxyflurane should not

   exceed _____ ppm.
   a. 0.2
   b. 2
   c. 20
   d. 200
5. The odor of halothane may be detected by a person when the levels reach a

   minimum of _____ ppm.
   a. 5
   b. 33
   c. 200
   d. 5000
6. Rooms in which animals are recovering from anesthesia may be highly contaminated with waste gas.
   True   False
7. It is recommended that for a passive scavenger system, the hose be no longer

   than _____ feet if it discharges into the room ventilation exhaust.
   a. 1
   b. 10
   c. 20
   d. 50
8. How often should a test for low-pressure leaks be conducted?
   a. Each time the machine is used
   b. At least once per week
   c. At least once per month
   d. When the anesthetist smells anesthetic gases
9. The safest way to transport a high-pressure tank, such as an oxygen tank, is by:
   a. Carrying it
   b. Rolling it along the floor
   c. A handcart
   d. Dragging it by the neck

10. Rooms in which waste anesthetic gases are at risk of being released should have a minimum of _____ air changes per hour.
   a. 5
   b. 10
   c. 15
   d. 20

For the following questions, more than one answer may be correct.

11. Long-term hazards that may occur from exposure to high levels of anesthetic waste gases include:
   a. Reproductive disorders
   b. Liver damage
   c. Kidney damage
   d. Nervous system dysfunction
12. A technician may reduce the amount of waste gases by:
   a. Using cuffed endotracheal tubes
   b. Ensuring the anesthetic machine has been tested for leaks
   c. Using an induction technique other than mask or chamber
   d. Using high fresh gas flows
13. To conduct a low-pressure test on an anesthetic machine (circle system), you must:
   a. Close the pop-off valve and occlude the end of the circuit
   b. Turn off the oxygen tank
   c. Compress the reservoir bag
   d. Pressurize the circuit with a volume of gas

ANSWERS FOR CHAPTER 5

1. False	**2.** True	**3.** a	**4.** b	**5.** b
6. True	**7.** b	**8.** a	**9.** c	**10.** c
11. a, b, c, d	**12.** a, b, c	**13.** a, c, d		

Selected Readings

American College of Veterinary Anesthesiologists: Commentary and recommendations on control of waste anesthetic gases in the workplace, *J Am Vet Med Assoc* 209(1):75-77, 1996.

American Society of Anesthesiologists Task Force on Trace Anesthetic Gases: www.asahq. org/ProfInfo/wasteanesgases.html.

Burkhart JE, Stobbe TJ: Real-time measurement and control of waste anesthetic gases during veterinary surgeries, *Am Ind Hyg Assoc J* 51(12):640-645, 1990.

Gross ME, Branson KR: Reducing exposure to waste anesthetic gas, *Vet Tech* 14(3):175-177, 1993.

Hoerauf K, Lierz M, Wiesner G, et al: Genetic damage in operating room personnel exposed to isoflurane and nitrous oxide, *Occupational and Environmental Medicine* 56(7):433-437, 1999.

Johnson JA, Buchan RM, Reif JS: Effect of waste anesthetic gas and vapor exposure on reproductive outcomes in veterinary personnel, *Am Ind Hyg Assoc J* 48:62-66, 1987.

Lietzemayer DW: Current methods for removal of anesthetic gas, Vet Tech 11(4):213-220, 1990.

McKelvey D: *Safety handbook for veterinary hospital staff,* Lakewood, Colo, 1999, American Animal Hospital Association Press.

Meyer RE: Anesthesia hazards to animal workers. In Lanley RL, editor: *Occupational medicine state of the art reviews,* Philadelphia, 1999, Hanley and Belfus.

OSHA Office of Science and Technology Assessment: Anesthetic agents—workplace exposures, OSHA Instruction TED 1.15 (H-2), 1996.

Short CE, Hargvey RC: Anesthetic waste gases in veterinary medicine, *Cornell Vet* 73(4): 363-374, 1983.

CHAPTER 6

Anesthetic Problems and Emergencies

PERFORMANCE OBJECTIVES

After completion of this chapter, the reader will be able to:

- List the most common reasons why anesthetic emergencies occur, including problems arising from human error, equipment failure, and the adverse effects of anesthetic agents.
- Explain how anesthesia of geriatric and pediatric patients differs from anesthesia of healthy adult dogs and cats.
- Describe the problems involved in anesthetizing each of the following: brachycephalic dogs; sighthounds; obese animals; and patients with trauma or cardiovascular, respiratory, central nervous system (CNS), hepatic, or renal disease.
- Describe the role of the veterinary technician in responding to anesthetic emergencies.
- List the most common causes of the following anesthetic problems: inadequate anesthetic depth, excessive anesthetic depth, pale mucous membranes, prolonged capillary refill, dyspnea, and tachypnea.
- Describe the appropriate response to common emergencies, including dyspnea, hypotension, hypoventilation, respiratory arrest, and cardiac arrest.
- List the most common problems that may arise in the recovery period and the appropriate action that can be taken to prevent or treat these problems.

General anesthesia poses minimal risk to most patients when performed by capable personnel using an anesthetic protocol appropriate for the animal. Emergencies are uncommon, and the overwhelming majority of patients recover from anesthesia with no lasting ill effects. After successfully anesthetizing hundreds of patients, the technician can be easily lulled into a false sense of security. However, it is vitally important that the anesthetist remember that every anesthetic procedure has the potential to cause the death of the animal. Anesthesia is not a normal physiologic state: the patient is not "asleep." The anesthetist must remain watchful for problems that may arise in even the most routine anesthetic procedure.

A survey of British veterinary clinics revealed a mortality rate of one death for every 870 anesthetic procedures in healthy dogs and one death for every 552 procedures in healthy cats. The same study found a mortality rate of 1 in 30 patients where systemic disease was present. An American study of 3239 cases found the incidence of anesthetic complications to be 12% in dogs and 10.5% in cats, with a mortality rate of 0.43% (4.3 per 1000) in both dogs and cats.* A Canadian study of 16,000 anesthetized animals found the incidence of cardiac arrest to be approximately 1 in 900 patients. Of the dogs with anesthetic complications, bulldogs, Pekingese, and other brachycephalic breeds; weimaraners; and Jack Russell terriers were disproportionately represented.

Risk not only varies with patient breed but also depends on the patient's health, the experience and skills of the anesthetist and surgeon, the surgical procedure, and the circumstances that make the anesthesia necessary. Emergency anesthesia is associated with a much greater risk than elective anesthesia. For each procedure, the benefits must outweigh the risk to the patient.

This chapter describes problems that may arise during anesthesia, ranging from routine (such as maintaining appropriate anesthetic depth) to major (including respiratory arrest and cardiac arrest). Appropriate responses to various anesthetic emergencies are presented, and the reasons why the anesthetic problems may arise (and procedures for their prevention) are emphasized. The challenges associated with anesthesia of patients with special problems such as heart disease or brachycephalic conformation are also discussed.

REASONS WHY ANESTHETIC PROBLEMS AND EMERGENCIES ARISE

Although an awareness of the correct response to an anesthetic emergency is essential, it is even more important to understand why emergencies arise and how they may be prevented. Most anesthetic emergencies are the result of one or more of the following factors: human error, equipment failure, the adverse effect of anesthetic agents, and patient-related factors.

Human Error

Human error is, unfortunately, a contributing cause in some anesthetic deaths. Common human errors committed by anesthetists in veterinary practice include the following:
1. Failure to obtain an adequate history or physical examination on the patient
2. Inadequate experience with the anesthetic machine or anesthetic agents being used
3. Incorrect administration of drugs
4. Failure to devote sufficient time or attention to the anesthetized patient
5. Fatigue
6. Failure to recognize and respond to early signs of patient difficulty

Failure to obtain an adequate history or to perform a physical examination

Ideally, every patient scheduled for anesthesia should have a complete physical examination, and a thorough history should be obtained with the owner present. In some clinical situations, however, this is sometimes difficult to achieve. Animals are sometimes dropped off at the veterinary clinic by owners who are in a hurry and reluctant to stop and answer questions about their pet. Animals may be brought in by neighbors or friends of the owner or by other persons unfamiliar with the animal's

---

*The mortality rate related to general anesthesia in human patients has been variously estimated to be as high as 1.5 per 1000 and as low as 1 per 10,000 patients.

history. The receptionist or other person admitting the animal to the hospital may fail to ask important questions or may not transmit the information to the anesthetist or veterinarian. The physical examination is sometimes cursory or omitted entirely. The net result is that significant information may be overlooked. For example, the anesthetist may be unaware that a patient has not been fasted or that an animal scheduled for surgery is dehydrated as a result of vomiting and diarrhea. An anesthetic protocol that is safe for a healthy patient could be inappropriate for these animals, and an anesthetic problem or even death of the patient could result.

Lack of familiarity with the anesthetic machine or drugs used

It is the responsibility of the veterinarian to ensure that his or her personnel are sufficiently trained and have the knowledge to perform competently all required procedures. Some simple anesthetic tasks, such as adjusting a vaporizer setting, can be done by unskilled personnel working under a veterinarian's direct supervision. More demanding tasks, such as inducing anesthesia and monitoring anesthetized patients, are best assigned only to personnel (veterinarians or technicians) who have sufficient training, knowledge, and experience to recognize abnormalities and danger signals and to respond appropriately.

Incorrect administration of drugs

Many anesthetic agents have a narrow margin of safety between therapeutic and toxic doses. The incorrect administration of drugs may have serious or even fatal consequences and may arise from any of the following:
- Failure to weigh the patient and calculate an accurate dose.
- Mathematical errors (particularly decimal errors, which can result in a tenfold or 100-fold error in the amount of drug given).
- Use of the wrong medication (for example, calculating a dose of atropine and drawing up xylazine instead).
- Use of the wrong concentration of a medication. This is a common problem with drugs that are available in several different concentrations (for example, atropine or acepromazine). The anesthetist must ensure that the concentration used in calculating the dose is the same as that drawn up into the syringe.
- Administration of anesthetics by the incorrect route (for example, administration of the intramuscular [IM] dose of ketamine by the intravenous [IV] route).
- Confusion between syringes drawn up for two different patients. This involves either a failure to label the syringes or a failure to read the labels correctly.
- Use of a syringe that is too large for the volume drawn up, leading to inaccurate doses (for example, 0.3 ml drawn up in a 3- or 6-ml syringe, instead of a 1-ml syringe).

Personnel who are preoccupied or are in a hurry

Although efficiency is desirable in any anesthetic procedure, it is not necessary or advisable for the anesthetist to feel hurried. A technician who is feeling rushed is more likely to inject barbiturates perivascularly or to insert an endotracheal tube into the esophagus. Unfortunately, it is common for the technician working in a busy practice to feel pressured and distracted. The technician responsible for anesthesia may be called on to restrain patients for examination or procedures, answer the phone, perform laboratory tests, take radiographs, discharge animals, and carry out other similar tasks. However, when an animal is anesthetized, the technician's first priority must be monitoring that patient because failure to satisfactorily perform this duty may result in the animal's death.

In a busy practice, the technician usually does not have the luxury of being constantly by the animal's side throughout the procedure. If periodic absences are necessary, the anesthetist should return to check the patient at least once every 5 minutes or more frequently if the patient's status requires close monitoring. If necessary, other tasks must be temporarily set aside to allow the anesthetist to return to the patient.

Fatigue

Fatigue is an ailment common to many veterinarians and technicians, particularly at the end of a busy day. Anesthetic emergencies may arise when personnel are tired and less alert than normal, possibly because minor problems are not detected and corrected at an early stage. If possible, operations that are lengthy or difficult should be scheduled early in the day.

Inattentiveness

One of the most serious human errors in anesthesia is the failure to monitor and recognize danger signals. It is obviously better for the patient—and easier for the anesthetist—to detect and address anesthetic problems early, rather than late. For example, an animal experiencing respiratory depression when under an inhalation anesthetic will show a gradually decreasing respiratory rate, from 12 breaths per minute to 8 breaths per minute (at which point the anesthetist should consider adjusting the vaporizer to a lower setting); then from 8 breaths per minute to 4 (at which point the vaporizer should be turned off and the animal bagged with oxygen); then from 4 breaths per minute to 0 (at which point cardiac arrest is likely to occur).

The anesthetist's attitude toward patient care is a key factor in the safety of anesthesia. The conscientious anesthetist will monitor the animal often to ensure that the patient is not in trouble. A brief check of the vital signs and depth indicators listed on p. 57 takes less than 1 minute and gives the anesthetist a good assessment of the patient's status. The best attitude is one of low-level anxiety, which is relieved only when a quick examination of the patient reveals that all vital signs and depth indicators are within acceptable limits.

Equipment Failure

Equipment failure is an uncommon cause of anesthetic emergencies, but it does occur. In many cases the failure of the anesthetic machine is in fact a failure of the operator to maintain and monitor the machine properly. The importance of a preanesthetic check of the anesthetic machine, as described in Chapter 4, cannot be overemphasized.

The following anesthetic machine problems are occasionally encountered in routine anesthesia.

Carbon dioxide absorber exhaustion

Patients connected to a rebreathing system rely on the carbon dioxide (CO_2) absorber to remove expired CO_2 from the circuit and prevent inhalation of excessive levels of this toxic gas. If CO_2 is not removed from the circuit, the patient will experience hypercapnia (elevated blood CO_2). Signs of this disorder include tachypnea (rapid respiration), sweating, brick red mucous membranes, tachycardia, and cardiac arrhythmias. If exhaustion of the CO_2 absorber crystals has occurred, examination of the crystals will reveal an obvious color change. Hypercapnia may also be seen in patients connected to a nonrebreathing system such as a Bain, if the gas flow is too low and significant rebreathing of expired gases occurs.

Insufficient oxygen flow

Failure to deliver oxygen to the patient is one of the most serious and yet one of the most easily prevented mistakes that an anesthetist can make. Before starting an anesthetic procedure, the anesthetist must ensure that the tank contains sufficient oxygen for the duration of the surgery and that the flowmeter indicates that an adequate flow rate can be achieved. (For information on calculating the amount of oxygen present in a tank, refer to p. 177.) During the procedure, the oxygen tank pressure and flowmeter should be checked every 5 minutes. At the end of a procedure, the patient should be disconnected from the machine before the oxygen flowmeter is turned off.

Oxygen flow to the patient may be disrupted in several ways. The oxygen tank may run out, the regulator valves may jam in a closed position, the flowmeter float may become lodged in the tube, a hose may become disconnected, or a serious obstruction or leak may develop between the tank and the patient. However it happens, being able to recognize when the machine is no longer delivering oxygen to the patient is vital. If the oxygen flowmeter reads zero flow, the system is not receiving any oxygen, regardless of the oxygen tank pressure. Occasionally, the situation arises in which the oxygen tank pressure gauge reads zero, but the flowmeter indicates some oxygen flow; in this case the tank is still delivering a small amount of oxygen, but loss of oxygen pressure is imminent and the tank should be changed immediately.

The anesthetist must be aware of the proper response when oxygen delivery to the patient is stopped, because of machine malfunction or the tank's lack of oxygen. If the oxygen flow stops (that is, the flowmeter reads zero despite the efforts of the anesthetist to establish flow) and the patient is connected to a nonrebreathing system, the anesthetist should disconnect the hose from the endotracheal tube, allowing the patient to breathe room air until the oxygen delivery is reestablished. If a circle system with a full reservoir bag is in use, the patient can remain connected for a short period of time, provided the reservoir bag remains inflated.

Misassembly of the anesthetic machine

It is essential that the person handling the anesthetic machine be familiar with every connection, hose, dial, and component of the machine. Before using an unfamiliar machine, the anesthetist should take a few minutes to examine it carefully for the location of the controls and to learn the direction and path of gas flow within the machine. Every time a connection such as a Bain system is added or removed, the anesthetist must trace the flow of gas, ensuring that the correct pattern of flow is maintained and that all connections are secure. Failure to do so can result in the patient rebreathing expired CO_2 or not receiving anesthetic gases.

Endotracheal tube problems

Although the endotracheal tube is, strictly speaking, not a part of the anesthetic machine, it is a critical component of the anesthetic delivery system and is subject to many problems. Endotracheal tubes may become blocked during anesthesia, cutting off the flow of anesthetic gas and oxygen to the patient. Blockages may be the result of twisting or kinking of the tube; accumulation of material such as blood, mucus, saliva, or excess lubricant within the tube; or inappropriate positioning of the tube (as may occur when the neck is flexed). The endotracheal tube should be premeasured from the incisor teeth to the midneck, and it should be advanced no further than the point of the shoulder. If the tube is accidentally advanced into a bronchus, the patient may become hypoxic and hypercapnic.

Endotracheal tube blockage (if complete) results in a cessation of oxygen flow to the patient and retention of carbon dioxide. The patient may become dyspneic and progress to respiratory arrest. The anesthetist may become aware of the problem by observing the patient's exaggerated breathing pattern or by noting that the reservoir bag no longer inflates and deflates with the patient's respirations. If a problem is suspected, the anesthetist should quickly check the endotracheal tube function in the following two ways:

1. Attempt to bag the patient and observe if the chest rises. If the endotracheal tube is blocked, no chest movement will be seen, and there will be considerable resistance to the passage of air into the patient.
2. If the patient cannot be bagged, disconnect the animal from the machine. With the endotracheal tube still in place, feel for air coming out of the tube when the patient's chest is compressed. If no air movement is felt, a blockage may be present. In this case, the tube should be removed and another endotracheal tube or mask used to deliver oxygen to the patient.

If accumulation of blood, mucus, or similar material within the trachea is causing the obstruction, it may be helpful to suction with a 20-ml syringe through a cut-down feeding tube inserted into the endotracheal tube.

Vaporizer problems

There are several problems commonly associated with vaporizers.

- A potentially disastrous problem can arise if the wrong anesthetic is put into a vaporizer. In particular, the inadvertent use of isoflurane, sevoflurane, or halothane in a nonprecision vaporizer designed for methoxyflurane may result in delivery of extremely high concentrations of anesthetic gas to the patient. (The use of isoflurane or halothane in this type of vaporizer is safe if special techniques are used, as discussed in Chapter 4 under low-flow closed system anesthesia.)
- Vaporizers should not be tipped. Tipping may lead to leakage of anesthetic into the oxygen bypass, which may result in delivery of uncontrolled amounts of anesthetic.
- Occasionally, a vaporizer dial may stick or become jammed. If the dial cannot be adjusted, the patient should be transferred to another machine.
- Anesthetic machines equipped with two vaporizers in series should be monitored carefully to ensure that both vaporizers are not turned on at the same time.
- If a vaporizer that is not temperature compensated is used, the anesthetist must be aware that high room temperatures will result in increased anesthetic delivery.

- Vaporizers should not be overfilled. If too much anesthetic is put into the vaporizer, it should be drained until the fluid level is at, or below, the indicator line.

Pop-off valve problems

Occasionally, an anesthetist inadvertently leaves the pop-off valve in a closed position. If the pop-off valve is closed and the oxygen flow rate is greater than the patient's oxygen requirement, pressure within the circuit will rapidly rise. (An example of this situation is a closed system in which the oxygen flow rate is greater than the metabolic oxygen consumption, approximately 10 ml/kg/min.) As pressure rises in the circuit, the reservoir bag will expand, as will the patient's lungs. This prevents exhalation and also decreases the venous return to the heart. This in turn may decrease cardiac output, cause blood pressure to fall rapidly, and lead to death within a short time.

To detect the problem at an early stage, the anesthetist should frequently monitor the reservoir bag size and ensure that it does not overfill. If pressure rises within the circuit and the bag is full and tight, the anesthetist should attempt to open the pop-off valve and/or decrease the oxygen flow rate. If this does not alleviate the problem, the patient should be disconnected from the circuit.

Anesthetic Agents

Every injectable or inhalation agent has the potential to harm a patient and, in some cases, cause death. A detailed description of the pharmacologic and physiologic effects of preanesthetic and general anesthetic agents is given in Chapter 1 (preanesthetic agents) and in Chapter 3 (general anesthetic agents).

The following strategies are used to reduce anesthetic risk:

- The anesthetic protocol must be chosen to reflect the special needs of the patient. For example, acepromazine may be harmful in patients with low blood pressure because this agent may cause vasodilation, further decreasing the blood pressure. Similarly, halothane is not the preferred inhalation agent for patients with cardiac arrhythmias. In each case, the veterinarian might choose to use an alternative agent.
- The anesthetist must be familiar with the side effects and contraindications associated with each of the preanesthetic and general anesthetic agents used in the hospital. For example, the anesthetist who administers xylazine should be aware of its potential to cause bradycardia, cardiac arrhythmias, hypotension, vomiting, bloat, abortion, and respiratory depression.
- Multidrug use to achieve balanced anesthesia can be safer than anesthesia with a single drug, provided that the doses of the individual drugs are appropriately reduced. For example, the concentration of halothane needed to anesthetize an animal is significantly reduced if the animal is premedicated with acepromazine and butorphanol, as compared with an animal given halothane without premedications. If the same halothane concentration was used in both situations, the multidrug regimen could be dangerous for the patient.

Patient Factors

Animals that are to undergo anesthesia may have systemic abnormalities that considerably increase anesthetic risk. Patients with a preoperative status of class IV or class V are particularly difficult to anesthetize successfully. Challenging patients routinely encountered in veterinary practice include geriatric animals, neonates, brachycephalic animals, sighthounds, and obese animals. Cesarean delivery of puppies or kittens also places unique demands on the anesthetist because the response of both the dam and the offspring to anesthetic agents must be considered. Animals with recent trauma may be presented for emergency surgery, and the anesthetist must be prepared to deal with shock, head injuries, respiratory difficulties, and cardiac arrhythmias in these patients. Animals with cardiac problems such as heartworm disease or congestive heart failure may require anesthesia for diagnostic or therapeutic procedures. Similarly, animals may require anesthesia despite the presence of renal or hepatic disease. Although a detailed discussion of the anesthetic challenges posed by these and other patients is beyond the scope of this book, it is desirable that the technician be familiar with some of the special problems encountered when anesthetizing these animals. These are summarized in Table 6-1.

Geriatric patients

A geriatric patient is one that has reached 75% of the average life expectancy for that species and breed. In these patients the functions of critical organs such as the heart, lungs, kidneys, and liver are reduced in comparison with the healthy, young patient. As a result, geriatric animals have less functional reserve than younger animals and a relatively poor response to stress. Often they are less able to adequately maintain their state of hydration than younger patients can. In addition, geriatric animals may suffer from disorders such as diabetes mellitus, chronic renal disease, cancer, or mitral valve insufficiency, all of which are of concern to the anesthetist. Unfortunately, a geriatric animal that appears to be in good health may actually have impaired function of one or several vital organs that only becomes apparent when the animal is stressed by anesthesia, surgery, disease, or hospitalization.

Because of the high incidence of health problems in these animals, the importance of a thorough history and physical examination cannot be overemphasized. Preoperative tests such as a blood chemistry panel, urinalysis, chest radiographs, and an electrocardiogram (ECG) may be advisable for selected patients.

Geriatric animals typically have reduced anesthetic requirements, and doses of injectable anesthetic agents are often decreased by one half to one third compared with the healthy, young patient. In the case of barbiturates, dose requirements may be as little as one twentieth of the normal dose. Response to drugs is slower, and the technician should allow more time for IV injections to take effect. Some injectable drugs that are well tolerated by healthy, young patients may be less well tolerated by geriatric patients (for example, alpha-2 agonists such as medetomidine or xylazine, high doses of acepromazine, and barbiturates). Atropine and ketamine may cause undesirable tachycardia. Other drugs (for example, diazepam, opioids, propofol, and etomidate) are suitable for use in most geriatric patients. The minimum alveolar concentration (MAC) for inhalation agents is reduced in most geriatric patients, and therefore lower concentrations of inhalation anesthetics are often sufficient for maintenance of anesthesia. Recovery from general anesthesia may be prolonged in geriatric animals, partly because of decreased renal and hepatic function (and thus decreased ability to excrete drugs).

Geriatric patients also have a tendency to develop hypothermia because they have a reduced ability to regulate body temperature. Respiratory function is also

TABLE 6-1

Patient Factors That Increase Anesthetic Risk

PATIENT FACTOR	ANESTHETIC PROBLEMS ENCOUNTERED	STRATEGIES USED TO DECREASE RISK
Geriatric patients	Reduced organ function; poor response to stress; degenerative disorders common; increased risk of hypothermia and overhydration	Reduce anesthetic dosages by 30% to 50%; allow longer time for response to drugs; administer fluids at reduced rate; keep patient warm; select agents with minimal cardiovascular effect; preoxygenate
Pediatric patients	Increased risk of hypothermia and overhydration; inefficient excretion of drugs; difficult intubation and intravenous catheterization	Avoid heat loss; avoid prolonged fasting; administer 5% dextrose in lactated Ringer's solution using delivery; weigh accurate methods of accurately; dilute injectable drugs; reduce anesthetic dosages; inhalant agents preferred to injectable agents
Brachycephalic dogs	Conformational tendency toward airway obstruction; abnormally high vagal tone	Include anticholinergic in anesthetic protocol; preoxygenate; induce rapidly using intravenous agents; delay extubation; observe closely during recovery period
Sighthounds	Increased sensitivity to barbiturates	Use alternative agents
Obese animals	Accurate dosing difficult; poor distribution of anesthetics; may have respiratory difficulties	Dose according to ideal weight; preoxygenate; induce rapidly; assist ventilation if necessary; delay extubation; observe closely in recovery period
Cesarean patients	Dam: increased workload to heart; respiration may be compromised; increased tendency to vomit or regurgitate; increased risk of hemorrhage Offspring: anesthetic agents cross placenta and may reduce respiratory and cardiovascular function	Dam: administer intravenous fluids; clip patient before induction; preoxygenate; use lowest effective dose of general anesthetic; avoid pentobarbital and ketamine/diazepam Offspring: use reversing agents and doxapram; administer oxygen by face mask; administer atropine for bradycardia

TABLE 6-1		
Patient Factors That Increase Anesthetic Risk—cont'd		
PATIENT FACTOR	ANESTHETIC PROBLEMS ENCOUNTERED	STRATEGIES USED TO DECREASE RISK
Trauma patients	Respiratory distress common; cardiac arrhythmias seen for 72 hours after incident; shock and hemorrhage common; internal injuries often present	Stabilize before anesthesia; obtain thoracic radiographs and ECG; thorough physical examination necessary to check for concurrent injuries
Cardiovascular disease	Circulation is compromised; pulmonary edema common; increased tendency to develop arrhythmias and tachycardia	Alleviate pulmonary edema with diuretics; preoxygenate for 5 minutes before induction; avoid agents that depress myocardium or cause arrhythmias; avoid overhydration
Respiratory disease	Poor oxygenation of tissues; patient may be anxious and difficult to restrain; respiratory arrest common	Avoid stress and unnecessary handling; preoxygenate; avoid nitrous oxide; induce with injectable agents; intubate rapidly and control ventilation if necessary; monitor closely during recovery
Hepatic disease	Delayed metabolism of anesthetic agents; decreased synthesis of blood clotting factors; may be hypoproteinemic; dehydration common; may be anemic and/or icteric	Preanesthetic blood chemistry tests; may omit preanesthetic medication; inhalation agents preferred over injectable agents; expect prolonged recovery
Renal disease	Delayed excretion of anesthetic agents; electrolyte imbalances common, including hyperkalemia, hyperphosphatemia, and metabolic acidosis; dehydration usually present	Rehydrate before surgery; obtain renal function tests and electrolyte values; reduce dosages of anesthetic agents; use caution with barbiturates; may require intraoperative intravenous fluids
Urinary obstruction	Dehydration, acidosis, azotemia, and hyperkalemia common; bradycardia may be present	Avoid barbiturates and IM ketamine; treat for hyperkalemia if present

impaired, and even mild respiratory depression may lead to severe hypoxia and hypercarbia. Cardiac output, blood volume, and arterial blood pressure are often reduced compared with the younger patient.

The routine use of IV fluids is generally advocated in geriatric animals because they have less tolerance for hypotension and often have reduced kidney function. Anesthesia itself may adversely affect renal function by decreasing renal blood flow as much as 40%, which is of particular concern in a patient that already has renal disease. Geriatric animals are at increased risk for overhydration problems such as pulmonary edema, however, and IV fluids should be given with care.

Geriatric patients often have impaired hearing and vision and are commonly anxious or easily startled. Gentle handling and quiet reassurance may be preferable to the use of sedative drugs in some patients.

Pediatric patients

Special considerations apply when anesthetizing veterinary patients younger than 3 months. Potential problems in this age group include excitement during induction, difficult intubation and IV access, hypoglycemia, bradycardia, hypotension, and hypoxia.

Preoperative fasting of the pediatric patient may not be advisable because hypoglycemia and dehydration can occur after even a short period of fasting. Oral fluids are usually allowed up to 1 hour and food up to 2 hours before induction. To prevent hypoglycemia during surgery, many veterinarians administer 5% dextrose in lactated Ringer's solution to anesthetized pediatric patients. (This can be formulated by adding 100 ml of 50% dextrose to 900 ml of lactated Ringer's solution.) Blood glucose should be regularly monitored if anesthesia is prolonged. The fluid administration rate should not exceed 10 ml/kg/hr in dogs and 5 ml/kg/hr in cats (unless shock or dehydration is present) because very young animals are prone to overhydration if fluid administration is rapid. The use of an infusion pump, pediatric minidrips (60 drips per milliliter), or a burette is helpful in preventing inadvertent overinfusion of fluid. Air should be removed from IV lines to avoid the risk of air embolism.

To calculate drug dosages, obtain an accurate weight. For animals weighing under 5 kg, a pediatric or lab animal scale gives more reliable weights than does a conventional scale. Injectable agents may require dilution; otherwise, the dose may be too small to measure or administer accurately. The dose of injectable anesthetics given to pediatric animals is often one half to two thirds of the dose given to mature animals because young animals have less plasma protein binding of drugs and lack an efficient mechanism to metabolize drugs within the liver. Injectable anesthetic agents that require liver metabolism for inactivation (for example, thiopental and pentobarbital) can be expected to have a prolonged effect in puppies or kittens younger than 8 weeks and should be avoided. Renal function is also inefficient in animals younger than 4 weeks, and excretion of drugs by this route may be slow. Xylazine or medetomidine may cause significant bradycardia in animals younger than 4 weeks and should be avoided. Injectable agents used for chemical restraint should be short acting and administered at low doses. Examples include acepromazine (0.03 mg/kg) plus butorphanol (0.2 mg/kg) or meperidine (4 mg/kg) given IM. If the patient is still nursing, acepromazine is normally unnecessary. Atropine (0.04 mg/kg SQ) is commonly used to prevent bradycardia, but response to this agent is unpredictable in animals younger than 14 days.

Many veterinarians prefer to anesthetize patients younger than 3 months with inhalant agents (particularly sevoflurane or isoflurane) because administration and elimination of these agents is accomplished without IV injections and patient recovery tends to be rapid. Intubation may be difficult in pediatric patients because of their small body size. The larynx is difficult to see, and use of a laryngoscope may be required. It is often necessary to cut endotracheal tubes short to avoid bronchial intubation or excessive dead space.

Apart from obvious differences in size, monitoring of pediatric patients during anesthesia is similar to adults. The anesthetist should be particularly watchful for bradycardia, which is associated with poor cardiac output in the anesthetized animal younger than 4 weeks. Another common problem during anesthesia of neonatal patients is hypoxia. A Bain or other low-resistance nonrebreathing system may be preferred in small patients.

Pediatric patients are prone to hypothermia because of their lack of subcutaneous fat, their relatively large surface area, and their inability to shiver. Hypothermia, if severe, may cause cardiac arrest. Heat loss during surgery can be avoided by using warmed IV fluids and circulating warm water heating pads.

Brachycephalic dogs

Technicians are often called on to anesthetize brachycephalic dogs such as the English bulldog, pug, Boston terrier, and Pekingese. Because of their conformation, these animals may have one or more anatomic characteristics that impede air exchange. These include very small nasal openings, an elongated soft palate, and a small-diameter trachea. Any anesthetic agent that depresses respiration or reduces muscle tone in the pharyngeal and laryngeal area may cause increased respiratory difficulty in these animals. In some cases this may be fatal, particularly if the animal is not intubated and if an open airway cannot be maintained. These problems are most evident in animals undergoing an operation to correct conformation defects in the larynx or pharynx (for example, soft palate resection) because postoperative swelling or hemorrhage often increases the risk of respiratory difficulty.

In addition to their respiratory problems, many brachycephalic animals also have abnormally high parasympathetic tone, which may cause bradycardia. Use of atropine or glycopyrrolate in these patients may help to increase heart rates before surgery. Acepromazine is also useful as a preanesthetic agent, particularly in young and healthy dogs, although opioids may be preferable in calm or sick animals. Butorphanol is commonly used because it depresses the cough reflex (allowing prolonged intubation into the recovery period) and causes less respiratory compromise than other opioids.

The induction period is particularly difficult for brachycephalic dogs. If possible, the anesthetist should preoxygenate brachycephalic patients for 5 minutes before induction. This is done by gently restraining the animal and administering oxygen through a face mask. This procedure helps maintain adequate blood oxygen levels and gives the animal an extra margin of safety during the induction period that follows.

Induction should be rapid, and for this reason IV induction agents are generally preferred over mask induction. Agents that are rapidly metabolized (for example, propofol, ketamine/diazepam, and methohexital) are preferred. The dog must be deeply enough anesthetized to allow rapid and efficient intubation. Difficulties may be encountered during intubation because of the large amount of redundant tissue in the pharynx. This reduces visibility of the laryngeal opening, and the use of a laryngoscope is helpful in these patients. The anesthetist may find that the endotracheal tube that fits the trachea is smaller than that expected, considering the size and weight of the dog. For example, a 35-kg bulldog may not accommodate a tube greater than 6 mm in diameter.

Anesthesia usually can be safely maintained through the use of an inhalation anesthetic. With the help of an endotracheal tube, breathing during anesthesia may in fact be superior to that of the healthy, awake brachycephalic animal. Because dyspnea is common in these dogs early in the recovery period, it is better to use anesthetics that allow rapid recovery (particularly isoflurane and sevoflurane) so that these animals can quickly regain normal respiratory function.

After surgery, the patient should be observed closely until it is extubated and is breathing well. Vigilance is necessary well into the recovery period because patients have had airway obstructions even after attempting to stand. The endotracheal tube should be left in place as long as possible (until the patient begins to chew) because the animal will maintain an open airway as long as the tube is in place. Oxygen should be delivered until the patient is extubated. Once the endotracheal tube is removed, the animal's head and neck should be extended, and the animal should be watched closely for dyspnea and cyanosis. If dyspnea is seen, the mouth should be kept open with a mouth gag and the tongue pulled forward. Administration of oxygen by mask or even reinduction (with ketamine/diazepam, propofol, or other IV induction agent) and reintubation are occasionally necessary. It is advisable to have supplemental oxygen and supplies for reintubation (that is, a laryngoscope, endotracheal tube, and the appropriate dose of an inducing agent) readily available in the recovery area in case dyspnea occurs after extubation. After reinduction, anesthesia with an inhalation agent can be continued for an additional 15 minutes, at which time the patient can be awakened and evaluated. Administration of dexamethasone (0.25 to 0.5 mg/kg IV) is helpful to reduce swelling in the laryngeal area.

Excitement and stress should be minimized as much as possible in the recovery period, especially if airway surgery was carried out. Some patients may require mild tranquilization or the use of opioid analgesics to reduce the rapid respirations that can aggravate laryngeal swelling.

Sighthounds

Several canine breeds (including the greyhound, saluki, Afghan hound, whippet, and Russian wolfhound) show increased sensitivity to anesthetic agents, particularly barbiturates such as thiopental. The reason for this increased sensitivity is not well understood, but it may involve a lack of body fat for redistribution of the drug and inefficient hepatic metabolism of many drugs. Fortunately, many other agents (including diazepam and ketamine, methohexital, propofol, isoflurane, and sevoflurane) can be safely used in these animals.

Obese animals

Some patients presented for anesthesia have a high percentage of body fat. Because the blood supply to fat is relatively poor, anesthetics are not efficiently distributed to fat stores. Obese dogs, therefore, require less injectable anesthetic on a per kilogram basis than do healthy dogs. It is advisable to decrease the dose of preanesthetic and injectable anesthetic agents so that the animal is dosed according to a weight halfway between the normal breed weight and the actual weight.

Obese animals also may have some degree of respiratory difficulty, further complicating the anesthetic process. Dogs that show respiratory difficulties should receive oxygen by face mask for 5 minutes before induction. They may also require the use of induction techniques similar to those used in brachycephalic dogs.

Obese dogs often exhibit rapid shallow respirations during anesthesia because they have less compliant chest walls compared with nonobese animals and cannot increase tidal volume. Instead, they compensate for increasing blood CO_2 levels and decreasing oxygen levels by increasing the respiratory rate. The anesthetist who observes persistent rapid and shallow respirations should assume control over respiration by bagging the patient with oxygen and anesthetic, once every 5 seconds, until slower respirations are observed.

Cesarean sections

The anesthetist for animals undergoing cesarean operation must be aware of the special needs not only of the patient undergoing the surgery, but also of the neonates being delivered. Anesthetic drugs administered to the pregnant patient (with the exception of neuromuscular blocking agents and local anesthetics) will readily cross the placenta and affect the newborn. Although it is essential that the patient receive adequate anesthetic agent to provide immobilization and analgesia for the surgery, it is advisable to use minimal doses of those agents that depress respiration in the puppies or kittens.

The pregnant female patient is at increased anesthetic risk for several reasons. Advanced pregnancy greatly increases the workload of the heart, particularly when the patient is in dorsal recumbency. Additionally, the pressure of the abdominal organs on the diaphragm compromises respiratory function. Pregnant animals are prone to vomiting or reflux of gastric contents because of pressure from the uterus on the stomach. (Studies of human cesarean procedures have shown that aspiration of vomit causes approximately 50% of maternal anesthetic deaths.) Additionally, the patient may be exhausted before the operation begins, particularly if the owner has delayed bringing the animal in for veterinary attention.

Hemorrhage from the uterus is a common complication of cesarean surgery, and even nonhemorrhaging patients have an increased risk of shock. It is therefore advisable that an IV catheter and intraoperative fluid administration be routinely used in cesarean patients. In dogs, a fluid administration rate of 10 ml/kg is adequate if the patient is not dehydrated or hemorrhaging. Dehydrated patients require 20 to 30 ml/kg (given over a half hour), and patients with ongoing hemorrhage may require shock dosages (50 to 90 ml/kg in the first hour).

It is helpful to do most of the shaving and other presurgical preparation of the patient before induction to reduce the anesthesia time. Whether the patient is awake or anesthetized, it is advisable that patient clipping and surgical preparation be done as much as possible with the patient gently restrained in left lateral recumbency rather than in dorsal recumbency. The latter position may cause the heavy uterus to compress the vena cava, decreasing venous return to the heart.

The administration of oxygen through a mask for 5 minutes before induction is called *preoxygenation*. This technique helps to prevent neonatal hypoxia. After induction, all patients should be intubated to protect the airway from obstruction in case of regurgitation or vomiting. Intubation also allows assisted ventilation, should the patient demonstrate hypoventilation.

The following various anesthetic techniques are used for cesarean operations, depending on the preference of the veterinarian:

- Epidural analgesia (Chapter 7) combined with a tranquilizer or neuroleptanalgesic is popular because this technique, once mastered, provides inexpensive but effective anesthesia with minimal depression of the patient or the neonates. IV fluids and oxygen should be administered in conjunction with epidural analgesia.
- General anesthesia with a variety of injectable and inhalant agents is also commonly used, with anesthetics given at the lowest effective dose to maintain anesthesia without unnecessarily depressing pediatric respiration. Preanesthetic tranquilizers such as acepromazine or alpha-2 agonists should be used at minimal doses or not at all. Recent studies and clinical experience indicate that premedications are often not needed in these patients, because they are usually amenable to catheterization, preoxygenation, and other procedures without these drugs. Propofol, low-dose thiopental, or mask induction with an inhalation agent is commonly used to induce these patients. If mask induction is used, the head should be elevated to avoid regurgitation. Because of the dam's increased sensitivity to medications, the dose of inhalant anesthetic required for maintenance is often reduced by up to 40%.
- The use of nitrous oxide may be helpful to supplement opioids or inhalation agents because it reduces the amount of other agents required and has minimal effects on respiration in the newborn animal. The anesthetist should be aware of the possibility of diffusion hypoxia in newborn animals delivered from mothers receiving nitrous oxide, and oxygen should be administered to each puppy or kitten immediately after delivery.
- Pentobarbital is considered to be a high-risk agent and should be avoided because pediatric mortality may approach 100%.
- Use of diazepam as a preanesthesia or induction agent should be avoided because puppies and kittens are depressed by this agent and may hypoventilate.
- Opioid agents are used by many veterinarians to provide analgesia in patients undergoing cesarean surgery. They should be reversed if significant respiratory depression is seen in either the dam or the neonate.

Puppies or kittens delivered by cesarean section often show signs of reduced respiratory and cardiovascular function when first delivered. *If no heartbeat can be detected,* external chest massage should be undertaken. The animal should be placed in the palm of the hand, and the chest compressed between the thumb and fingers approximately 120 times per minute. The newborn animal can be intubated with a 16- or 18-gauge IV catheter and gently bagged with oxygen every 5 seconds. The administration of epinephrine, reversing agents, and/or doxapram (injected into the root of the tongue) is helpful in some situations. Aspiration of fluid from the mouth and nose with an eyedropper or bulb syringe can also be attempted. *If a slow heartbeat is detected,* a drop of dilute atropine (0.25 mg/ml) can be placed under the tongue or injected into the tongue. The chest can be gently rubbed to stimulate breathing. If breathing appears inadequate or if cyanosis is seen, oxygen should be administered by face mask.

Newborn animals are prone to hypothermia and should be wrapped in a warm towel or placed in an incubator. They should be placed with the mother and encouraged to nurse as soon as the mother appears to be recovered from anesthesia (or, with supervision, during the recovery period). The dam may be disoriented and should be closely watch to ensure the safety of the puppies or kittens. Anesthetic agents and analgesic secreted in the milk appear to have little effect on nursing ability or neonatal viability.

Trauma patients

Animals that have recently undergone trauma, such as being hit by a car, may have numerous ailments that greatly increase anesthetic risk. Respiratory difficulties are common and may be the result of pneumothorax, pulmonary contusions and hemorrhage, airway obstruction, or diaphragmatic hernia. Cardiac arrhythmias are often seen in the first 12 to 72 hours after chest trauma. Shock is also common in animals that have undergone significant trauma, particularly if hemorrhage has been severe. Serious internal injuries such as fractures and herniated or ruptured organs may pose further difficulties for the veterinarian and anesthetist. Animals with head injuries may show altered responses to anesthetic agents and analgesics (see following section).

Few trauma patients require anesthesia immediately after the accident, and as a general rule it is wise to stabilize these animals before anesthesia. Delaying anesthesia offers two advantages: (1) it allows time for a thorough workup to assess the extent of the injuries, and (2) it provides some time to stabilize the animal's condition (which reduces anesthetic risk). The patient should be closely monitored for signs of dyspnea, cardiac arrhythmias, cardiovascular shock, and decreased response to outside stimuli such as talking or petting.

It is advisable to obtain thoracic radiographs before repair of fractures and other injuries resulting from trauma. Studies have shown that one third of patients with traumatic forelimb, hind limb, or pelvic injuries have concurrent thoracic injuries that could jeopardize the safety of anesthesia. It is obviously advisable to identify and treat a disorder such as pneumothorax before anesthetizing an animal for the repair of a fractured femur. The veterinarian may also request an ECG as part of the preanesthetic workup. Fortunately, many thoracic injuries improve with cage rest, and if anesthesia can be delayed for 24 to 72 hours after the traumatic incident, the anesthetist may encounter fewer problems.

Central nervous system disease

Patients with central nervous system (CNS) disorders such as epilepsy, head injury, or spinal cord trauma are occasionally presented for anesthesia. Diagnostic procedures such as cerebrospinal fluid (CSF) taps or myelograms usually require general anesthesia to achieve adequate patient restraint. Comatose patients and animals with a reduced level of consciousness, however, may require little or no anesthetic agent for these procedures.

Some anesthetics should be avoided or used with extreme caution in animals with CNS disorders. These include agents that lower the seizure threshold or cause seizures (ketamine, tiletamine, methohexital) and agents that can increase intracranial pressure (ketamine, morphine). Some agents are considered relatively safe, including diazepam and midazolam (both of which help to prevent postoperative seizures) and low doses of opioids, thiopental, and propofol. General anesthetics (particularly isoflurane) can be used; however, the anesthetist must be aware that inhalation agents have the potential to increase intracranial pressure, which leads to decreased brain perfusion and may result in brain damage. This can be prevented by ensuring that the patient's blood carbon dioxide levels remain in the low to normal range (ideally, end tidal CO_2 of 28 to 32 mm Hg, corresponding to a $Paco_2$ of 30 to 35 mm Hg). Patients' lungs are often manually ventilated at a rate of 15 breaths per minute (at 15 cm pressure for small dogs and 20 cm pressure for large dogs) for the first few minutes of anesthesia to ensure that carbon dioxide is blown off.

Cardiovascular disease

Common cardiovascular disorders found in patients scheduled for anesthesia include shock, cardiomyopathy (primary or secondary to hyperthyroidism), cardiac arrhythmias, congestive heart disease (often resulting from mitral valve insufficiency), and congenital heart defects such as a patent ductus arteriosus. In some areas, heartworm disease is also common, although affected animals may be asymptomatic. Signs of heart disease may include a rapid heart rate, irregular pulse, respiratory problems (coughing, panting, dyspnea), poor tolerance for exercise, syncope (fainting), cyanosis (particularly when stressed), and ascites.

Animals with severe cardiac disease are challenging anesthetic patients. A heart that is struggling to maintain function even in a rested, unstressed dog may be unable to respond to the stress of hospitalization, anesthesia, and surgery. Some preanesthetics and general anesthetics may cause further deterioration of cardiac function. However, many of these animals have serious problems (such as severe dental disease) that require anesthesia. The decision of whether to proceed with anesthesia in the compromised cardiac patient is sometimes a difficult one for the veterinarian and client to make.

As with patients that have undergone recent trauma, it is generally advisable to stabilize the patient's condition before anesthesia by treating cardiovascular and respiratory disease to alleviate the symptoms as much as possible. Many animals with heart disease have concurrent pulmonary disease, particularly pulmonary edema, which further complicates anesthesia. Diuretics such as furosemide (Lasix) may be helpful in alleviating pulmonary edema before anesthesia.

Anesthetic risk can be reduced in several ways. Premedications should be avoided or used at low doses only as needed to minimize pain and excitement (which causes epinephrine release and may lead to arrhythmias). Atropine may not be given initially but is sometimes used intraoperatively if bradycardia is seen. Preoxygenation with a face mask or oxygen chamber for 5 minutes immediately before induction is extremely helpful in reducing anesthetic risk in animals with cardiovascular or respiratory difficulties, provided it does not stress the patient. Ventilatory support (bagging or the use of a ventilator) may be required throughout anesthesia. Anesthetic agents that depress the myocardium or increase the workload of the heart or exacerbate arrhythmias (for example, xylazine, medetomidine, atropine, thiopental, ketamine, and halothane) are avoided as much as possible in these animals. Opioid agents, diazepam, etomidate, and isoflurane offer the advantage of relative lack of toxicity to the heart.

Animals with cardiac disease may have increased circulation times, and injectable drugs may take longer than expected to exert their effects. Additionally, some cardiac medications may affect the patient's response to anesthetic agents or analgesics. For example, angiotensin-converting enzyme (ACE) inhibitors such as enalapril and benazepril may reduce the effectiveness of some nonsteroidal antiinflammatory drugs.

When anesthetizing animals with cardiovascular problems, the anesthetist should be aware of the increased risk of overhydration through excessive or too rapid administration of IV fluids. Even an infusion rate of 10 ml/kg/hr may be excessive for these animals. It is advisable to frequently monitor the anesthetized patient for signs of overhydration such as ocular or nasal discharge, increased lung sounds (moist rales), and increased respiratory rate. Central venous pressure monitoring, if available, is useful to detect overhydration.

Respiratory disease

Of all the animals that undergo anesthesia, those with respiratory problems are perhaps the most challenging for the anesthetist. Because of the importance of this problem, all patients that are to undergo anesthesia should be carefully evaluated for the rate, depth, and nature of respiration. Patients showing signs of dyspnea must be handled cautiously to avoid stress or excitement, which may greatly exacerbate the breathing difficulty.

Before anesthesia, thoroughly evaluate the animal and, if possible, find the cause of the respiratory distress. Radiographs and thoracocentesis may be particularly helpful. Thoracocentesis is not only useful in diagnosis but also may be therapeutic if large volumes of air or fluid can be removed from the chest.

Examples of respiratory disorders include pleural effusion (that is, free fluid present in the chest cavity), diaphragmatic hernia, pneumothorax, pulmonary contusions resulting from trauma, pneumonia, tracheal collapse, and pulmonary edema. Patients with these disorders are often hypoxic and may show signs of tachypnea, dyspnea, and cyanosis.

If possible, anesthesia should be delayed until respiratory function has improved. If surgery is absolutely required (for example, to place a chest tube), local analgesia and gentle manual restraint may be preferable to general anesthesia. In the awake patient, administration of oxygen through a nasal line or other means (described in Chapter 2) is helpful in alleviating hypoxia.

Nitrous oxide should be avoided in patients with respiratory distress because the administration of 100% oxygen is usually necessary to maintain adequate oxygenation. In animals with diaphragmatic hernia, nitrous oxide may also cause distention of the stomach and intestines.

One of the most common procedures requiring anesthesia of an animal in respiratory distress is surgical repair of a diaphragmatic hernia. When these patients are being prepared for anesthesia, it is advisable to preoxygenate for 5 to 10 minutes before induction. Head-down positions should be avoided before and during anesthesia because they may result in further movement of abdominal organs into the thorax. If possible, an induction method that allows rapid intubation (that is, use of an injectable agent) is preferred over mask induction. Administration of the IV induction agent should be stopped as soon as the patient loses consciousness and is able to be intubated. During induction, some patients may show signs of respiratory depression and even respiratory arrest, and the anesthetist must be prepared to intubate rapidly and assist or control ventilation. Ventilatory assistance may be provided by periodic or continuous "bagging" of the patient, or a ventilator may be used. A respiratory rate of 8 to 20 breaths per minute is adequate, with a pressure of 10 to 20 cm water (H_2O) and a tidal volume of 10 to 15 ml/kg. The animal should be closely observed for cyanosis. Pulse oximetry, capnography, and arterial blood gas determination are helpful aids for assessing ventilation. Before closure, gentle ventilation may help to inflate collapsed lung tissue; however, this must be done cautiously to avoid pulmonary trauma (starting with an inflation pressure of 5 to 10 cm H_2O and increasing up to 20 cm H_2O if necessary). The surgeon should watch the lungs reinflate and advise the anesthetist accordingly. The inspiratory pressure should be held for 1 to 2 seconds at a time, then the pressure returned to zero before reinflating.

These patients require close observation during the recovery period. Administration of oxygen should be continued if signs of respiratory distress are seen. Pneumothorax is common after chest surgery, and affected patients may require chest tube placement or removal of air from the pleural space with a syringe and needle.

Hepatic disease

Animals with liver disease are at increased anesthetic risk because of that organ's central role in drug metabolism, synthesis of blood clotting factors and serum proteins, and carbohydrate metabolism. Some animals with liver disease are hypoproteinemic, which may lead to increased potency of barbiturate agents. Patients with chronic liver failure are also commonly dehydrated, thin, and icteric, and may be anemic and/or hypoglycemic. Ideally, the patient with hepatic disease that is undergoing anesthesia and surgery should have a packed cell volume greater than 25% (or a hemoglobin level greater than 8 g/dl) a total protein level over 3.5 g/dl, and normal clotting times.

Injectable drugs should be given with caution or omitted from the protocol because most of these agents require hepatic metabolism before they can be excreted. Recovery from anesthesia is often slow in patients with liver disease, in part because of the impaired metabolism of drugs. Xylazine, medetomidine, and acepromazine in particular may have long-lasting effects in patients with compromised hepatic function. In dogs, the use of ketamine and diazepam should also be avoided because both agents require liver metabolism. Preanesthetic sedation and analgesia, if required, can be accomplished by administration of low doses of opioids.

If severe hepatic disease is present, induction and maintenance of anesthesia are best achieved with isoflurane or propofol, which require little or no hepatic function for elimination. Halothane, although not directly hepatotoxic, is metabolized to free radicals that may be harmful to the liver.

The anesthetist should take special care to closely monitor the patient to ensure that it does not become hypotensive, hypothermic, or hypoxic during surgery. Patients with hepatic disease also are prone to hypoglycemia, and it is helpful to administer glucose-containing fluids such as 2.5% dextrose in a balanced electrolyte solution during anesthesia.

Renal disease

The kidneys are the organs most involved in maintaining the volume and electrolyte composition of body fluids. This helps explain why animals with renal disease are often dehydrated and may have severe electrolyte or acid-base imbalances, including metabolic acidosis and hyperkalemia. Animals with renal disease also may have elevated levels of waste products in their blood, including urea and creatinine. Hypertension, anemia, and hypoproteinemia are also seen in some patients with renal disease. Tests such as urinalysis (especially urine-specific gravity), blood urea nitrogen (BUN), and creatinine may be useful in obtaining an accurate picture of renal function. Normal urine production is no less than 1 ml/kg/hr in dogs and should be considerably greater if the patient is receiving IV fluids.

Preoperative water deprivation may not be advisable in patients with renal disease because dehydration may occur rapidly after withdrawal of oral fluids. Water should be offered up to 1 hour before premedication. The patient with renal disease should be rehydrated with parenteral fluids as much as possible before surgery, and electrolyte problems should be identified and addressed. Administration of IV fluids is often continued throughout the anesthetic and postanesthetic period (at a rate of 10 ml/kg/hr) until the animal is fully hydrated and able to drink unassisted.

If possible, blood pressure should be monitored during anesthesia of renal patients to ensure that hypotension (which may result in reduced blood supply to the kidneys) does not occur. Use of injectable nonsteroidal antiinflammatory drugs such as ketoprofen during anesthesia may further compromise renal function, especially if hypotension is present.

Many preanesthetic and anesthetic agents and their metabolites are eliminated from the body by renal excretion. For this reason, animals with compromised renal function may show prolonged recovery after anesthesia if conventional dosages are used. It is prudent to avoid or reduce dosages of injectable anesthetic drugs (including acepromazine, medetomidine, xylazine, diazepam, ketamine, and barbiturates) in these patients. Barbiturates, in particular, have increased potency in acidotic and uremic animals and should be used with great caution in patients with renal disease. Inhalation agents (particularly isoflurane and sevoflurane) have some advantages over injectable agents, although halothane and methoxyflurane can produce fluoride ions, which are damaging to the kidneys.

Animals with urinary blockages (including male cats with urethral obstructions due to struvite crystals) pose similar problems to the anesthetist. Many of these cats are depressed, dehydrated, uremic, acidotic, and hyperkalemic. Hyperkalemic animals are at particular risk of cardiac arrest.[*] Hyperkalemic patients may sometimes be identified by auscultation because bradycardia is often present if plasma potassium levels exceed 6 mEq/L. Treatment of hyperkalemia may require the use of sodium bicarbonate, 10% calcium gluconate, and/or dextrose, and it should be done only with close supervision and guidance from the veterinarian. Conditions stressful to the animal should be avoided as much as possible because the release of epinephrine from the adrenal glands may potentiate cardiac arrhythmias.

---

[*]If possible, anesthesia should be delayed for any patient with a blood potassium level of 5.5 mEq/L or greater until the potassium concentration is within the normal range.

The administration of inhalation agents (particularly isoflurane) to cats with urinary blockages may be less hazardous than the use of injectable drugs because renal excretion is not required for patient recovery. Propofol or ketamine/diazepam may be used IV with caution and at reduced dosages, provided normal kidney function is present. Obstructed cats showing extreme depression may not require general anesthesia, particularly if a local anesthetic such as lidocaine gel or 0.5 ml of 2% lidocaine is administered as part of the urethral catheterization procedure.

RESPONSE TO ANESTHETIC PROBLEMS AND EMERGENCIES

Despite every precaution, the veterinary technician is likely to encounter anesthetic emergencies several times during the course of a career. The nature of the technician's response may mean the difference between life and death for the anesthetized patient.

Role of the Veterinary Technician in Emergency Care

Ideally, emergency response is a team effort involving the veterinarian, technician, and other hospital staff. Normally the veterinarian acts as the team leader, directing the staff in emergency procedures. However, the veterinarian may be performing surgery on the patient when an anesthetic emergency arises and therefore may have other pressing concerns besides anesthesia. The technician must be prepared to take an active role in resuscitating the patient and not rely solely on the veterinarian, who is already busy. Constant communication between the veterinarian and the technician is obviously important under these circumstances.

It is a good idea to conduct periodic "dress rehearsals" or mock resuscitations in which all staff members participate. Everyone in the hospital should be familiar with the location of the crash kit and IV fluids. Procedures such as warming towels in a clothes dryer, making up hot water bottles, and drawing up drugs into a syringe can be readily taught to all hospital staff and, once mastered by them, will free the veterinarian and technician to perform more demanding tasks.

Occasionally an emergency arises when the veterinarian is absent from the hospital or unavailable to assist. For example, seizures may occur in the postoperative recovery period. Most state and provincial regulations allow the technician to undertake emergency care if the veterinarian is absent. It is advisable to discuss in advance the procedures that the veterinarian authorizes the technician to do in an emergency to protect the veterinarian and technician from liability and to ensure optimum patient care. It is helpful to have written instructions available in the form of an emergency protocol authorized by the veterinarian.

When responding to an emergency, the technician should bear in mind the principles of emergency care listed in Procedure 6-1.

It cannot be assumed that every anesthetic emergency should be treated in the same way. For example, the veterinarian and animal owner may choose not to resuscitate a severely ill or debilitated animal that undergoes cardiac arrest during anesthesia. Cost considerations may influence the treatment given in some cases. Emergency care is labor intensive, and treatment costs may be considerable. Most veterinarians, however, will not stop to consider cost if the emergency arises during a routine operation, such as a spay, and will do everything possible to revive the animal.

PROCEDURE 6-1	Responding to an Emergency

1. The technician should take a few seconds to think before doing anything. After consulting with the veterinarian, the technician should mentally list the most important things to be done and undertake them in order of priority.
2. Every veterinary practice should have a well-stocked crash kit for use in emergency situations within the hospital. A list of supplies that may be useful in a crash kit is given in Appendix C.
3. Useful emergency drugs are listed in Tables 6-3 and 6-4. Doses for emergency drugs should be posted or listed on a paper kept in the crash kit. Emergency drugs kept in the crash kit should be periodically checked to ensure that they have not expired. In particular, epinephrine has a short shelf life and should not be used if a brown discoloration is present.
4. Above all, the technician should do no harm. In an emergency it is easy to panic and do things that are not only unnecessary but also potentially harmful to the animal, including performing cardiac compressions or giving epinephrine to an animal whose heart is still beating. Sometimes the best course of action is to watch, monitor, and wait.
5. After an anesthetic emergency, the technician, veterinarian, and hospital staff should discuss the reasons why the emergency arose and determine what could be done to prevent the same thing from happening again. The adequacy of the resuscitation efforts should be analyzed, and if a problem exists, it should be addressed.

Emergency Situations that May Arise during Anesthesia

Although anesthetic emergencies are by their nature unpredictable, certain problems occur with some frequency. The following situations are addressed in detail:
- Animals that will not stay anesthetized
- Animals that are too deeply anesthetized
- Pale mucous membranes
- Hypotension
- Hypoventilation
- Cyanosis and dyspnea
- Tachypnea
- Respiratory arrest
- Cardiac arrest

Intervention guidelines for these emergencies are summarized in Table 6-2.

Animals that will not stay anesthetized

Occasionally, the anesthetist will have difficulty in maintaining a patient at sufficient anesthetic depth. Often the veterinarian becomes aware of the problem when the patient shows signs of movement in response to surgical stimulation. If depth appears inadequate, the anesthetist should check the following:
- Has the vaporizer been turned off, or is the setting too low to maintain an adequate depth of anesthesia?
- Is the oxygen on?

TABLE 6-2

Intervention Guidelines for Anesthetized Dogs and Cats

VITAL SIGN	NORMAL (ANESTHETIZED)		REQUIRES TREATMENT		CRITICAL LEVEL	
	DOG	CAT	DOG	CAT	DOG	CAT
Respiratory rate (breaths per minute)	8-15	12-18	<8	<10	<4	<6
Heart rate* (beats per minute)	70-120	130-170	<60 or >140	<110 or >200	<40 or >175	<100 or >225
Arterial blood pressure (mm Hg)	100 (Mean)	120 (Systolic)	<60 (Mean)	<100 (Systolic)	<50 (Mean)	<80 (Systolic)
Temperature	100°-102° F 38°-39° C		<98° F/37° C >103°F/39° C		<95° F/36° C >104° F/40° C	

Modified from Brock N, Anesthesia Northwest.
*Note that heart rates vary between breeds of dog, with toy breeds generally having higher rates than larger dogs. Value will vary for animals given preanesthetic agents such as atropine or alpha-2 agonists.

- Does the vaporizer contain anesthetic?
- Is the endotracheal tube in the esophagus? This can be easily determined by checking to see if the reservoir bag expands and contracts with the appropriate tidal volume as the animal breathes. If so, the endotracheal tube is likely in the trachea. Movement of the reservoir bag also tells the anesthetist that the endotracheal tube is connected to the Y piece and that the tube is not blocked. Other procedures used to determine the location and patency of the endotracheal tube include palpation of the neck and gentle compression of the reservoir bag to see if the chest expands.
- Is the end of the endotracheal tube located within a bronchus? Animals with endobronchial intubation are difficult to maintain at adequate anesthetic depth. To determine if endobronchial intubation is present, use a second endotracheal tube of the same length as the one in the patient and lay it against the patient to verify that the distal tip does not extend past the first rib.
- Is air leaking around the endotracheal tube? If so, the patient may be breathing room air, which dilutes the anesthetic gas entering the lungs. Air leakage can be detected by closing the pop-off valve, inflating the reservoir bag, and gently pressing on the bag while listening for the sound of air escaping from the animal's mouth. A soft hiss of escaping air is acceptable, but a large gush of exiting air should warn the anesthetist that either the endotracheal tube is too small or the cuff is not sufficiently inflated. If this is the case, the cuff can be further inflated, the tube replaced, or the pharyngeal area packed with damp gauze.
- Is the animal holding its breath? This is most commonly seen immediately after the intubated animal is connected to the machine, particularly if propofol or ketamine/diazepam was used for induction. Prolonged breath holding may lead to arousal from anesthesia because vaporized anesthetic is not entering the lungs

or the bloodstream. If arousal appears imminent, it may be necessary to periodically bag the animal with a mixture of oxygen and anesthetic until adequate depth of anesthesia is achieved.

- Are the patient's respirations too shallow to draw sufficient anesthetic into the lungs? Rapid, shallow respiration, commonly seen in toy dogs and obese animals, may be associated with insufficient anesthetic depth. The anesthetist should assist ventilation by bagging these patients (with vaporizer on) every 5 seconds.
- Is the anesthetic machine assembled correctly and are all connections tight? Occasionally, hoses become detached from the machine or the endotracheal tube, in which case the patient obviously does not receive any anesthetic from the machine.
- Is the oxygen flow rate adequate to vaporize anesthetic? For some precision vaporizers, a minimum flow rate of 500 ml/min is necessary for accurate delivery of anesthetic (although some vaporizers may function at rates as low as 100 to 200 ml/min). Very high oxygen flow rates or excessive use of the oxygen flush valve may also result in unpredictable vaporization of anesthetic.
- Is the anesthetic machine functioning correctly? Repeated episodes of awakening during anesthesia may indicate poor vaporizer function. If a halothane or isoflurane vaporizer setting of 3% to 4% seems necessary to maintain anesthesia in many patients, cleaning and recalibration of the vaporizer are probably necessary.
- Is the exaggerated respiratory movement actually an agonal (near death) phenomenon, indicating dangerous anesthetic depth rather than a light plane? If this is a possibility, the patient's heart rate, pulse strength, mucous membranes, and depth indicators should be immediately assessed.

If none of the reasons just listed can explain the patient's arousal, the anesthetist should consult with the veterinarian. It may be necessary to increase the vaporizer setting or administer an analgesic or injectable inducing agent to achieve the desired anesthetic depth.

Animals that are too deeply anesthetized

An animal that is too deeply anesthetized will usually show the following signs:
- Respiration rate is 8 breaths per minute or less; respirations may be shallow or the patient may be breathing with difficulty.
- Mucous membranes are pale and may be cyanotic.
- Capillary refill may be greater than 2 seconds.
- The heart rate is bradycardic (less than 60 to 70 bpm in a dog or 100 bpm in a cat).
- The pulse is weak; systolic blood pressure is less than 80 mm Hg (indirect measurement).
- Cardiac arrhythmias may be present; QRS complexes (ventricular contractions) are irregular on the ECG, or abnormal complexes such as ventricular premature contractions (VPCs) may be present.
- The animal's extremities and ears are cold; body temperature is often less than 35° C.
- Reflexes are completely absent, including palpebral and corneal reflexes.
- Muscle tone is flaccid.
- Pupils may be dilated, and pupillary light reflex is absent.

The anesthetist should use judgment in interpreting these signs. The presence of one or two signs may not indicate excessive depth, provided the other signs are normal.

| PROCEDURE 6-2 | Treating Excessive Anesthetic Depth |

1. After concluding that the anesthetic depth is excessive, the anesthetist should immediately decrease the vaporizer setting (to zero, if necessary) and inform the veterinarian.
2. If the veterinarian decides that the animal's condition has deteriorated so that resuscitation efforts are warranted, the anesthetist should begin to bag the animal with pure oxygen. (This assumes that the patient is intubated and is undergoing gas anesthesia. If an injectable agent has been used, intubation and oxygen delivery by means of an anesthetic machine should be initiated immediately.)
3. To bag the animal, the anesthetist should close the pop-off valve part way, fill the reservoir bag with oxygen, and gently squeeze the bag until the animal's chest rises slightly (watch the pressure manometer, 15-20 cm H_2O).
4. This procedure should be repeated every 5 seconds until the animal shows signs of recovery (such as increased heart rate, stronger pulse, and improved mucous membrane color and refill).
5. The use of IV fluids, external heat, and drugs (as directed by the veterinarian) may also expedite recovery.
6. Occasionally the anesthetist may be unsure of whether a patient's anesthetic depth is excessive. If the veterinarian is not immediately available to advise on the patient's condition, it is safest to assume that the animal is too deep and to decrease the vaporizer setting, while observing the animal carefully for signs of arousal.

Vital signs also vary depending on the preanesthetic and general anesthetics used (for example, atropine may affect heart rate and pupil dilation). The more variables that the anesthetist considers, the more accurate the assessment of anesthetic depth is likely to be.

There are several reasons why anesthetic depth may be excessive. In most cases, the vaporizer setting is too high for the patient being anesthetized, or in the case of injectable agents, too high of a dose has been given. Occasionally, the animal may have a preexisting problem such as shock or anemia that increases susceptibility to anesthetic overdose.

Treatment of animals that are at an excessively deep plane of anesthesia is outlined in Procedure 6-2.

Pale mucous membranes

Pale mucous membranes may arise from several causes. Some patients have preexisting anemia resulting from diseases such as feline leukemia, hemolytic anemia, acute or chronic blood loss, neoplasia, or chronic renal disease. In other cases blood loss may have occurred during surgery. Some anesthetic agents (particularly inhalation agents, xylazine, and acepromazine) may cause vasodilation and decrease blood pressure, resulting in poor perfusion of capillary beds and pale mucous membranes in some animals. Hypothermia or pain can also reduce blood supply to the tissues and cause pale mucous membranes.

If pale mucous membranes are observed during surgery, follow Procedure 6-3.

PROCEDURE 6-3	Treating Pale Mucous Membranes

1. The anesthetist should ascertain the animal's anesthetic depth and monitor vital signs, including heart rate, respiration, pulse strength and coordination with heartbeat, and capillary refill time.
2. The veterinarian should be consulted because it may be necessary to initiate IV fluid therapy or a blood transfusion to stabilize the patient's condition.

Hypotension

Hypotension was the most common anesthetic complication found in a recent study of dogs and cats (Gaynor et al, 1999). Hypotension may be present before the induction of anesthesia, as in the case of animals undergoing emergency surgery after trauma. Hypotension or shock also may arise as a result of blood loss during surgery or may occur in patients that are at a very deep plane of anesthesia or in patients that have cardiac arrhythmias. Acepromazine and the inhalation agents may also cause hypotension in susceptible patients.

Monitoring of blood pressure is discussed in Chapter 2. In some hypotensive animals, capillary refill may be prolonged (that is, greater than 2 seconds), although this is seen also with decreased perfusion due to vasoconstriction or other causes. Transitory decreased perfusion is a common effect of alpha-2 agonists such as medetomidine. However, prolonged capillary refill should prompt the anesthetist to check blood pressure (by palpating the pulse or measuring blood pressure), monitor the heart rate, and check the temperature of the extremities. If hypotension is suspected, follow Procedure 6-4.

In some cases, hypotension is a symptom of an even more serious disorder, circulatory shock. The treatment for shock in the anesthetized patient is similar to that in the conscious patient and should be done under the supervision of a veterinarian.

Hypoventilation

Because of the respiratory depression induced by many preanesthetics and general anesthetics, it is common for anesthetized patients to hypoventilate. Other causes of hypoventilation include pulmonary disease, impaired circulation to the lungs, inadequate oxygen flow rates, obesity, head-down positions, abdominal distention (from ascites, pregnancy, or other causes), and airway obstruction. The anesthetist must be alert for signs of hypoventilation, including shallow excursions of the reservoir bag (if a rebreathing system is being used), mucous membrane discoloration, a deeper than expected plane of anesthesia, and pulse oximeter readings less than 95%. If this progresses to severe hypoxia, the animal may show cardiac arrhythmias, bradycardia, cyanosis, labored or rapid breathing, hypotension, and pulse oximeter readings less than 85%.

If hypoventilation is present, the anesthetist should inform the veterinarian and take steps to correct the cause, if known (for example, increase the oxygen flow rate and discontinue nitrous oxide administration). Breathing should be assisted by gently squeezing the reservoir bag (manual ventilation is further discussed in Chapter 7). If this is ineffective or if severe hypoxia is present, consult with the veterinarian and follow the steps outlined in Procedure 6-5.

PROCEDURE 6-4	Treating Hypotension

1. The anesthetist who observes a prolonged capillary refill time should immediately check the animal's pulse quality, heart rate, and blood pressure reading (if available). In an anesthetized dog or cat, a systolic blood pressure under 80 mm Hg or a mean arterial pressure less than 60 mm Hg indicates hypotension and poor perfusion.

2. If blood pressure readings are unavailable, the anesthetist can roughly estimate the systolic pressure by palpating a peripheral pulse. As a general rule, the absence of a palpable pulse at the metatarsal artery suggests a systolic pressure under 60 mm Hg, and the absence of a palpable pulse at the femoral artery suggests a systolic pressure under 40 mm Hg.

3. If pulse pressure is reduced, the anesthetist should closely observe the animal for other signs of shock, including hypothermia and tachycardia (or bradycardia in later stages of shock). As circulation to the extremities deteriorates, the surface temperature of the ears and paws is reduced. The heart may respond to the fall in blood pressure by increased rate and force of contraction, although this effect may not be present in deep anesthesia.

4. If shock is present, IV fluids should be administered at a rapid rate. Over the first 15 minutes, 20 ml/kg should be given, and the animal should be observed closely for a response. The maximum fluid administration rate for a patient in shock is 90 ml/kg for the first hour in the dog (or 65 ml/kg in the cat). The use of colloid therapy (plasma, dextran, hetastarch) or blood transfusions may be appropriate in some situations.

5. Anesthetic depth should be reduced, if possible, and 100% oxygen should be administered.

6. The patient must be kept warm through the use of supplemental heat in the form of warm towels, circulating warm water heating pads, hot water bottles, or similar devices.

7. Various drugs are recommended for the treatment of shock, including corticosteroids (prednisone sodium succinate, dexamethasone), sodium bicarbonate, and cardiac inotropes such as dopamine, ephedrine, or dobutamine. Administration of oxygen is helpful for both awake and anesthetized patients. Drugs that cause vasodilation (for example, acepromazine) should be avoided.

Dyspnea and/or cyanosis

Any patient showing dyspnea or cyanosis during the administration of an anesthetic should be immediately brought to the veterinarian's attention. The presence of dyspnea (respiratory difficulty) indicates that the animal is unable to obtain sufficient oxygen or remove adequate CO_2 using normal respiratory movements. Cyanosis (a bluish coloration of the mucous membranes) indicates that tissue oxygenation is inadequate. Pulse oximetry readings are usually less than 80% in these animals. Dyspnea and cyanosis often are seen together and may be followed by respiratory arrest, in which respiratory efforts cease and the amount of oxygen available to the tissues rapidly declines. Severe dyspnea is often accompanied by cardiac arrhythmias, hypotension, and bradycardia.

PROCEDURE 6-5	Treating Dyspnea

1. The anesthetist must first ensure that oxygen is being delivered to the patient. If the oxygen tank has run out, the patient must be disconnected from a nonrebreathing apparatus. If the patient is connected to a circle system and the rebreathing bag is moderately full, the animal can remain connected for 1 to 2 minutes while another oxygen source is secured.

2. Once oxygen flow has been established, the vaporizer should be turned off and the animal should be bagged with 100% oxygen. If the anesthetic machine is unavailable, an Ambu bag (Fig. 6-1) can be used to deliver room air to the patient. While initiating bagging, the anesthetist should observe the chest for movement. If the chest does not rise when the animal is bagged, the endotracheal tube or airway may be blocked, and the blockage must be relieved. Suspected endotracheal tube blockage can be confirmed by disconnecting the endotracheal tube from the Y piece and feeling for air passage through the tube when the patient breathes or the chest is gently compressed. Capnography, if available, will confirm if blockage has occurred. A blocked endotracheal tube must be removed and replaced.

3. If the chest does rise when the reservoir bag is squeezed, oxygen is being delivered to the lungs and bagging should be continued until the mucous membrane color improves or pulse oximeter readings rise to 90% to 95%. It is best to watch the

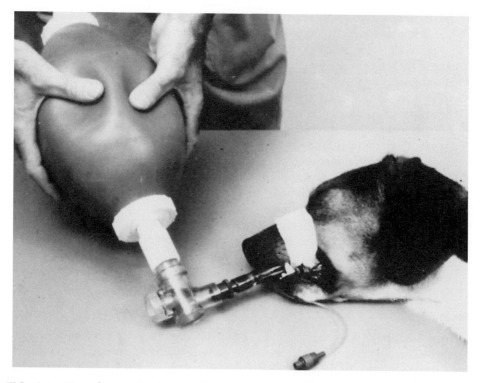

FIG. 6-1 Use of an Ambu bag to deliver room air to an intubated patient. (*From Muir WW III, Hubbell JAE, Skarda RT: Handbook of veterinary anesthesia, ed 3, St Louis, 2000, Mosby.*)

Continued

PROCEDURE 6-5   **Treating Dyspnea—cont'd**

anterior thorax for chest rise movement in the area of the heart, so as not to be misled by passive movement of the chest because of distention of the stomach by a misplaced endotracheal tube.

4. On rare occasions, dyspnea and cyanosis may result from complete airway obstruction. If intubation is not possible under these circumstances, the veterinarian may choose to perform an emergency tracheostomy, a surgical opening of the trachea to allow the insertion of a breathing tube. Alternatively, a 14-gauge IV catheter can be placed through the cricothyroid membrane and into the trachea. The catheter is connected to the barrel of a 3-ml syringe, which is in turn attached to the Y piece of an anesthetic machine for oxygen delivery.

5. Administration of IV fluids or emergency drugs may be helpful in reviving patients with respiratory depression or arrest.

6. The anesthetist should closely observe the patient during resuscitative efforts to ensure that cardiac arrest does not occur. If a pulse or heartbeat cannot be detected, cardiac compressions should be initiated in conjunction with continued bagging.

7. If necessary, supplemental oxygen should be continued into the recovery period, with a mask, oxygen cage, or intranasal insufflation.

The most common sources of respiratory distress during anesthesia are as follows:

- The animal is unable to obtain oxygen from the anesthetic machine because the oxygen supply has run out, the flowmeter has been turned off, or the flow of oxygen through the anesthetic machine or breathing system is blocked.

- The animal is unable to breathe normally because of airway obstruction or respiratory disease. Causes of airway obstruction include endotracheal tube blockage, accumulation of mucus in the trachea or endotracheal tube, excessive flexion of the head and neck, kinked endotracheal tube, laryngospasm, bronchoconstriction, aspiration of stomach contents after vomiting or regurgitation, or brachycephalic conformation. Common causes of respiratory disease include pneumothorax, pleural effusion, broken ribs, lung contusions, asthma, pulmonary edema, diaphragmatic hernia, and pleural effusion. Use of heavy surgical drapes or constricting bandages also may impair normal respiration.

- The reservoir bag is excessively full or empty.

- The animal is too deeply anesthetized, to the point that respiration and other vital functions are adversely affected.

Respiratory problems are potentially life threatening and should be addressed as discussed in Procedure 6-5.

Tachypnea

Tachypnea, or rapid respirations, must be differentiated from dyspnea, in which respiratory distress is present. Tachypnea may arise at any time during anesthesia and may be disconcerting to the anesthetist. It is particularly common during procedures in which opioids such as oxymorphone are used. If anesthetic depth is inadequate, tachypnea may occur in response to surgical stimulation, in which case it is often accompanied by tachycardia and spontaneous movement. Paradoxically, tachypnea

---

PROCEDURE 6-6   Treating Tachypnea

1. The anesthetist should assess the anesthetic depth and check the CO_2 absorber granules and capnograph reading (if available) to ensure that hypercapnia is not present. Signs of hypercapnia include tachycardia, hyperventilation, sweating, increased blood pressure, and brick-red mucous membranes.
2. Consider opioid-induced panting if patient has received morphine or another opioid drug.
3. If anesthetic depth, body temperature, and vital signs appear to be within acceptable limits, the anesthetist should refrain from changing the vaporizer setting because the condition will usually correct itself within 1 to 2 minutes.
4. If tachypnea arises as a result of surgical stimulation and the perception of pain, slow IV injection of an analgesic such as oxymorphone, hydromorphone, or butorphanol may be helpful.
5. Obese patients are prone to tachypnea, which may result in inefficient ventilation. It may be necessary to assist or control ventilation in these patients.

---

also may occur in deep anesthesia as a response to low blood oxygen and high blood carbon dioxide levels. Tachypnea is also seen in hyperthermic patients, including animals with malignant hyperthermia. If tachypnea is seen, follow Procedure 6-6.

Respiratory arrest

Respiratory arrest is the cessation of respiratory efforts by the patient. It may lead to cardiac arrest and is therefore a potentially fatal condition.

Not all cases of respiratory cessation require immediate action by the anesthetist. Respiratory efforts may temporarily cease after the IV injection of ketamine, barbiturates, propofol, and other induction agents. Minimal respiratory efforts may also be seen after a period of prolonged bagging with oxygen and, in this case, reflect low blood carbon dioxide and high blood oxygen levels. In both types of ventilatory arrest (whether the result of drug administration or bagging with oxygen) the anesthetist must be sure that other vital signs, particularly heart rate, mucous membrane color, and pulse strength are normal. If the heart rate is greater than 80 bpm and no arrhythmia is present, the pulse is strong, and mucous membranes are pink, the patient does not usually require immediate treatment for respiratory arrest. Pulse oximeter readings are helpful in indicating if the patient's oxygenation status is adequate (that is, a reading of 95% or greater usually indicates that bagging is not necessary). To be safe, the anesthetist can deliver occasional "breaths" of oxygen (one every 30 seconds) to the patient during this period to prevent hypoxia and hypercarbia. However, premature bagging with oxygen may extend the period of apnea by removing carbon dioxide from the blood, which is a stimulus for the patient to resume breathing. The anesthetist who suspects that respiratory efforts have temporarily ceased because of administration of drugs or ventilation with oxygen should closely monitor the patient's heart rate, pulse quality, and mucous membrane color for 1 to 2 minutes before assuming that a serious condition exists. If spontaneous respiration does not resume within this time (or if pulse oximeter readings fall below 95%), the veterinarian should be consulted, and it may be advisable to begin bagging the patient with oxygen while trying to determine the reason for the hypoxia.

True respiratory arrest is a serious emergency and requires immediate attention, because it will quickly lead to cardiac arrest if not effectively treated. This condition may arise because of anesthetic overdose, cessation of oxygen flow, or preexisting respiratory disease such as pneumothorax or diaphragmatic hernia. Affected animals may show warning signs such as dyspnea and/or cyanosis before respiratory arrest occurs. Other vital signs, such as heart rate, capillary refill, pulse strength, and pupil dilation, are often abnormal. Pulse oximetry values rapidly fall below 90%.

The treatment of respiratory arrest involves the steps outlined in Procedure 6-7.

Bagging should continue until the heart rate, pulse quality, mucous membrane color, and pulse oximeter values have been restored to normal. Once this is achieved, the anesthetist should discontinue bagging for 15 to 30 seconds and closely observe the patient for respiratory efforts. If no respiratory efforts are seen, bagging should resume.

On occasion, the anesthetist may be faced with a patient in respiratory arrest in the absence of an anesthetic machine. It is possible to substitute an Ambu bag or

---

PROCEDURE 6-7   Treatment of Respiratory Arrest

1. Inform the veterinarian.
2. Turn off the anesthetic vaporizer and nitrous oxide flow. Discontinue injectable anesthetic agents.
3. If the patient is not intubated, an endotracheal tube should be immediately inserted and the patient connected to an anesthetic machine delivering 100% oxygen. If a tube cannot be passed and the animal is severely hypoxic and unconscious, a tube tracheostomy should be performed. In this procedure, an endotracheal tube or tracheostomy tube is inserted directly into the trachea through a longitudinal incision immediately caudal to the larynx. The skin is incised over the ventral neck and the underlying muscle is separated such that the tracheal rings are seen. A transverse incision is made between tracheal rings, and the tube is inserted through this incision.
4. Check the heart rate to ensure that cardiac arrest has not occurred. Monitor patient with ECG if possible.
5. Ensure oxygen flow is adequate by checking the tank pressure gauge and flowmeter.
6. Ensure the airway is not obstructed by bagging the patient and observing that the chest rises on inspiration.
7. Bag with oxygen at a rate of once every 5 seconds. Continue bagging until vital signs improve (particularly mucous membrane color, heart rate, and pulse oximeter readings).
8. If an IV catheter is present, administer IV fluids at a rate suitable for treatment of shock.
9. The veterinarian may advise that doxapram, reversing agents, or other drugs be given.
10. Ensure that the patient is kept warm.

even institute mouth-to-endotracheal tube or mouth-to-muzzle resuscitation in these cases (see Fig. 6-1). An Ambu bag is a manually operated and self-filling reservoir bag used to assist breathing. The bag has a one-way valve that can be used to control air flow. Ambu bags may be attached to an oxygen source or may use room air (21% oxygen). Mouth-to-endotracheal tube resuscitation delivers approximately 14% oxygen and can be attempted if another oxygen source is unavailable.

Cardiac arrest

Cardiac arrest is defined as the sudden cessation of effective ventilation and circulation. Cardiac arrest may occur at any time during anesthesia. In many cases the anesthetist receives some warning that arrest is imminent, in the form of a short period in which cyanosis, dyspnea or respiratory arrest, tachycardia or bradycardia, cardiac arrhythmias, or prolonged capillary refill is evident. If cardiac arrest appears imminent, the anesthetist should immediately alert the veterinarian and the hospital staff while continuing to monitor the heart by auscultation, by palpation of the chest, or (preferably) through the use of an ECG. A patient with cardiac arrest rapidly has the following signs:

- In the awake animal, loss of consciousness within 10 to 15 seconds.
- No heartbeat can be auscultated or palpated.
- There is no palpable arterial pulse, and blood pressure readings are 25 mm Hg or less.
- The ECG tracing may be abnormal and can be used to classify the type of cardiac arrest. In *asystole* the ECG is a flat line, whereas in *ventricular fibrillation,* a wavy pattern is seen (Chapter 2). In *electromechanical dissociation,* normal QRS complexes may be present on the ECG, although there are no effective cardiac contractions.
- Mucous membranes are gray or cyanotic.
- Capillary refill may be prolonged or normal.
- Pupils are widely dilated with no response to light within 30 to 45 seconds of arrest.
- Respiration is absent except for intermittent, abrupt gasps.

Coordinated action by all hospital staff members is essential to reverse cardiac arrest. Once cardiac arrest occurs, permanent brain damage may result if oxygen delivery to the brain is not reestablished within 4 minutes, either by cardiopulmonary resuscitation or restoration of cardiac function. Ideally, at least four staff members should participate in the resuscitative efforts as follows: (1) performs chest compressions, (2) bags the animal, (3) assesses the pulse during compressions and checks the pulse or ECG when compressions are temporarily suspended, and (4) draws up and administers drugs on the veterinarian's orders and maintains a record of patient status and resuscitative treatments.

The essential steps in responding to a cardiac arrest may be summarized with the mnemonic ABCDEF (*a*irway, *b*reathing, *c*irculation, *d*rugs, *E*CG, *f*luids).

Airway and breathing. One staff member should note the time of arrest and immediately call for help. If the animal is intubated and connected to an anesthetic machine, initiate respiratory support by turning off the vaporizer and nitrous oxide flow and bagging the animal with 100% oxygen at the rate of one breath every 3 to 5 seconds. Mask administration of oxygen is inadequate; if an endotracheal tube is not in place, it is essential that the animal be intubated immediately. Additionally, the anesthetist must ensure that the patient's chest rises slightly during bagging, indicating that the airway is not blocked. The volume of chest expansion should be the same as expected for the animal when breathing normally: do not overinflate.

Circulation. Cardiac compressions should be initiated. The animal should be turned on its right side with its feet toward the person doing compressions and the head tilted down, if possible.

- *Cardiac compressions for a large dog:* A firm object such as a book, sandbag, or rolled-up towel should be placed under the dog's chest just behind the elbow. The heel of the compressor's hand should compress the chest against this object, with the pressure applied at the point where the chest is widest. Both hands should be used to compress the chest. The chest wall should be allowed to bounce back rapidly after each compression. Alternatively, the animal can be placed in dorsal recumbency and compression applied to the caudal one third of the sternum.
- *Cardiac compressions for a medium-sized dog:* One hand should be placed under the chest and the other hand placed at the fifth intercostal space, just over the heart itself (Fig. 6-2). The chest is then compressed between the two hands.
- *Cardiac compressions for a cat or small dog:* With the animal in lateral recumbency, compression is applied using the thumb to compress the chest against the fingers of the same hand.

The rate of compressions should be 1 to 2 times per second, depending on the size of the animal (for example, 80 times per minute for a large dog and up to 120 times per minute for a small dog or cat). The chest should be compressed by approximately one third the diameter of the chest wall. The aim of the compressions is to manually force blood through the heart and ultimately to the tissues. It is thought that compressions also may assist circulation by increasing pressure in the chest, indirectly inducing blood flow. Each compression should result in a palpable femoral pulse, which should be periodically monitored by another staff member, if possible. If a pulse is not detected and the mucous membrane color or pulse oximeter reading does not improve, the method of compression should be adjusted by changing the rate or intensity, by repositioning the resuscitator's hands or the patient, or by assigning the compression task to another staff member.

If two people are administering cardiopulmonary resuscitation (CPR), one person should bag every 3 to 5 seconds, while the other compresses the chest. Bagging and compressions should be delivered simultaneously. In the case of a technician working alone, 10 compressions should be given alternately with two breaths. Once CPR is initiated, it should not be discontinued for longer than 20 to 30 seconds at a time.

If external cardiac compressions are not effective, as shown by failure to achieve a palpable pulse or pink mucous membranes within 2 minutes, internal compressions may be attempted. In the case of dogs that weigh more than 20 kg or animals that have diaphragmatic hernia, rib fractures or flail chest, pericardial effusion, or severe hypovolemia, some authorities suggest that internal compressions should be initiated immediately after cardiac arrest is identified. Investigators have shown that external chest compression in dogs weighing more than 20 kg results in less than 30% of normal cardiac output, whereas internal massage results in an output of up to 70% of normal. Internal massage also achieves better cerebral perfusion and

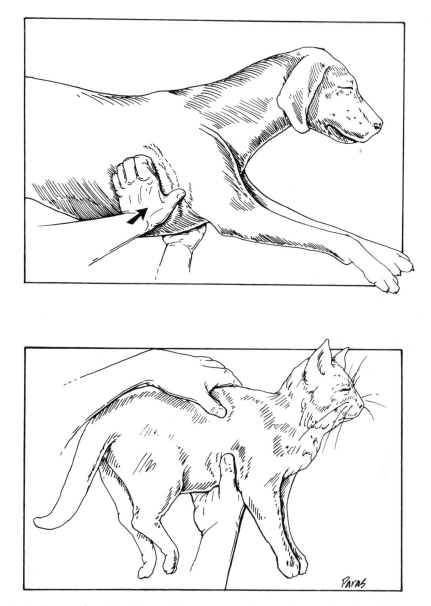

FIG. 6-2 Correct location for cardiac compressions for a medium-sized dog or a cat. (*From Muir WW III, Hubbell JAE, Skarda RT:* Handbook of veterinary anesthesia, *ed 3, St Louis, 2000, Mosby.*)

ultimately, better neurologic recovery. There is understandable reluctance on the part of many veterinarians and technicians to enter the chest to perform internal massage; however, controlled studies have demonstrated that the success rate for resuscitation of large dogs is much greater if internal cardiac massage is performed.

Internal compressions are performed by quickly shaving the lateral thorax and rinsing with alcohol, applying a self-adhering sterile drape to the prepared area, and making a skin incision between the seventh and eighth ribs, with a scalpel or scissors.* The incision is extended through the muscle until the chest cavity is encountered. Care should be taken to avoid incising lung tissue, which lies immediately below the pleura. A gloved hand is advanced into the chest by gently pushing between the ribs (the use of a retractor may be necessary to separate the ribs adequately). The heart is grasped in the hand (not with the fingertips), and gentle but firm pressure is applied to the ventricles at a rate of 80 times per minute. Care should be taken not to twist or rotate the heart. If resuscitation efforts are successful, a palpable heartbeat may return within seconds or minutes. The chest cavity is lavaged with warm sterile saline and surgically closed. Antibiotic therapy is essential.

Once compressions are started, it is necessary to stop periodically to determine whether the heart has resumed spontaneous contractions. This is easy to ascertain by palpation when doing internal compressions, but more difficult with external compression methods. Spontaneous contractions can be detected by discontinuing external compression and either palpating for a spontaneous pulse or observing for an ECG for QRS complexes.

If spontaneous contractions are not observed, external or internal compressions can be resumed, although after 15 minutes they are unlikely to be successful in establishing a heartbeat. Use of a defibrillator is helpful in some situations but should be authorized and directly supervised by a veterinarian.

If spontaneous contractions are observed, cardiac compressions should be discontinued, although bagging must be maintained until spontaneous breathing is established, which may require up to several hours. The anesthetist should periodically check the capillary refill, mucous membrane color, blood pressure, and heart rate and should discontinue bagging only if these vital signs appear normal. If mucous membrane color deteriorates or if spontaneous respiration does not occur within 1 minute after bagging is discontinued, bagging should be resumed.

Monitoring equipment, if available, is extremely helpful in measuring the effectiveness of CPR. Capnography indicates the efficacy of cardiac compressions, because high levels of expired carbon dioxide indicate that compressions are effectively pumping blood and tissues are being perfused. The ECG machine is almost indispensable for effective CPR because it allows differentiation between the three forms of arrest: asystole, ventricular fibrillation, and electromechanical dissociation. Each of these requires different drug treatment for the best chance of success. For example, lidocaine and electrical defibrillation are helpful for ventricular fibrillation but not in electromechanical dissociation. Asystole responds best to epinephrine, atropine, and sodium bicarbonate.

Drugs and fluids. Drugs are commonly administered to aid recovery. In all cases, the veterinarian, if present, should authorize the dosage, route, and nature of drugs to be administered.

---

*In the case of animals undergoing a laparotomy at the time of arrest, the surgeon may immediately initiate internal compressions by opening the diaphragm, entering the thorax, and compressing the heart.

If an IV catheter is present, the drugs are normally given through it, followed by rapid infusion of IV fluids at a dose of 20 ml/kg (cats) or 40 ml/kg (dogs) as rapidly as possible. Dextrose solutions should not be used because saline or balanced electrolytes are more effective in maintaining blood pressure. Caution should be used when administering fluids to patients in cardiac arrest because overhydration and pulmonary edema are common sequelae.

If IV access is difficult, drugs may be given by injection into the base of the tongue (intralingual) or by intratracheal administration. Intratracheal administration may involve injection of the drug directly into the tracheal lumen, or the drug may be administered by means of a urinary catheter passed through the endotracheal tube. For intratracheal administration, the dose of emergency drug given should be twice the recommended IV dose.

Intracardiac injections should be avoided in dogs and cats because injections by this route require the interruption of cardiac compressions and may damage the myocardium.

Commonly administered agents include epinephrine, prednisolone sodium succinate (Solu-Delta Cortef), dopamine, dobutamine, doxapram, atropine, lidocaine, sodium bicarbonate, and anesthetic-reversing agents. The current recommended doses of emergency drugs are given in Tables 6-3 and 6-4.

Epinephrine is the drug most commonly used for initial treatment of cardiac arrest, because it stimulates heart contractions and increases blood flow to the vital organs. The currently recommended dose is 1 mg/10 kg, which is approximately equal to 0.5 ml for cats, 1 ml for small dogs, 2 ml for medium-sized dogs, and 3 ml for large dogs, all drawn up from a 1:1000 solution. These doses should only be given to animals in cardiac arrest because rapid IV administration may cause fatal cardiac arrhythmias in a healthy animal. Epinephrine should be stored in a cool place away from light.

Many authorities also advise dopamine or dobutamine infusions because these drugs increase the force and rate of cardiac contractions. Bicarbonate administration is no longer recommended unless the animal is hyperkalemic or if cardiac arrest has been present for more than 10 minutes. Calcium injections are also no longer advocated, except in hyperkalemic animals.

Aftercare. Successful cardiac resuscitation often depends on the quality of nursing care given to the patient. Continued monitoring of respiratory rate and depth, level of consciousness, urine output, and temperature is vital. Oxygen administration should be continued if it can be done without stressing the patient. As with any recovering patient, restoration of body temperature is important. Other procedures, such as the installation of ophthalmic lubricant and regular repositioning of the patient, are similar to those outlined in Chapter 2 under anesthetic recovery.

Return of normal cerebral and cardiac function is the ultimate goal of CPR, but this may be difficult to achieve. Even after successful resuscitation, serious complications may arise, including repeated cardiac arrest, disseminated intravascular coagulation, and acute renal failure. Cerebral edema is a common problem and is manifested by seizures, failure to return to consciousness, and temporary or permanent neurologic damage. Treatment includes the administration of oxygen, corticosteroids, mannitol, furosemide, and dimethyl sulfoxide (DMSO). Ice packs placed around the animal's head and neck during resuscitation may be helpful in preventing

TABLE 6-3

Management of Anesthetic Complications

COMPLICATION	TREATMENT	DOSAGE	SIDE EFFECTS
Hypoventilation	1. Ventilate with oxygen	—	—
depression	2. Doxapram	1-2 mg/kg IV	2. Excitement, respiratory
Dyspnea	1. Ventilate with oxygen		
	2. Tracheostomy		
Pneumothorax	1. Oxygen		
	2. Chest tube or thoracentesis		
Tachycardia	1. IV fluids	10-20 ml/kg/hr IV	—
	2. Propranolol	0.05-0.10 mg/kg IV	2. Bradycardia, hypotension
Bradycardia	Glycopyrrolate or atropine		Tachycardia
Ventricular arrhythmia	Lidocaine	0.5 mg/kg IV	Bradycardia
Hypotension	1. IV fluids	10-20 ml/kg/hr IV	—
	2. Dopamine or dobutamine	1-5 µg/kg/min IV	2. Arrhythmias, hypertension, CNS toxicity
Blood loss	Lactated Ringer's solution IV	20-90 ml/kg/min IV to effect	
Hypothermia	Warmed IV fluids, external heat source, insulating wraps		Overhydration, edema Burns, hyperthermia
Hypoglycemia	Dextrose 50%	1-2 ml/kg IV	
Metabolic acidosis	Sodium bicarbonate	0.5-1.0 mEq/kg/10 min IV	
Hyperkalemia	1. Sodium bicarbonate	0.5-1.0 mEq/kg/10 min IV	
	2. Sodium chloride (0.9%)	10-40 ml/kg/hr IV	Hyperosmolality
	3. Calcium chloride	0.5 ml/kg IV	
Prolonged recovery	1. Doxapram	1-2 mg/kg IV	1. CNS excitement
	2. Specific reversing agents (atipamezole, naloxone, etc)		
Cardiac arrest	ABCDEF (see text)		

Modified from Muir WW: Anesthesia for dogs and cats with cardiovascular disease, part II, *Compendium* 20(4):481, 1998.

TABLE 6-4

Doses of Emergency Drugs Used in Cardiopulmonary Resuscitation of Cats and Dogs

EMERGENCY DRUG	DOSE	3 KG 6.6 LB	5 KG 11 LB	10 KG 22 LB	15 KG 33 LB	20 KG 44 LB	25 KG 55 LB	30 KG 66 LB	40 KG 88 LB	50 KG 110 LB
Epinephrine 1:1000 (1 mg/ml)	0.1 mg/kg	0.3 ml	0.5 ml	1 ml	1.5 ml	2 ml	2.5 ml	3 ml	4 ml	5 ml
Atropine 0.5 mg/ml	0.025 mg/kg	0.15 ml	0.25 ml	0.5 ml	0.75 ml	1.0 ml	1.2 ml	1.5 ml	2.0 ml	2.5 ml
Lidocaine 20 mg/ml	2 mg/kg	0.3 ml	0.5 ml	1 ml	1.5 ml	2 ml	2.5 ml	3 ml	4 ml	5 ml
Sodium bicarbonate 1 mEq/ml	1 mEq/kg	3 ml	5 ml	10 ml	15 ml	20 ml	25 ml	30 ml	40 ml	50 ml
Prednisolone sodium succinate (Solu–Delta Cortef)	30 mg/kg	90 mg	150 mg	300 mg	450 mg	600 mg	750 mg	900 mg	1200 mg	1500 mg

From Robello CD, Crowe DT: Cardiopulmonary resuscitation: current recommendations, *Vet Clin North Am Small Anim Pract* 19(6):1129, 1989.
For intratracheal epinephrine, 0.2 mg/kg (double doses given above).

neurologic injury. Despite therapy, patients that do not regain consciousness within 15 to 30 minutes of the arrest have a poor prognosis for full return to function.

Problems that May Arise in the Recovery Period
Regurgitation and vomiting during and after anesthesia

Regurgitation and vomiting are not the same. Vomiting is the active expulsion of stomach contents and is often accompanied by retching. Regurgitation is a passive phenomenon in which stomach contents exit through the cardiac sphincter, move up the esophagus, and enter the pharynx, nasopharynx, and oral cavity. Unlike vomiting, regurgitation is not accompanied by retching or other outward signs, and the only sign apparent to the anesthetist may be a small amount of fluid draining from the animal's mouth or nose. Regurgitation is most common in animals placed in a head-down position during surgery because this places increased pressure on the stomach.

Stomach contents that reach the pharynx through vomiting or regurgitation may be aspirated into the respiratory tract. This is a serious hazard in animals that are unconscious and in which the airway is not protected with an endotracheal tube. In this situation, the stomach contents may be easily aspirated into the trachea and airways. Aspiration of vomitus may cause immediate signs of dyspnea and cyanosis as a result of airway obstruction and bronchospasm. If the patient survives this episode, signs of aspiration pneumonia (including fever, increased respiratory rate, and increased lung sounds) may appear over the next 24 to 48 hours.

The appropriate response to regurgitation or vomiting in the patient will vary depending on whether the patient is conscious or unconscious and whether an endotracheal tube is in place.

- *Unconscious patient with no endotracheal tube:* If vomiting or regurgitation is suspected in the unconscious patient, the anesthetist must make every effort to prevent the accumulation of vomitus within the oral cavity and the subsequent aspiration of this material into the air passages. For this to be achieved, an endotracheal tube should be immediately inserted if time allows. If this is not possible, the animal's head should be placed at a lower level than the rest of its body (for example, over the edge of the surgery or prep table). This helps prevent passive flow of liquid material into the trachea. When the vomiting stops, the oral cavity should be cleaned, with suction if available. If respiratory arrest occurs because of airway blockage, the animal should be intubated and bagged with oxygen.

- *Unconscious patient with endotracheal tube in place:* Unconscious animals have a low risk of aspiration if a cuffed endotracheal tube is already in place during the vomiting episode. This is the reason why the endotracheal tube is customarily left in place until the patient regains the swallowing reflex and is close to consciousness. If vomiting is seen in an unconscious animal that has a cuffed endotracheal tube in place, the anesthetist should ensure that the cuff of the tube is inflated and position the animal's head lower than the rest of its body to prevent accumulation of vomitus within the oral cavity.

- *Conscious patient:* Fortunately, most vomiting episodes occur after the animal has regained consciousness and the ability to swallow. It is not usually necessary to intubate conscious animals during a vomiting episode; however, the anesthetist should ensure that the head is kept extended and as low as possible.

Occasionally the technician may be called on to anesthetize an animal that has not been fasted before induction. These patients may be at risk of vomiting and/or regurgitation during induction, maintenance, and recovery. The anesthetist can help avoid problems by ensuring that rapid induction and intubation techniques are used. A rapid-acting injectable agent is preferred over masking in these patients. A cuffed endotracheal tube with adequate diameter should be placed as soon as possible. If possible, head-down positions should be avoided during surgery to prevent excessive pressure on the stomach. The anesthetist should also ensure that suction is readily available in case of regurgitation or vomiting. Use of antiemetic drugs such as metoclopramide may be helpful in some cases.

Postanesthesia seizures and excitement

Seizures are occasionally seen in animals recovering from anesthesia. Seizures may be caused by the administration of drugs (such as methohexital), by diagnostic procedures such as myelography, or by patient disorders such as epilepsy or hypoglycemia.

The anesthetist should differentiate between seizures and confusion or excitement during recovery. Excitement most often appears as spontaneous paddling of the limbs and occasionally as vocalization. Geriatric animals may also vocalize and appear agitated and confused after anesthesia. Usually, treatment is unnecessary other than the calm reassurance of the patient. Sedatives are occasionally helpful, especially if the patient did not receive a sedative in the preanesthetic period. If the patient has undergone a potentially painful procedure and has not received analgesics, these should be administered immediately.

Occasionally, disorientation or excitement may be seen after the administration of high doses of opioids to animals that have not been tranquilized (particularly cats). Treatment with naloxone or another opioid-reversing agent may be helpful in these animals. Excitement is rarely observed in animals that receive opioids for moderate or severe pain.

In contrast to excitement, seizures appear as spontaneous twitching or uncontrolled, violent movements of the head, neck, and limbs and are often triggered by a stimulus such as sound or touch. Animals given cyclohexamines may show stiff forelimbs, opisthotonus, and exaggerated responses to touch or noise.

Animals undergoing postoperative excitement or seizures should be brought to the veterinarian's attention. Elimination of stimuli such as light, sound, and touch may be adequate to resolve the episode. Adequate postoperative analgesia should be provided. If seizures are present, many animals respond well to administration of IV or rectal diazepam at a dosage rate of 0.2 to 0.4 mg/kg. If diazepam is not effective or is unavailable, the animal may be anesthetized with pentobarbital in sufficient quantity to induce sedation and eliminate seizures (5 to 10 mg/kg).

Animals undergoing seizures or excitement during recovery require surveillance and nursing care to prevent self-injury. In the case of cats recovering from ketamine anesthesia, it may be necessary to trim the front claws or to bandage the paws to prevent the animal from scratching its face. Animals undergoing seizures also should be monitored for hyperthermia and cyanosis. Hyperthermia can be treated by the application of cool wet towels. Cyanosis should be treated by the administration of oxygen by face mask or by endotracheal intubation (if unconscious).

Dyspnea in cats during the recovery period

Dyspnea resulting from upper airway obstruction is the most common cause of death in the postanesthetic period. Dyspnea in cats is usually caused by laryngospasm, whereas dyspnea in dogs is most commonly associated with breed-related (for example, brachycephalic) soft tissue obstruction.

Laryngospasm is a condition in which the cartilages in the laryngeal area become so tightly closed that air is unable to enter the trachea. This condition commonly arises in cats because of this species' extremely active laryngeal reflex. In some recovering cats, the removal of the endotracheal tube may initiate reflex closure of the airway. This reflex is normally useful to the cat in that it prevents the aspiration of food or water into the larynx in the conscious animal; however, in the unconscious animal, it may well result in complete airway blockage.

Laryngeal edema may result from repeated attempts to intubate during light anesthesia. Clinically, this resembles laryngospasm.

Cats undergoing laryngospasm or laryngeal edema may breathe with an audible stertor or wheeze. They typically show exaggerated thoracic movements, gasping, and upward movement of the head during inspiration. If conscious, the animal usually appears anxious or excited. Laryngospasm must be differentiated from growling, which is common in cats recovering from anesthesia.

If a cat shows signs of laryngospasm during recovery from anesthesia, the anesthetist should check the mucous membrane color and pulse oximeter readings (if available). If the cat's mucous membranes appear pink and the SaO_2 is greater than 90%, the obstruction is likely partial rather than complete. In this case, the situation may resolve without treatment, although administration of oxygen by face mask may be helpful provided it does not stress the cat. It may be helpful to extend the neck. If cyanosis is present or SaO_2 readings are less than 90% and the cat is losing consciousness—and these signs are not alleviated by the administration of oxygen by face mask—the animal must be intubated. If intubation is impossible, the veterinarian may choose to perform a tracheotomy to reestablish airflow. The animal should be kept anesthetized while furosemide and corticosteroids are given to reduce swelling. The cat can be extubated once the vocal cords appear less rounded and swollen. Nasal oxygen is useful during extubation.

Laryngospasm is easier to prevent than to treat. When cats are anesthetized, gentle intubation technique is essential to avoid unnecessary laryngeal trauma. Use of lidocaine spray and/or gel is also helpful during intubation. Early extubation is recommended in cats so that the tube is removed before the laryngeal reflex returns.

Dyspnea in dogs during the recovery period

Postoperative dyspnea is common in brachycephalic breeds of dogs, because the airway is easily obstructed by the soft palate or by other redundant tissue in the pharynx. However, there are many other potential causes of obstruction, including foreign objects such as blood clots, gauze sponges, or even extracted teeth. Allergic reactions may cause acute swelling and laryngeal edema. Fluid or mucus in the area may also cause a functional obstruction. Animals that have undergone an operation of the pharynx or larynx often undergo postoperative tissue swelling that may lead to airway obstruction. Tracheal collapse is also seen, especially in small dogs.

However it arises, airway obstruction will usually not become evident until after the endotracheal tube is removed. At this point the patient may show the following signs: stridor (loud noises on inspiration, may be similar to snoring), excessive movement of the abdomen and chest wall during inspiration, anxious behavior, low pulse oximeter readings, and (if severe) cyanosis. Strategies to prevent and treat postoperative dyspnea in brachycephalic dogs are outlined on pp. 247-248.

If supplemental oxygen is deemed necessary during the recovery period, it can be administered by face mask, nasal cannula, or oxygen cage/tent (see Chapter 2). The flow rate used to deliver supplementary oxygen will depend on the patient's size and the method of administration. As a general rule, the flow rate should be at least 100 ml/kg/min. If possible, oxygen being delivered to an awake animal should be humidified (for example, by directing the flow of oxygen through a bottle of distilled water before delivery to the patient).

Prolonged recovery from anesthesia

Animals experiencing prolonged recovery from anesthesia should be examined by the veterinarian. There are many possible reasons why a patient may be slow to recover, including impaired renal or hepatic function, hypothermia, hypoglycemia, individual susceptibility to a particular anesthetic, breed variation (particularly sighthounds), or the presence of a disorder such as shock, hemorrhage, or portocaval shunt. Excessive anesthetic depth or prolonged anesthesia may also result in delayed recovery. Some agents (including methoxyflurane, IM ketamine, or repeated injections of barbiturates) may be associated with prolonged recovery even in healthy animals.

If delayed recovery is seen, follow Procedure 6-8.

PROCEDURE 6-8   Expediting Recovery from Anesthesia

1. The patient should be placed in a location where frequent observation is possible. Emergency and monitoring equipment and oxygen should be available in the immediate area.
2. It is often helpful to administer IV fluids that support circulation and thus, hasten renal and hepatic elimination of anesthetics. The recommended rate of fluid administration for most intensive care patients is 3 to 5 ml/kg/hr.
3. Good nursing care is important. The patient should be turned frequently and kept warm. If the patient's temperature is less than 37° C, active warming procedures should be instituted, including the use of fan heaters, reflective blankets, circulating warm water pads, heat-producing "oat bags," chemical warmers, or towels warmed in a dryer. One-liter fluid bags can be heated in a microwave and used as hot water bottles.
4. The animal must be periodically monitored for vital signs, reflexes, and urine production (which should be at least 2 ml/kg/hr).
5. Reversing agents and analeptics are used occasionally to hasten anesthetic recovery. However, the anesthetist whose patients consistently demonstrate slow recoveries should not rely on pharmacologic solutions to solve what may be a problem of technique. The anesthetist should reexamine the anesthetic protocol and consult with the veterinarian to determine whether more appropriate agents or means of administration should be used. It is important to ensure that animals are not maintained at excessively deep levels of anesthesia for routine procedures.

KEY POINTS

1. Although anesthetic complications are uncommon, the technician must be able to anticipate and respond to emergencies in an efficient and knowledgeable fashion.
2. Human error may result in anesthetic problems. Such errors may include the failure to obtain an adequate history or physical examination, a lack of familiarity with the anesthetic machine or drugs used, the incorrect administration of drugs, fatigue, inattentiveness, or distraction.
3. Examples of equipment failure or operator carelessness include carbon dioxide absorber exhaustion, failure to deliver sufficient oxygen to the patient, misassembly of the anesthetic machine, failure of the vaporizer or pop-off valve, or endotracheal tube blockage.
4. Anesthetic agents may be associated with significant side effects. The anesthetic protocol must be chosen to reflect the special needs of each patient to avoid these. The anesthetist must be familiar with the adverse effects associated with the use of each agent in the anesthetic protocol.
5. Some patients are at increased risk of anesthetic complications because of preexisting factors such as old age, pregnancy, organ failure, recent trauma, or breed-related conformation.
6. Geriatric patients have less reserve than younger patients and have reduced anesthetic requirements. Pediatric patients also require reduced dosages of injectable agents and are prone to hypothermia and hypoglycemia.
7. Brachycephalic dogs have anatomic characteristics that make respiration difficult, particularly during the recovery period. Preoxygenation before induction, rapid induction and intubation, and close monitoring during recovery are essential.
8. Thiopental should not be used in sighthounds. Alternative agents, such as propofol, are preferable.
9. Pregnant animals presented for cesarean section are at increased anesthetic risk. Various anesthetic techniques (including epidural anesthesia, balanced anesthesia, and neuroleptanalgesia) are sometimes used as alternatives to inhalation anesthesia in these patients. Almost all anesthetic agents may cause depression of fetal respiration and/or circulation, and the use of reversing agents may be advisable.
10. If possible, patients that have undergone recent trauma should be stabilized and thoroughly evaluated before anesthesia.
11. Animals with cardiovascular or respiratory disease may require special anesthetic techniques such as preoxygenation and manual control of ventilation. Anesthetic agents that depress respiration and cardiovascular function may exacerbate the patient's condition and should be avoided.

KEY POINTS—cont'd

12. Hepatic or renal disease may delay excretion of injectable agents, and prolonged recovery times may be seen.

13. Emergency care is ideally a team effort involving all hospital personnel. It is helpful to have preauthorized emergency protocols and periodic "dress rehearsals."

14. It may be difficult to maintain adequate anesthetic depth in some patients. Incorrect placement of the endotracheal tube, incorrect vaporizer setting, inadequate endotracheal tube size, and many other factors may contribute to this problem.

15. Excessive anesthetic depth may result from excessive administration of anesthetic agents or from preexisting patient problems. It may be necessary to discontinue the general anesthetic and bag the patient with 100% oxygen to achieve a lighter plane of anesthesia.

16. Pale mucous membranes may be the result of anemia, hemorrhage, or poor perfusion. Prolonged capillary refill suggests that inadequate perfusion or hypotension may be present.

17. Cyanosis is a critical emergency and arises because of insufficient delivery of oxygen to the tissues. It may result from a machine problem, airway or endotracheal tube blockage, or respiratory difficulties resulting from excessive depth, pneumothorax, or respiratory disease. Oxygen delivery to the patient must be reestablished through masking, intubation, or tracheostomy.

18. Respiratory arrest that is accompanied by cyanosis and/or bradycardia is an emergency and must be treated by ventilation with 100% oxygen.

19. Cardiac arrest should be treated according to the principles of ABCDEF: establish a patent *airway, bag* the patient with 100% oxygen, initiate internal or external *cardiac massage*, and administer epinephrine and other *drugs*, monitor by *ECG*, and administer *fluids*.

20. Regurgitation and/or vomiting may be dangerous in the anesthetized animal because of the danger of airway obstruction and aspiration pneumonia.

21. Postanesthesia seizures may be treated by eliminating external stimuli and administering diazepam.

22. Dyspnea caused by laryngospasm or brachycephalic airway obstruction may be treated by administration of oxygen by mask, reintubation of the patient, or tracheostomy.

23. Animals experiencing prolonged recovery from anesthesia require close observation and nursing care. An effort should be made to determine the reason for delayed arousal of each patient.

REVIEW QUESTIONS

1. When an animal scheduled for a surgical procedure is brought in by a neighbor who is in a hurry, the best thing to do is:
   a. Instruct the receptionist to have the neighbor sign the consent form
   b. Ask the neighbor to take the animal back home
   c. Ask the neighbor some quick questions about the animal
   d. Have the neighbor sign the consent form and ensure that the owner is called before the procedure is initiated

2. In preparation for an anesthetic procedure, you have drawn up a syringe of barbiturate and an identical syringe of saline. You are then called to the examination room to assist the veterinarian. About 10 minutes later you return to prepare the animal for induction. With the IV catheter in place, you are just about to inject some saline into the animal when you realize that you are not sure if the syringe contains saline. The best thing to do would be to:
   a. Inject a small amount of the solution and see what effect it has
   b. Discard both syringes and start over
   c. Ask the person who was holding the animal which syringe had saline in it
   d. Discard both syringes, label some new syringes, and start over

3. You are about to use the anesthetic machine and notice that although the flowmeter is working, the pressure gauge on the oxygen tank reads close to zero. The best thing to do would be to:
   a. Assume that the pressure gauge may be faulty and wait and see if the flowmeter stops working
   b. Change the oxygen tank
   c. Call the repair person to have the pressure gauge checked
   d. Use low-flow anesthesia techniques and ignore the pressure gauge reading

4. While monitoring a patient that is connected to an anesthetic machine, you realize that the oxygen tank has become empty. The best thing to do would be to:
   a. Leave the patient connected and put on a new oxygen tank, if the reservoir bag is full
   b. Remove the circuit from the patient to allow him to breathe room air for the remainder of the procedure
   c. Resuscitate the patient with an Ambu bag
   d. Switch to an injectable anesthetic

5. If the pop-off valve is inadvertently left shut, it will:
   a. Stop the oxygen flow from entering the circuit
   b. Convert the circuit to low-flow anesthesia
   c. Cause a significant rise of pressure within the circuit
   d. Cause the flutter valves to malfunction

6. You look at the oxygen tank and note that 1000 psi of pressure is left in the tank, but the flowmeter now reads 0 and you cannot obtain a flow by twisting the knobs. The best thing to do would be to assume:
   a. The oxygen tank pressure gauge is malfunctioning and you need to recheck the flowmeter
   b. The oxygen pressure is adequate and the flowmeter just is not registering the flow
   c. The animal is not getting oxygen, and you need to remove the animal from the circuit until a new machine is found or the problem is corrected
7. A geriatric patient is considered to be one that:
   a. Is older than 10 years
   b. Is older than 12 years
   c. Has reached 50% of its life expectancy
   d. Has reached 75% of its life expectancy
8. Brain damage may occur when there is inadequate oxygenation of the tissues for longer than _____ minutes.
   a. 2
   b. 4
   c. 6
   d. 8
   e. 10
9. When a technician is performing CPR alone, the ratio of cardiac compressions to ventilation should be:
   a. 5:1
   b. 10:1
   c. 5:2
   d. 10:2
10. To ensure that the benefit an animal obtains from CPR is not lost, one should not discontinue the CPR for longer than:
    a. 30 seconds
    b. 60 seconds
    c. 90 seconds
    d. 120 seconds
11. Respiratory arrest is always fatal.
    True   False

For the following questions, more than one answer may be correct.

12. One may suspect that the endotracheal tube is malfunctioning even if it is in the trachea because:
    a. Compression of the reservoir bag does not result in the raising of the chest
    b. The animal is dyspneic
    c. The animal cannot be kept at an adequate plane of anesthesia
    d. The reservoir bag is not moving or is moving very little

13. One may suspect that the pop-off valve has been closed or that it is malfunctioning if the:
    a. Reservoir bag is distended with gas
    b. Patient has difficulty exhaling
    c. Patient wakes up
    d. Flow rate starts to drop
14. Administration of the normal rate of fluids (10 ml/kg/hr) during an anesthetic procedure may result in overhydration in the:
    a. Patient with cardiac disease
    b. Obese patient
    c. Pediatric patient
    d. Brachycephalic patient
15. Brachycephalic dogs may be an increased anesthetic risk because of their:
    a. Physical size
    b. Excess tissue around the oropharynx
    c. Increased vagal tone
    d. Small trachea in comparison with their physical body size
    e. Increased susceptibility to barbiturates
16. To decrease the anesthetic risk associated with a brachycephalic dog, the anesthetist may choose to:
    a. Use atropine as part of the anesthetic protocol
    b. Preoxygenate the animal before giving any anesthetic
    c. Use an injectable anesthetic to hasten induction rather than masking
    d. Intubate as soon as possible after induction
17. Animals that undergo cesarean section are at increased risk during anesthesia because of:
    a. Decreased respiratory function
    b. Increased chance of aspiration vomitus
    c. Possibility of hemorrhage from the uterus
    d. Increased workload of the heart
18. Anesthetic agents or drugs that one may want to avoid in the animal with cardiovascular disease include:
    a. Halothane
    b. Isoflurane
    c. Xylazine
    d. Opioids
19. An animal that has liver dysfunction may be hypoproteinemic and therefore requires _____ for induction compared with that needed for a normal dog.
    a. More barbiturate
    b. Less barbiturate
    c. The same amount of barbiturate

20. Too light a plane of anesthesia may be the result of:
   a. Endotracheal tube cuff not inflated
   b. Incorrect vaporizer setting
   c. Incorrect placement of the endotracheal tube
   d. Use of an anesthetic with a low MAC

21. Tachypnea may result from:
   a. Increased levels of arterial oxygen
   b. Increased levels of arterial CO_2
   c. The use of ketamine
   d. Too light a plane of anesthesia

ANSWERS FOR CHAPTER 6

1. d	**2.** d	**3.** b	**4.** a	**5.** c
6. c	**7.** d	**8.** b	**9.** d	**10.** a
11. False	**12.** a, b, c, d	**13.** a, b	**14.** a, c	**15.** b, c, d
16. a, b, c, d	**17.** a, b, c, d	**18.** a, c	**19.** b	**20.** a, b, c
21. b, d				

Selected Readings

Bedford PGC: *Small animal anaesthesia: the increased-risk patient,* London, 1991, Balliere Tindall.

Clarke KW, Hall LW: A survey of anaesthesia in small animal practice: AVA/BSAVA report, *J Assoc Vet Anaesth* 17:4-10, 1990.

Dodman NH, Lamb LA: Survey of small animal anesthetic practice in Vermont, *J Am Anim Hosp Assoc* 28:439-445, 1992.

Dyson DH, Mathews K: Recommendations for intensive care management in small animals following anaesthesia, *VCOT* 5:66-70, 1992.

Dyson DH, Maxie MG: Morbidity and mortality associated with anesthetic management in small animal veterinary practice in Ontario, *J Am Anim Hosp Assoc* 34(4):325-335, 1998.

Evans AT: New thoughts on cardiopulmonary resuscitation, *Vet Clin North Am Small Anim Pract* 29(3):819-829, 1999.

Gaynor JS, Dunlop CI, Wagner AE, et al: Complications and mortality associated with anesthesia in dogs and cats, *J Am Anim Hosp Assoc* 35(1):13-17, 1999.

Haskins SC: Opinions in small animal anesthesia, *Vet Clin North Am Small Anim Pract* 22(2), 1992.

Holland M: Anesthesia for feline cesarean section, *Vet Tech* 12(5):397-402, 1991.

Mathews K: *Veterinary emergency and critical care manual,* New York, 1996, Lifelearn, Inc.

Muir WW: Anesthesia for dogs and cats with cardiovascular disease, *Compendium* 20(4): 473-483, 1998.

Sawyer DC: Anesthesia for problem and high-risk patients, *Vet Tech* 15(2):61-69, 1994.

Wittnich C, Belanger MP, Salerno TA, et al: Canine cardiopulmonary resuscitation: external versus internal cardiac massage, *Compendium* 13(1):50-56, 1991.

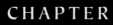

Special Techniques

T he anesthetic agents and techniques used for routine procedures on most small animal patients have been described in previous chapters. Occasionally, however, a specialized technique such as local anesthesia, mechanical ventilation, and/or the use of neuromuscular blocking agents may be indicated for a patient. This chapter describes these techniques and indicates the circumstances in which they may be useful.

LOCAL ANESTHESIA

The term *local anesthesia* (also referred to as *local analgesia*) can be defined as the use of a chemical agent on sensory neurons to produce a disruption of nerve impulse transmission, leading to a temporary loss of sensation. Motor neurons also may be affected, and the patient may lose voluntary motor control of the affected body part.

Although less commonly used than general anesthetics, local anesthetics are an effective and practical alternative in many canine and feline patients. Local anesthesia offers the advantages of low cardiovascular toxicity, low cost, excellent pain control in the immediate postoperative period, and minimal patient recovery time. The choice between local anesthesia and general anesthesia is made by the veterinarian on the basis of such factors as the temperament, age, and physical status of the patient; cost; the nature of the operation to be performed; and the anesthetist's skill in performing the local anesthesia procedure.

Local anesthetics are sometimes used in conjunction with general anesthesia to enhance pain control during and after surgery. The dose of the general anesthetic required may be significantly reduced because of the excellent analgesia provided by the local anesthetic.

Agents

Many local anesthetic agents are available. These agents vary in strength, duration of effect, and method of use (Table 7-1). Lidocaine (Xylocaine), bupivacaine (Marcaine), mepivacaine (Carbocaine), and procaine (Novocain) are the agents most commonly used for skin infiltration and application to mucous membranes. Tetracaine (Pontocaine) and proparacaine (Ophthaine) are reserved chiefly for ophthalmic use.

Of the various local anesthetic agents available, lidocaine and bupivacaine are most commonly used in veterinary medicine. Lidocaine is administered at a concentration of 0.5% to 2% and bupivacaine as a 0.25% or 0.5% solution. Both agents can be diluted with sterile saline (not water) if a lower concentration is desired. Bupivacaine has a slower onset of action (20 minutes) and a longer duration (6 hours) compared with lidocaine (almost immediate onset, duration 1 to 2 hours).

Characteristics

Local anesthesia differs from general anesthesia in several important respects:
- Local anesthetics are not general anesthetics. The term *general anesthetic* is reserved for those drugs such as barbiturates, ketamine, propofol, or inhalation anesthetics that primarily affect neurons in the brain. Like general anesthetics, local anesthetics exert their effect on neurons, but the target is the peripheral nervous system and spinal cord. Because local anesthetics normally do not affect the brain, they have no sedating effect. The patient remains fully conscious unless other agents such as tranquilizers, neuroleptanalgesics, or general anesthetics are used.
- If the appropriate dose and route of administration are used, local anesthetics have relatively few effects on the cardiovascular or respiratory systems. In contrast, preanesthetics and general anesthetics may have significant cardiovascular and respiratory effects. For this reason, local anesthesia may be preferable to general anesthesia in certain high-risk patients. However, local anesthetics are not without risk of toxicity, and the anesthetist should use caution to avoid overdosage, especially in small patients.
- Whereas general anesthetics are widely distributed throughout the body, local anesthetics primarily exert their effects in the area closest to the site of injection. Effective use of local anesthetics requires precise placement of the drug immediately adjacent to the target nerve. The veterinarian or technician performing

TABLE 7-1

Local Analgesics

AGENT (GENERIC NAME)	AGENT (TRADE NAME)	POTENCY (PROCAINE = 1)	DOSAGE	ONSET AND DURATION OF ACTION
Lidocaine	Xylocaine	2	0.5%-2% for injection 2%-4% for topical use Do not exceed 10 mg/kg SC or 2 mg/kg IV in dogs 4 mg/kg SC or 0.5 mg/kg IV in cats	Immediate onset, duration 1-2 hours with epinephrine; 1 hour without
Mepivacaine	Carbocaine	2.5	1%-2% for injection Do not exceed 5 mg/kg in dogs or 2.5 mg/kg in cats	Immediate onset, duration 90-180 minutes
Tetracaine	Pontocaine	12	0.1% for injection 0.2% for topical use	Onset 5-10 minutes, duration 2 hour
Bupivacaine	Marcaine	8	0.25%-0.5% for injection Give SC only Do not exceed 2 mg/kg in dogs or 1 mg/kg in cats	Onset 20 minutes, duration 4-6 hour
Procaine	Novocain	1	1%, 2%, 10%	Immediate onset, 1 hour duration

From Skarda RT: Local and regional analgesia. In Short CE, *Principles and practices of veterinary anesthesia,* Baltimore, 1987, Williams and Wilkins.

the procedure must be familiar with the technique involved for each type of nerve block. For example, it is possible to block the sensory nerve of a tooth in a dog to perform a dental procedure; however, accurate and detailed knowledge of the neuroanatomy of the oral cavity is necessary. Local anesthetics are relatively ineffective in areas where drug diffusion is impeded by fat, bone, cartilage, fascia, tendon, and other connective tissues.

- Unlike general anesthetics, local anesthetics are not normally transferred across the placenta to the fetus. For this reason, local anesthesia is sometimes used for cesarean sections and obstetric manipulations.

Mechanism of Action

The peripheral nervous system and spinal cord are made up of many types of neurons. The primary targets of local anesthetic drugs are the neurons that convey sensations (that is, pain, heat, cold, and pressure) from the skin, muscles, and other peripheral tissues to the brain. These neurons (called *sensory neurons*) are affected by even small amounts of local anesthetic, provided the drug is deposited in proximity to the neuron. Another type of neuron (called a *motor neuron*) conveys impulses from the brain to muscle fibers and is responsible for initiating and controlling voluntary movements. Motor neurons are also sensitive to the effect of local anesthetics, and administration of a local anesthetic may cause temporary paresis (weakness) or paralysis (loss of voluntary movement) in the area served by the affected motor neurons.

Loss of sensation and loss of motor ability are seen concurrently. For example, use of a local anesthetic near the terminal end of the spinal cord (called an *epidural block*) will result in loss of sensation and voluntary movement to all areas innervated by the affected sensory and motor neurons. The patient sensations that are lost include (in order of loss) pain, cold, warmth, touch, joint sensation, and deep pressure in the caudal abdomen and pelvic limbs. After an epidural block, the patient also will be unable to move the pelvic limbs, and the muscles will appear relaxed.

Local anesthetics also affect the neurons of the autonomic nervous system. These neurons convey impulses between the brain and the blood vessels and internal organs (including the heart). If these neurons are exposed to local anesthetics, there may be a temporary loss of function. This is most important in the sympathetic nervous system, and the loss of function of these neurons is called a *sympathetic blockade*. The main effect in the peripheral tissues is vasodilation, resulting in flushing and increased skin temperature of the affected area. If severe, vasodilation may cause blood pressure to fall, leading to hypotension. A sympathetic blockade can also be seen after epidural blocks with lidocaine and other local anesthetics, because sympathetic ganglia adjacent to the vertebrae are affected by the local anesthetic. If a sympathetic blockade occurs within the thoracic spinal cord (as may occur if local anesthetic is allowed to diffuse into the thoracic spinal canal), sympathetic innervation to the heart may be blocked, resulting in bradycardia and impaired ventricular contractions.

The mechanism of action of local anesthetics is not fully understood but appears to involve a loss of transmission of electrical impulses along the nerve fiber. The local anesthetic appears to block the membrane channels through which sodium flows into the neuron. A local anesthetic drug therefore acts as a membrane stabilizer, stopping the process of nerve depolarization. The result is a loss of nerve conduction. Reversal of this effect occurs as the drug is absorbed into the local circulation. Local anesthetics are then redistributed to the liver, where they are metabolized.

Route of Administration of Local Anesthetics

Local anesthetic techniques are often used in conjunction with neuroleptanalgesics, tranquilizers, or other injectable medications. This helps to ensure adequate restraint, allowing accurate and safe injection of the local anesthetic and preventing patient movement during the surgical procedure.

Local anesthetics can be used by a variety of routes, including topical application, infiltration (injection), or introduction into a joint, nerve plexus, vein, or the epidural space.

Topical use

Local anesthetics such as lidocaine are usually ineffective when applied directly to intact skin because the drug molecules are unable to penetrate the epidermis and reach the dermis, where the peripheral nerves are located. However, local anesthetics can be used for topical analgesia in some clinical situations:

- Ethyl chloride sprayed on intact skin provides partial, short-term (less than 3 minutes) analgesia by significantly cooling the skin. It is occasionally used for skin biopsies and other superficial procedures. There is some risk of frostbite if a large area is sprayed.
- A cream formulation containing a mixture of 2.5% lidocaine and 2.5% prilocaine (EMLA cream) can be used to desensitize intact skin for superficial minor procedures such as catheterization. A thick layer of cream is applied to intact shaved skin in the area to be anesthetized and covered with an occlusive dressing for 10 minutes. Duration of effect is 1 to 2 hours. EMLA cream is available in 5-g or 30-g tubes and in single-dose anesthetic discs. It should not be applied to the eyes or to inflamed or broken skin. The patient should be prevented from licking treated areas.
- Wounds or open surgical sites (for example, lateral ear resections, dewclaw removals) can be treated with topical anesthetic sprays such as 10% lidocaine, or by direct application of 0.25% bupivacaine. Sterile gauze sponges soaked with a mixture of local anesthetic and saline can also be placed on an open surgery site. The use of sprays or soaked gauze sponges is called a *splash block*. The efficacy of this technique has not been well established, but it appears to be most effective if the surgical field is relatively dry, with minimal bleeding. Care must be taken to avoid local anesthetic overdose, which is a particular concern with small patients (see pp. 300-301). The dose of lidocaine given by this route should not exceed 4 mg/kg for the dog (2 mg/kg for the cat). For bupivacaine, the dose should not exceed 2 mg/kg in dogs and 0.5 mg/kg in cats.
- Bupivacaine can be instilled through a chest tube placed during thoracic surgery. Local anesthetic administration should be delayed until the patient is awake, because instillation of bupivacaine into the chest cavity of an anesthetized patient may cause cardiac arrhythmias.
- Local anesthetics can be absorbed by mucous membranes, including the conjunctiva, nose, mouth, larynx, and lining of the urethra. They can be administered as topical sprays, drops, or ointment applied to these areas. For example, lidocaine spray is used to desensitize the larynx and prevent laryngospasm in cats. Another example of topical use of local anesthetics is the application of 0.5% proparacaine or tetracaine to the surface of the eye. This procedure desensitizes the cornea and conjunctiva, allowing procedures such as conjunctival scraping or tonometry. Gel containing local anesthetic (lidocaine, tetracaine, or amethocaine) can be applied to a urinary catheter to ease the catheterization process. In each case, analgesia of the mucous membrane results within 60 to 90 seconds and allows procedures to be performed with less discomfort to the patient. Analgesia lasts for 10 to 15 minutes.

Although topical anesthetics are useful in some situations, they generally offer less pain relief and shorter duration of effect than local anesthetics given by infiltration.

Infiltration

Local anesthetics may be infiltrated (injected) into tissues, preferably in proximity to the target nerve. The local anesthetic can be given intradermally, subcutaneously, or between muscle planes. Infiltration techniques are used to provide analgesia for surgery involving superficial tissues, including skin biopsies, removal of small skin tumors, and repair of minor lacerations.

The procedure used for infiltration of local anesthetics is relatively simple. The area must be clipped and a skin antiseptic applied in a manner similar to a surgical prep. This prevents inadvertent contamination of the tissues with skin bacteria when the local anesthetic is injected. A small needle (23- or 25-gauge) is often used to prevent tissue damage and allow for more precise placement of the drug. The amount of the drug to be injected varies with the location and procedure used and may be as little as 0.1 ml or as much as several milliliters in a dog. The onset of analgesia is usually 3 to 5 minutes after the injection of lidocaine.

Before surgery commences it is advisable to test the effectiveness of the block by gently pricking the skin with a 22-gauge needle. If sensation is still present, the anesthetist should wait several minutes longer and consider repeating the injection or using another anesthetic protocol if the block does not take effect.

The infiltration of local anesthetics is not universally effective. Deep tissues such as muscles are unlikely to be affected when only superficial neurons are blocked. Additionally, obstacles such as scar tissue or fibrous tissue, fat, edema, and hemorrhage impede diffusion of local anesthetic. Local anesthetics are also relatively ineffective when injected into inflamed areas. In areas of active inflammation, tissue pH is acidic, resulting in rapid inactivation of the drug. For this reason and also for the prevention of contamination of other tissue, local anesthetics should not be infiltrated into infected tissues.

Once the local anesthetic reaches the neuron, the duration of effect depends on the type of drug being used and the rate of absorption by local blood vessels (see Table 7-1). This in turn depends on whether epinephrine is used with the local anesthetic. Lidocaine, the drug most commonly used for local injection, may be purchased with or without epinephrine. The concentration of epinephrine used is 0.01 mg/ml of lidocaine.

Epinephrine is added to lidocaine for two reasons:
1. Epinephrine causes constriction of blood vessels in the area of the injection. This decreases the rate of drug absorption and thereby prolongs the effect of the lidocaine by approximately 50%.
2. By causing vasoconstriction, epinephrine reduces the concentration of local anesthetic that enters the circulation at any given time, thereby reducing toxicity of the drug. This is most effective for short-acting drugs such as lidocaine and less helpful for long-acting drugs such as bupivacaine.

Lidocaine without epinephrine may be preferred to lidocaine with epinephrine in some situations. A solution containing epinephrine should not be used at an incision site because it may impair tissue perfusion and healing. Lidocaine with epinephrine should not be used on the ears, tail, or digits, because circulation to these areas may be compromised. Epinephrine also increases the risk of ventricular arrhythmias (particularly in animals anesthetized with halothane) and should be used with caution in animals with known cardiac disease. Lidocaine without epinephrine is used for intravenous techniques (see p. 300).

Local anesthetic injections may be painful in the awake patient. Some anesthetists add sodium bicarbonate* to decrease pain on injection.

Two techniques are commonly used for infiltration of local anesthetics: nerve blocks and line blocks.

Nerve blocks. A nerve block is achieved by injecting local anesthetic in proximity to a nerve to desensitize a particular anatomic site. One familiar example is the use of Novocain in human dentistry. Nerve blocks are used commonly in anesthesia of large animals and also may be used in small animals provided the location of the target nerve is known exactly. Reference texts contain illustrations that indicate the location of nerve blocks for different species and particular areas of the body. Before placing a nerve block, the nerve is palpated to determine its location, although this may not always be possible if the nerve is small.

Once the location of the nerve supplying the surgical site is known, the procedure is straightforward. After skin preparation, a small amount of local anesthetic is injected immediately adjacent to the nerve. Lidocaine, bupivacaine, or a 1:1 mixture of the two is most commonly used in small animals. The drug diffuses through the tissues to reach the target nerve. Caution should be used to avoid injecting directly into the nerve because temporary or permanent loss of nerve function can occur. Also, avoid intravenous injection of the local anesthetic, which may cause unwanted central nervous system and cardiovascular effects. To avoid intravenous injection, aspirate before injecting a local anesthetic. If blood appears in the syringe, the location of the injection should be changed.

Clinical situations in which nerve blocks can be used include the following:

- Lameness examinations in horses
- Cornual blocks for dehorning cattle
- Paravertebral blocks for abdominal surgery or cesareans in cattle
- Dental blocks in dogs and cats (infraorbital, mental, mandibular, and maxillary nerve blocks)
- Intercostal or intrapleural nerve blocks in animals undergoing chest surgery
- Infiltration of nerves during amputation of a limb (0.5 ml of 0.5% bupivacaine, injected into and around the nerve during the operation)

Specialty textbooks and journal articles provide complete descriptions of these and other nerve blocks. Regardless of the technique used, it is important to allow sufficient time for the tissues to absorb the drug (15 to 20 minutes) before starting the surgical or dental procedure. When properly performed, these blocks not only decrease the amount of general anesthetic required, but also provide excellent short-term analgesia after the procedure.

Line blocks. Often the veterinarian will perform an operation on an area of tissue that is served by numerous small nerves. One example of this type of surgery is a declaw operation in a cat. In this situation, a line block consisting of a continuous line of local anesthetic can be placed in the subcutaneous or subcuticular tissues immediately proximal to the target area. If the line of local anesthetic completely encircles an anatomic part, such as a digit or teat, it is called a *ring block*.

---

*Sodium bicarbonate (8.4%, 1 mEq/ml) is used as follows: add 0.8 ml bicarbonate to 10 ml of 2% lidocaine or 0.08 ml of bicarbonate to 20 ml of 0.5% bupivacaine.

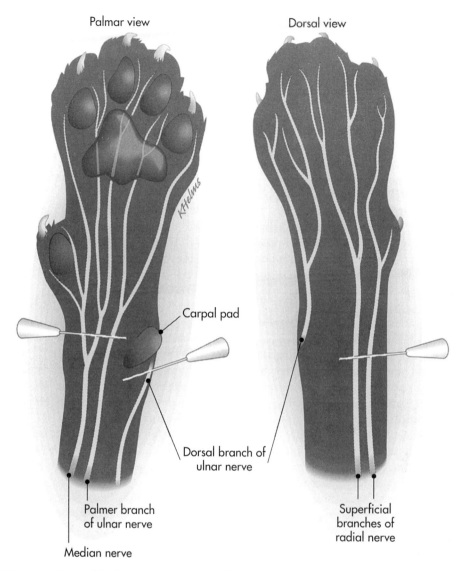

Palmar view

Dorsal view

Carpal pad

Dorsal branch of
ulnar nerve

Palmer branch
of ulnar nerve

Superficial
branches of
radial nerve

Median nerve

FIG. 7-1 Nerve block for feline declaw (distal radial, ulnar, and median nerve blocks). (*From Tranquilli WJ, Grimm KA, Lamont LA:* Pain management for the small animal practitioner, *Jackson, Wyo, 2000, Teton New Media.*)

Line blocks should be positioned between the target area and the spinal cord because this will block the sensory neurons most effectively. As with nerve blocks, the area is clipped and the skin prepped. A line block is placed by inserting the needle along the proposed line of infiltration, then gradually withdrawing the needle while simultaneously injecting a small amount of local anesthetic (Fig. 7-1). If several injections are made, the needle should be inserted into a desensitized area of skin to avoid patient discomfort. Care should be taken to avoid inserting the needle into contaminated tissue (for example, an infected wound).

Line blocks and ring blocks are used extensively in food animal and equine surgery, particularly in cattle. Examples include teat surgery and wound repair.

Intraarticular administration

In certain circumstances, local anesthetics can be injected directly into a joint. For example, bupivacaine has been shown to provide significant analgesia when injected into the stifle joint at the conclusion of cruciate surgery. A dosage rate of 0.4 ml/kg of 5% bupivacaine, diluted with sterile saline (not water) to a volume sufficient to fill the joint, has been recommended. The drug is injected immediately after closure of the joint capsule.

Regional anesthesia

Regional anesthesia is a technique whereby a local anesthetic is injected into a major nerve plexus or in proximity to the spinal cord. This results in the blockage of nervous impulses to and from a relatively large area, such as an entire limb or the caudal portion of the body. Examples of regional anesthesia in veterinary and human medicine include epidural, spinal (intrathecal), and brachial plexus blocks.

Epidural anesthesia

Epidural anesthesia is a regional anesthesia technique that is commonly used in both large- and small-animal patients. The procedure is not difficult (Procedure 7-1) and, once mastered, allows the anesthetist to reliably block sensation and motor control of the rear, abdomen, pelvis, tail, pelvic limbs, and perineum. The technique is useful for tail amputation, anal sac removal, perianal surgery, urethrostomies, obstetric manipulations, cesarean sections, and some rear limb operations. Epidural anesthesia is most commonly used in three classes of patients:

1. Large animals, particularly cattle, in which procedures such as replacement of a vaginal prolapse can be undertaken with epidural anesthesia alone or in combination with a sedative. Epidural procedures are also useful to prevent straining during obstetric procedures, including cesarean sections.
2. Debilitated small-animal patients in which general anesthesia is problematic but that may tolerate sedation and a lidocaine or bupivacaine epidural block. One common example is cesarean sections.
3. Patients requiring profound pain control after surgical procedures involving the hind limbs, pelvis, or caudal abdomen. For example, morphine or lidocaine epidural blocks are useful for animals undergoing surgical repair of a fractured femur.

The choice of drug used for epidural anesthesia is governed by the reason for the epidural: if immobility and anesthesia for surgery are required, a local anesthetic such as 2% lidocaine, 0.5% bupivacaine, or 0.75% ropivacaine can be used at a dose of 1 ml/5 kg. Duration of effect is 1 to 2 hours for lidocaine and up to 6 hours for bupivacaine. If the main objective of the epidural anesthesia is to ensure postoperative pain control, an opioid such as morphine is used (see Chapter 8). Opioids and local anesthetics such as lidocaine are sometimes mixed together and delivered epidurally. Opioids are generally associated with fewer unwanted side effects than lidocaine or bupivacaine (less risk of sympathetic blockade and hypotension, less ataxia) but may cause pruritus and urinary retention in some patients.

Anatomic considerations. To understand the technique used for epidural anesthesia, the anesthetist must be familiar with the anatomy of the terminal spinal cord region (see Fig. 7-2). The spinal cord is made up of sensory, motor, and autonomic neurons and is surrounded by three membrane layers: the pia mater, arachnoid, and dura mater. The subarachnoid space, which is the area between the arachnoid and the pia mater, is filled with cerebrospinal fluid. This fluid surrounds the entire spinal cord and communicates with the cerebrospinal fluid in the ventricles of the brain. The spinal cord and its membrane layers are encased within the spinal canal. This canal consists of bony vertebrae (cervical, thoracic, lumbar, sacral, and coccygeal) that protect the spinal cord from injury. Several ligaments also protect the vertebral canal, including the supraspinous ligament (which lies directly under the skin), the ligamentum flavum (also called the *ligamentum interarcuatum*), and the interspinous ligament (see Fig. 7-2). Neurons that supply the tissues exit from the spinal cord at regular intervals, emerging between the vertebrae and ultimately ending in the skin and other tissues. The spinal cord itself terminates in a group of neurons collectively called the *cauda equina.*

When epidural anesthesia is performed, local anesthetic is deposited in the epidural space, between the dura mater and the vertebrae. This is a potential space that is often filled with fat. Spinal nerves cross through the epidural space as they exit through the intervertebral foramina and are affected by local anesthetics and other drugs deposited in this space. In dogs the location of the block is between the last lumbar vertebra (L7) and the sacrum (see Fig. 7-3). When properly performed, injection of local anesthetic into this area is unlikely to damage the spinal cord because the cord normally ends at the sixth or seventh lumbar vertebra (L6 or L7). In cats the spinal cord extends further caudally (as far as S1), and there is a slight risk of spinal cord damage when epidural anesthesia is performed.

Epidural anesthesia must be differentiated from spinal anesthesia, which is commonly performed in human patients. In spinal anesthesia, the local anesthetic is injected into the subarachnoid space, where it mixes with the cerebrospinal fluid. Inadvertent injection of local anesthetic into the subarachnoid space is more common in the cat than in the dog.

Because lidocaine and similar drugs block not only sensory nerves (including those that transmit pain sensation) but also motor neurons, a dog or cat that has undergone epidural anesthesia may be unable to walk until the block wears off. Opioids, on the other hand, have no effect on motor neurons, and movement of the legs and tail is unimpaired after morphine epidural anesthesia.

Intravenous regional anesthesia (Bier block)

Intravenous injection of local anesthetics is not performed routinely in dogs or cats but is fairly common in large animals. A calculated amount of lidocaine (not bupivacaine) is injected into the distal segment of a superficial vein. The procedure is as follows: a 22-gauge, 1.5-inch catheter is placed in a vein in the distal part of the limb (because the valves of the veins prevent the backward flow of local anesthetic if the drug is injected too proximally). Once the catheter is in place, an elastic bandage is wrapped around the extremity starting at its distal end and wrapping it proximally to drive blood out of the veins. A tourniquet is applied just proximal to the area requiring anesthesia (for example, immediately above the elbow if the foreleg is to be anesthetized). The tourniquet must be tight, or symptoms of local anesthetic toxicity may be evident after injection. The bandage is then removed and the drug injected into the vein via the catheter. The usual dose used is 2 to 3 ml of 1% lidocaine without epinephrine, not to exceed 4 mg/kg (in the dog). Within 3 to 5 minutes, there is total desensitization of the limb distal to the tourniquet, allowing 25 to 30 minutes of analgesia. An additional advantage of this technique is the relatively blood-free surgery site that it affords. As with other local anesthetic procedures, however, patient restraint may be a problem unless concurrent sedation or neuroleptanalgesia is provided.

Sensation returns to the affected area within a few minutes of release of the tourniquet. It is important to remove the tourniquet soon after the procedure is completed. If the tourniquet is in place more than 90 minutes, prolonged hypoxia of the tissues of the limb may result, leading to tissue necrosis. In all patients, removal of the tourniquet should be gradual (that is, over a 5-minute period) because this helps prevent an excessive concentration of local anesthetic reaching the heart and brain.

Lidocaine can also be administered by constant rate infusion to healthy anesthetized animals to reduce the dose of general anesthetic or analgesic required for painful operations and to prevent cardiac arrhythmias. The dose used is 0.02 to 0.05 mg/kg/min in dogs and 0.025 mg/kg/min in cats.

Toxicity of Local Anesthetics

The use of local anesthetics is not without risk, and several adverse effects have been reported, including the following:
1. If local anesthetic is injected into a nerve, temporary or permanent loss of function may result. Direct injection into a nerve should be avoided, except for animals undergoing an amputation.
2. Tissue irritation may occur after the injection of some local anesthetics. Some veterinarians prefer mepivacaine (Carbocaine) instead of other local anesthetics because it appears to cause less tissue irritation.
3. Paresthesia, an abnormal sensation of tingling, pain, or irritation, may be apparent during recovery from local anesthesia. (Human patients also experience this tingling sensation, for example during recovery from "freezing" of the oral cavity with Novocain.) Animals should be monitored during recovery because they may chew or otherwise traumatize affected areas.
4. Human and animal patients may exhibit allergic reactions to local anesthetics, usually in the form of a skin rash or hives. Anaphylaxis is also occasionally seen. Local anesthetics should not be used in patients in which an allergic reaction to these drugs has been previously observed.
5. Systemic toxicity may occur, particularly if a local anesthetic is inadvertently given intravenously without the use of a tourniquet. Systemic toxicity may be seen even if the drug is placed in the subcutaneous tissues, if a large amount of local anesthetic is injected.

   The most common signs of systemic toxicity originate in the central nervous system. The first sign of systemic toxicity is usually sedation, followed by nausea, restlessness, muscle twitching, hyperexcitability, seizures, respiratory depression, and eventually, coma. Treatment of central nervous system signs may include intravenous or rectal diazepam (0.2 to 0.4 mg/kg) and administration of oxygen.

PROCEDURE 7-1   Epidural Anesthesia in the Dog and Cat

1. Gather the necessary equipment. This includes a short-beveled spinal needle with a stylet (18- to 22-gauge, 1.5 inches for small or thin dogs, and 2 to 3 inches for large overweight dogs) and several sterile 3- or 5-ml syringes. If a catheter is to be placed, a thin-walled, 18-gauge, 3-inch needle is required.
2. Sedate the patient to achieve adequate restraint and place in sternal or lateral recumbency. The head is positioned higher than the spinal cord for at least the first 10 minutes of analgesia. This prevents forward migration of the drug into the region of the thoracic spinal cord, which could potentially affect the phrenic nerve (causing respiratory arrest) or cause a sympathetic blockade.
3. Identify the right and left cranial dorsal wings of the ilium, the spinous process of L7, and the sacral crest. Shave and surgically prepare the area (approximately 10 cm × 10 cm) surrounding the injection site between L7 and the sacral crest. Wear surgical gloves for the procedure.
4. Palpate the lumbosacral space (between L7 and the sacrum), which is midway between the dorsal iliac wings (Fig. 7-2). The lumbosacral space is the depression just caudal to the L7 process and immediately cranial to the sacral crest, which feels like a series of small bumps under the skin. Place the spinal needle in the area of greatest depression, perpendicular to the skin surface and exactly on the midline.

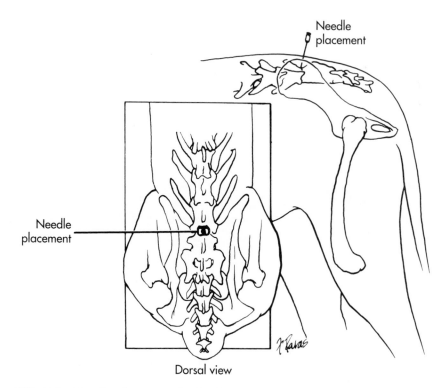

Dorsal view

FIG. 7-2 Needle placement for lumbosacral epidural anesthesia in the dog.

Continued

PROCEDURE 7-1   Epidural Anesthesia in the Dog and Cat—cont'd

The bevel should be directed cranially, and the stylet should be left in the needle to prevent introduction of skin into the epidural space. The needle is gently advanced perpendicular to the skin, passing through the skin, subcutaneous fat, supraspinous ligament, interspinous ligament, and ligamentum flavum (Fig. 7-3). Resistance may be encountered, and a distinct pop often can be felt as the needle is advanced through the ligamentum flavum. Immediately after the ligamentum flavum is penetrated, the needle enters the epidural space. This usually occurs at a needle depth of 1 to 3 cm, depending on the size of the animal. Occasionally, there is some difficulty in finding the intervertebral space, in which case the needle should be withdrawn, angled slightly caudally or cranially, and reinserted.

5. Remove the stylet and examine the needle hub for blood or cerebrospinal fluid (for 2 minutes). If cerebrospinal fluid is encountered, the needle is in the subarachnoid space. If this is the case, the procedure may be abandoned or the anesthetist may choose to administer 30% to 50% of the original dose, inducing spinal anesthesia, (provided the agent used has minimal spinal toxicity). If blood is encountered, the needle has entered the venous sinus, and the procedure should be abandoned. If blood and cerebrospinal fluid are not observed, the needle should be aspirated to ensure that neither is present. To further check for proper needle placement, inject 1 to 2 ml of air; no resistance to air passage should be felt. For large dogs, it may be easier to remove the stylet as it enters the skin. The hub can be filled with

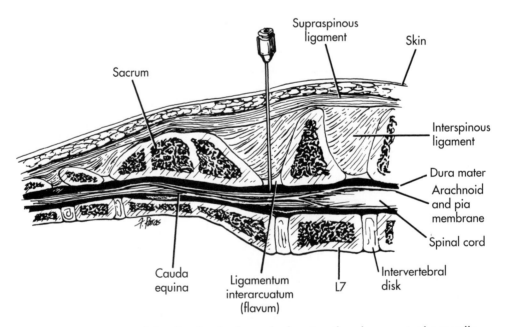

FIG. 7-3 Anatomy of the distal spinal canal, showing the placement of a needle for lumbosacral epidural analgesia. (*From Muir WW III, Hubbell JAE, Skarda RT: Handbook of veterinary anesthesia, ed 3, St Louis, 2000, Mosby.*)

Continued

saline, and as the needle penetrates the ligamentum flavum, the liquid will be drawn into the epidural space.

Surgical analgesia. If the epidural is performed for surgical analgesia and immobilization, lidocaine or bupivacaine is used. The dose of 2% lidocaine (without epinephrine) or 0.25% to 0.5% bupivacaine will vary with the extent of analgesia required. The anesthetist often will choose to produce anesthesia as far cranial as L2 (which is sufficient for most caudal abdominal procedures and all pelvic and rear limb procedures). The dose used in this case is 1 ml of 2% lidocaine for each 3.5 to 4.5 kg of body weight (cat or dog). The volume should be less than 0.25 ml/kg. Inject the calculated dose of lidocaine or bupivacaine over 1 minute. More rapid injection may cause pressure damage to the spinal cord and nerves or result in local anesthetic infiltrating too far forward along the spinal canal. Injection will be resistance-free if the needle is positioned correctly. If continuous epidural anesthesia is required, a polyethylene catheter may be advanced through the needle and the needle subsequently withdrawn, leaving the catheter in place. Advance the catheter only 1 cm into the epidural space.

Onset of analgesia is approximately 5 minutes after lidocaine injection or 20 minutes after bupivacaine injection. The block normally affects the most distal body parts (toes and tail) first. If a bilateral effect is desired, position the patient in dorsal recumbency for 20 minutes after the injection. If unilateral analgesia is required, place the patient in lateral recumbency, with the desired side positioned ventrally, allowing for gravitation of the local anesthetic within the epidural space to the targeted side of the spinal canal.

It has been reported that 12% of correctly performed epidural blocks are ineffective, perhaps because of individual variations in anatomy. Effectiveness of the block may be determined through a test with a needle prick or may become evident during patient preparation or application of towel clamps.

Duration of analgesia is 4 to 6 hours for bupivacaine with epinephrine and 1.5 to 3 hours for lidocaine. Lidocaine with epinephrine may have a longer duration.

Postoperative pain control. If the epidural is performed to provide postoperative analgesia, morphine or another opioid agent is used. The procedure used is the same as just described. It is advisable that single-use vials of preservative-free morphine (Duramorph) be used. See Chapter 8 for more information on the use of morphine epidurals for pain control.

Cardiovascular effects may also be observed, because of the direct effect of local anesthetics on the heart. Intravenous injection of lidocaine may inhibit the conduction of electrical impulses within the heart muscle and decrease the force of cardiac contractions. This is undesirable when performing local anesthesia but makes this drug of use in treating some types of ventricular arrhythmias. Bupivacaine is more cardiotoxic than lidocaine.

The dose of lidocaine given subcutaneously to dogs should not exceed 10 mg/kg and in cats should not exceed 4 mg/kg to avoid systemic toxicity. The smallest possible dose should be used. If given intravenously, the dose of lidocaine should not exceed 4 mg/kg in dogs and no more than 0.5 mg/kg in cats. The dose of bupivacaine given subcutaneously should not exceed 2 mg/kg in dogs and 1 mg/kg in cats. For the average (4-kg) cat, the maximum dose of 2% (20 mg/ml) lidocaine is 0.8 ml (16 mg) if given subcutaneously and 0.1 ml (2 mg) if given intravenously. For 0.5% (5 mg/ml) bupivacaine, the maximum subcutaneous dose for a 4-kg cat is 4 mg (0.8 ml). Bupivacaine should not be given by intravenous injection.

Dilution of the calculated dose of lidocaine or bupivacaine with sterile saline is helpful in small patients because it increases the volume and decreases the concentration of the solution to be injected.

6. Epidural or spinal injection may traumatize the spinal cord or cauda equina, particularly if the animal is struggling during placement of the needle. Inflammation and fibrosis have been reported after epidural infiltration of local anesthetics containing preservatives. Additionally, myelitis (spinal cord inflammation) and meningitis (inflammation of the pia mater, arachnoid, or dura mater) may occur if asepsis is not maintained.

7. If local anesthetics are permitted to infiltrate into the cranial portion of the spinal cord, serious toxicity and even death may occur. If the local anesthetic reaches the midthoracic vertebrae, innervation of the intercostal muscles may be blocked, interfering with normal respiration. If local anesthetic diffuses as far forward as the cervical spinal cord, the phrenic nerve may be affected. This nerve innervates the diaphragm, and loss of function may result in respiratory paralysis. Diffusion of local anesthetic into the cervical and thoracic spinal cord also may affect sympathetic nerves supplying the heart and blood vessels, resulting in a sympathetic blockade with symptoms of bradycardia, decreased cardiac output, and hypotension. If blood pressure measurement is unavailable, careful monitoring of the capillary refill time, heart rate, and pulse strength will alert the anesthetist to a fall in blood pressure. Treatment consists of intravenous fluid administration at a rate of 20 ml/kg over a 15- to 20-minute period.

When epidural anesthesia is performed, care should be taken to keep the patient's head elevated to avoid gravitational flow of the anesthetic into the anterior spinal canal around the thoracic and cervical spinal cord. The anesthetist should be prepared to intubate and artificially ventilate the lungs of any patient undergoing epidural anesthesia, because this may be necessary if intercostal and phrenic nerve function is impaired.

CONTROLLED VENTILATION

The anesthetist may be called on to assist or control patient ventilation during any anesthesia. In *assisted ventilation,* the anesthetist ensures that an increased volume of air is delivered to the patient, although the patient initiates each inspiration. In *controlled ventilation,* the anesthetist delivers all of the air that is required by the patient, and the patient does not make spontaneous respiratory efforts. The anesthetist controls the respiratory rate and the volume and pressure of gas that the animal breathes.

Any procedure by which the anesthetist assists or controls the delivery of oxygen and anesthetic gas to the patient's lungs may be termed *positive pressure ventilation*

(PPV). Whether achieved by bagging the patient or by mechanical ventilation, PPV is intended to ensure that the animal receives adequate oxygen and is able to exhale adequate amounts of carbon dioxide. This is a concern in veterinary anesthesia because the patient's own ventilation efforts may be inadequate to achieve these objectives.

Ventilation in the Awake Animal

To understand the use of PPV in anesthesia, it is necessary to review the mechanics of normal breathing and the reasons why they may be ineffective in the anesthetized animal. Ventilation is the physical movement of air and anesthetic gases into and out of the lungs and upper respiratory passageways. Ventilation has two parts: an active phase (inhalation) and a passive phase (exhalation). Inhalation is initiated by the respiratory center in the brain and is normally triggered by an increased level of carbon dioxide in the arterial blood ($Paco_2$). As $Paco_2$ rises above a threshold level, the respiratory center initiates the active inspiratory phase by stimulating the intercostal muscles and diaphragm to move, expanding the thorax. This creates a negative pressure (partial vacuum) within the chest, which causes the lungs to expand. As the lungs expand, air moves through the breathing passages and into the alveoli. When the lungs reach an adequate volume, nerve impulses feed back to the respiratory center, signaling the brain to stop the active phase of respiration. The intercostal muscles and diaphragm then relax, and exhalation takes place as the lungs deflate. Exhalation is passive, which means that no active muscle movement occurs. During exhalation, the carbon dioxide level in the blood begins to rise again, and after a short pause the respiratory center responds by initiating another inspiration.

Normally, exhalation lasts approximately twice as long as inspiration. For example, in an animal breathing 20 times per minute, each inspiration will last approximately 1 second and each exhalation will last approximately 2 seconds.

The amount of air that passes in or out of the lungs in a single breath is the tidal volume. Animals that are breathing deeply have a relatively large tidal volume, whereas animals that have shallow breathing or that are panting have a relatively small tidal volume. Normal tidal volume in the awake animal is 10 to 15 ml/kg.

The *respiratory rate* is the number of breaths that occur in 1 minute. The *respiratory minute volume* is the total amount of air that moves in and out of the lungs in 1 minute. This value can be found by multiplying the average tidal volume by the respiratory rate.

Ventilation in the Anesthetized Animal

Ventilation in the anesthetized animal differs significantly from normal ventilation just described. These differences include the following:

- Tranquilizers and general anesthetics may decrease the responsiveness of the respiratory center in the brain to carbon dioxide. This means that inspiration does not occur as often in the anesthetized animal as in the healthy awake animal, despite the fact that carbon dioxide may be significantly elevated. This explains the observation that a respiratory rate of 12 to 20 breaths per minute is normal in cats and dogs under inhalation anesthesia, whereas the same animal would be expected to have a respiratory rate between 20 and 30 breaths per minute when awake.

- Tranquilizers and general anesthetics relax the intercostal muscles and diaphragm, causing them to expand less than normal during the inspiratory phase. Because the chest does not expand fully, the tidal volume is reduced to 8 ml/kg or less (compared with the tidal volume in the healthy awake animal, 10 to 15 ml/kg). The anesthetist may become aware of the reduced tidal volume by noting that the reservoir bag does not collapse significantly during the inhalation phase (that is, the volume of gas inhaled is relatively small).

Because tidal volume and respiratory rate are decreased, respiratory minute volume is also decreased. As the amount of air entering and leaving the lungs in the anesthetized animal may be considerably reduced compared with the healthy awake animal, the anesthetist must be aware of the following potential problems:

1. *Hypercarbia.* Pa_{CO_2} may rise in the anesthetized patient, because carbon dioxide produced by the body is not eliminated as rapidly as in the awake animal. As the blood carbon dioxide level rises, it joins with water molecules in the bloodstream to form bicarbonate ions (HCO_3^-) and hydrogen ions (H^+) (see formula, p. 89). The accumulation of hydrogen ions causes the pH of circulating blood to fall, potentially leading to respiratory acidosis. Blood pH in the healthy awake animal is between 7.38 and 7.42, whereas in the anesthetized animal, blood pH may be as low as 7.20.

2. *Hypoxia.* If the anesthetized animal is breathing room air, Pa_{O_2} may fall below normal values as a result of the decreased respiratory minute volume. Less oxygen enters the lungs, and therefore less is available to be absorbed into the blood.

3. *Atelectasis.* Because tidal volume is reduced, the alveoli do not expand as fully as normal on inspiration. The alveoli in some sections of the lung may partially collapse (a condition called *atelectasis*).

Some patients are at increased risk of having these problems. Predisposing factors for hypercarbia, hypoxia, and atelectasis include the following:

- Prolonged anesthesia (more than 90 minutes).
- Obese patients.
- Animals given neuromuscular blocking agents (see following section).
- Animals with preexisting lung disease such as pneumonia.
- Animals that have undergone recent head trauma.*
- Animals undergoing surgical procedures involving the chest or diaphragm. These animals may have preexisting cardiovascular or pulmonary disease and are at significant risk of cardiovascular collapse or respiratory arrest if conventional anesthesia with unassisted ventilation is attempted.†

The anesthetist has several ways of compensating for these effects. The Pa_{O_2} can be elevated to normal levels (and, in fact, often above normal levels) if the patient is supplied with adequate oxygen. This is easily achieved because animals connected

---

*It is important to maintain Pa_{CO_2} less than 45 mm Hg in animals that have undergone recent head trauma. If the Pa_{CO_2} rises above 45 mm Hg, cerebral vascular resistance is decreased. This in turn increases cerebral blood flow, which may lead to increased intracranial pressure.
†In addition to assisted or controlled ventilation, these patients benefit from preoxygenation and intravenous induction techniques (rather than mask or chamber induction). In these and other patients, mechanical ventilation may be combined with the use of neuromuscular blocking agents. See the following section.

to anesthetic machines normally receive close to 100% oxygen (or a mixture of oxygen and nitrous oxide). The anesthetized patient connected to an anesthetic machine is unlikely to have a reduced PaO_2 unless a problem such as pulmonary edema or upper airway obstruction is present.

It is more difficult to prevent atelectasis or an increase in $PaCO_2$ and resulting respiratory acidosis. In each of these situations, it may be advisable to take active steps to assist or control patient ventilation.

Types of Controlled Ventilation

The following are two ways to assist or control patient ventilation:

1. Intermittent or continuous bagging of the patient, using the reservoir bag of the anesthetic machine. This technique is called *manual ventilation* or *bagging*. In this type of PPV, the lungs are filled with oxygen by the pressure of gas entering the airways as the anesthetist squeezes the reservoir bag. Exhalation is passive and occurs when the positive pressure is discontinued, allowing the lungs to empty. For most patients, intermittent bagging (one or two breaths every 5 minutes) is adequate to expand the lungs and reduce atelectasis, but some patients require continuous bagging throughout the anesthetic period.
2. Use of a ventilator (called *mechanical ventilation*). In this type of PPV, the lungs are filled with oxygen by the pressure of gas from a special apparatus called a *ventilator*. As with manual ventilation, exhalation is passive and occurs when the positive pressure is discontinued.

Whether the patient's lungs are to be ventilated by manual or mechanical means, the patient must first be intubated and connected to an anesthetic machine. Ventilating the patient's lungs through an ordinary anesthesia mask does not deliver adequate amounts of oxygen to the lungs and may cause the stomach to fill with air, increasing the risk of regurgitation.

Manual ventilation

Manual ventilation can be performed on an occasional basis (one or two breaths every 5 minutes) on any anesthetized patient. These periodic "sighs" help expand collapsed alveoli and reverse atelectasis. For the patient's lungs to be manually ventilated, the pop-off valve is closed and the reservoir bag is compressed until the lungs are inflated. When pressure is released on the reservoir bag, exhalation can occur. The anesthetist must use caution to ensure that the pressure used is not excessive: the patient's chest should only rise to the same extent as with normal awake respiration. When normal lungs are ventilated, the pressure manometer reading should not exceed 20 cm H_2O (14 mm Hg). The bag should be squeezed for 1 second or less. Excessive or prolonged pressure may damage lung tissue and impede venous return to the heart.

For some patients, respiratory depression is so severe that intermittent bagging does not provide the necessary level of ventilation. Animals with preexisting heart or lung disease or diaphragmatic hernias may go into respiratory arrest immediately after induction. Other patients continue to breathe under anesthesia but the tidal volume is small (shallow breaths) and/or the respiratory rate is 8 breaths per minute or less. These patients require more aggressive, continuous ventilation. Ventilation can be assisted starting immediately after induction, at which point the anesthetist should use the reservoir bag to superimpose positive pressure on the animal's own spontaneous breathing efforts. For many patients, it is adequate to give a few large tidal volumes manually, then connect the patient to a ventilator or initiate continuous manual bagging. The initial large tidal volumes depress the animal's urge to breathe by lowering the blood carbon dioxide levels. Once the patient is connected to a ventilator or is undergoing continuous manual ventilation, the patient usually stops spontaneous breathing efforts within 1 minute. Initially, the assisted ventilation rate should be 12 to 16 respirations per minute, at a manometer pressure of 15 to 20 cm H_2O (11 to 14 mm Hg). If, after 3 to 5 minutes, the patient still makes spontaneous breathing efforts, it may be necessary to use a neuro-muscular blocking agent, which paralyzes the muscles of respiration (see the following section).

Once control is established, a ventilation rate of 8 to 12 breaths per minute is usually adequate. A pressure of 15 to 20 cm H_2O is recommended, unless the chest is open, in which case pressures of 20 to 30 cm H_2O may be required depending on the degree to which the lungs are packed off by the surgeon to better expose the surgical field. When the reservoir bag is squeezed, the inspiratory time should be 1 to 1.5 seconds. Expiratory time should be twice as long as inspiratory time. The pop-off valve must be closed when the reservoir bag is squeezed; however, it should be opened briefly between every two to three breaths to allow gas to escape from the circuit. The anesthetist must allow the airway pressure to return to zero during expiration so that cardiopulmonary function can normalize (improving venous return of blood to the heart and increasing stroke volume).

When assisting or controlling ventilation, the anesthetist may find it difficult to evaluate the adequacy of the ventilation efforts. Pulse oximetry and end-tidal capnog-raphy are valuable aids. For example, if the pulse oximeter reading is 95% or less in a patient undergoing manual ventilation, the patient may need more frequent ventilation or ventilation at a greater pressure or volume.

When the surgical procedure is nearing completion, the anesthetist must "wean" the animal from the controlled ventilation procedure. This is accomplished by turn-ing off the anesthetic and nitrous oxide while continuing to ventilate the patient's lungs with oxygen. If a neuromuscular blocking agent has been used, it should be reversed, if possible. The anesthetist should gradually reduce the rate of inspirations to approximately five per minute, while observing the animal for evidence of spon-taneous breathing. When this is seen, the patient's ventilation can continue to be assisted by squeezing a small amount of air from the reservoir bag with each inspi-ration. Eventually, the animal regains the ability to maintain a normal rate and tidal volume, and ventilation assistance can be discontinued. This may take several minutes to reestablish, particularly in older, hypothermic, or debilitated patients and in patients in which ventilation has been controlled for a long time. Warm-ing the patient or stimulating the patient by pinching the toe pads or gently rub-bing the thorax and abdomen may help the patient regain spontaneous respira-tory movements.

Mechanical ventilation

Mechanical ventilation is similar to continuous manual ventilation in many respects. In mechanical ventilation, however, the patient's breathing is controlled by a ventilator, rather than by hand compression of the reservoir bag. When a ventilator is connected to the breathing circuit, it functionally replaces the reservoir bag and becomes a part of the breathing circuit. The ventilator automatically compresses a bellows, which forces oxygen and anesthetic gas into the patient's airways via an endotracheal tube.

There are many types of ventilators that can be used with a veterinary anesthesia machine, and they vary in the number and complexity of the controls (Fig. 7-4). The basic design is a bellows inside a housing, which is attached to the reservoir bag port of a circle breathing system. The bellows is compressed at a specified rate

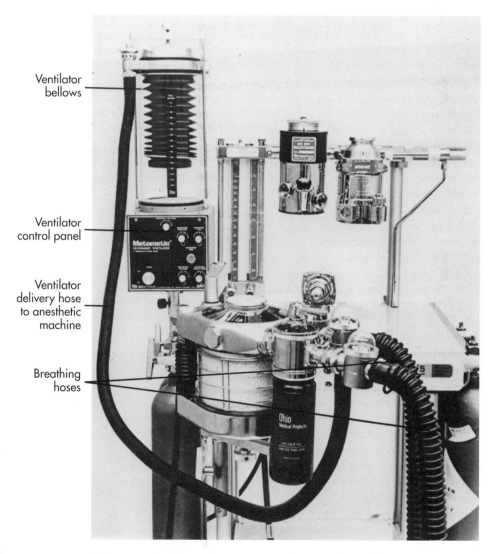

Ventilator bellows

Ventilator control panel

Ventilator delivery hose to anesthetic machine

Breathing hoses

FIG. 7-4   Ventilator for use in small-animal anesthesia.

and a specified volume by a driving gas. Most ventilators have a double gas circuit pattern, with one circuit providing oxygen and anesthetic for the patient, and the other circuit containing a separate gas (oxygen or air) to drive the bellows. Ventilators are available for either large-animal or small-animal use. In both cases, the scavenger should be attached to the exhaust port of the ventilator.

Depending on the type of ventilator used, the anesthetist may choose to deliver gases on inspiration according to a pressure cycle, volume cycle, or time cycle. A pressure-cycled ventilator (such as the Bird Mark 7 Respirator) will supply air until the pressure reaches a preset level. A time cycle ventilator (such as the Small Animal Ventilator by Drager) supplies air according to a set inspiratory time. A volume cycle type (such as the Ohio Metomatic) delivers a preset tidal volume regardless of the pressure required. In volume-cycled ventilators, the anesthetist must adjust the volume of gas to be delivered on inspiration (usually 10 to 15 ml/kg, less if respiration is to be assisted rather than controlled).

After connecting the ventilator to the breathing circuit, the anesthetist should closely observe the patient to ensure that the chest rises with each inspiration. Respiratory rate is usually 8 to 12 breaths per minute. Duration of inspiration is set at 1 to 2 seconds, and duration of expiration should be 2 to 4 seconds with an inspiratory/expiratory ratio of 1:2 to 1:3. If a pressure-cycled ventilator is used, a pressure setting of 12 cm to 20 cm is normally selected. These settings may be varied to adapt to the special needs of selected patients. For example, a dog with gastric dilation/volvulus may need higher airway pressures to deliver a minimal effective tidal volume. Obese cats and dogs often require normal rates but higher airway pressures to overcome the thoracic effects of obesity.

Like manual ventilation, mechanical ventilation is particularly indicated for patients with compromised respiration. It is not normally necessary in healthy anesthetized patients, in which intermittent manual bagging (once every 5 minutes) is usually sufficient. Mechanical ventilation is particularly helpful in animals undergoing a thoracotomy or other lengthy operation, in which continuous manual ventilation would be difficult for the anesthetist.

Technical consideration for continuous ventilation of anesthetized patients

Rebreathing versus nonrebreathing systems. Continuous manual bagging can be performed with either a rebreathing or a nonrebreathing system. Nonrebreathing systems usually lack a manometer, and the anesthetist must use sight and touch to determine the optimal tidal volume.

In-circle versus out-of-circle vaporizers. Patients connected to a circle system with an in-circle nonprecision vaporizer can be bagged every 5 minutes to assist ventilation. However, it is advisable to turn the vaporizer setting to zero before bagging the patient, to prevent sudden vaporization of large amounts of anesthetic as a result of the increased flow of carrier gas through the vaporizer. Continuous controlled ventilation with an in-circle vaporizer is difficult and may be dangerous, unless the vaporizer is turned down or off. Because of the increased gas flow associated with controlled ventilation and the lack of back pressure compensation in these vaporizers, the patient may receive excessive amounts of vaporized anesthetic.

In contrast, it is feasible to use continuous manual or mechanical ventilation on patients connected to a circle system with an out-of-circle precision vaporizer. If the vaporizer is compensated for gas flow and back pressure, it is not necessary to turn the concentration setting to zero during controlled ventilation. However, if continuous manual ventilation is used, it may be advisable to reduce the precision vaporizer setting, or the patient's level of anesthesia may become too deep because of increased delivery of anesthetic to the lungs. The anesthetist should closely monitor the patient and adjust the vaporizer setting according to the patient's depth.

Risks of Controlled Ventilation

Controlled ventilation, whether by manual ventilation with a reservoir bag or mechanical ventilation with a ventilator, has the potential to damage the animal's lungs if done incorrectly.

- Excessive airway pressure may rupture alveoli, causing pneumothorax or mediastinal emphysema.
- Cardiac output may be decreased if positive pressure is maintained throughout the respiratory cycle (during expiration and inspiration).
- If the ventilation rate is too high, excessive amounts of carbon dioxide may be exhaled, leading to respiratory alkalosis, which (if severe) can cause cerebral vasoconstriction and decreased cerebral blood flow.
- Mechanical ventilation is not intended to relieve the anesthetist of the necessity for patient monitoring. The anesthetist must closely monitor all animals in which ventilation is controlled or assisted to ensure that patient depth and vital signs are maintained within acceptable limits.

NEUROMUSCULAR BLOCKING AGENTS

Neuromuscular blocking agents (also called *muscle-paralyzing agents*) are often used in human anesthesia, but they have found only limited use in veterinary practice. Paralysis of the muscles of respiration is undesirable in conventional veterinary anesthesia; however, it is useful in the following situations:

- *Patients with mechanically ventilated lungs.* The use of neuromuscular blocking agents prevents spontaneous inspiratory efforts by the patient and allows more rapid and complete control of ventilation. This is particularly useful for thoracic or diaphragmatic surgery.
- *Orthopedic surgery.* Neuromuscular blocking agents provide excellent muscle relaxation, which is helpful in orthopedic procedures.
- *Ophthalmic surgery.* Neuromuscular blocking agents prevent movement of the eyeball.
- *Cesareans.* Neuromuscular blocking agents provide abdominal muscle relaxation and are not transferred across the placenta to the fetus.
- Neuromuscular blocking agents may be useful in facilitating difficult intubation (for example, reintubating animals with laryngospasm) because they allow rapid control of the airway without coughing or gagging.
- Occasionally muscle-paralyzing agents are used in "balanced anesthesia" techniques. In balanced anesthesia, different drugs provide the three components of general anesthesia (unconsciousness, muscle relaxation, and analgesia). Instead of using a high dose of a single agent such as thiopental to induce general

anesthesia, a balanced technique will include low doses of multiple agents (often an analgesic, a muscle-paralyzing agent, and an unconsciousness-inducing agent). The aim is to induce general anesthesia with a minimum of cardiovascular, respiratory, and other side effects.

Neuromuscular blocking agents should be administered only after the patient is unconscious and respiration has been controlled by means of continuous manual or mechanical ventilation. These agents should be considered to be an adjunct to, rather than a replacement for, anesthesia with other agents. Use of neuromuscular blocking agents in a conscious animal is inhumane because these agents have no tranquilizing, analgesic, or anesthetic properties. The patient given only these drugs will be fully conscious and have normal sensitivity to pain, but will be unable to move or otherwise resist the surgeon's efforts. Control of respiration is also essential after the administration of these drugs because the respiratory muscles will be paralyzed, making it impossible for the patient to breathe on its own.

Neuromuscular blocking agents act by interrupting normal transmission of impulses from motor neurons to the muscle synapse. The site of action is the nerve-muscle junction, where acetylcholine is released by the neurons in proximity to the muscle end plate. There are two ways in which muscle-paralyzing agents may disrupt nervous transmission, and neuromuscular blocking agents are classified as *depolarizing* or *nondepolarizing* according to which of the two mechanisms applies.

Depolarizing agents, such as succinylcholine, cause a single surge of activity at the neuromuscular junction, which is followed by a period in which the muscle end plate is refractory to further stimulation. Animals given these agents may show spontaneous muscle twitching, followed by paralysis. Succinylcholine has a fast onset (20 seconds) but short duration of effect. Potential adverse effects of succinylcholine include hyperkalemia and cardiac arrhythmias.

Nondepolarizing agents, such as gallamine, pancuronium, atracurium besylate, and cisatracurium, act by blocking the receptors at the end plates. As their classification suggests, they do not cause an initial surge of activity at the neuromuscular junction, and spontaneous muscle movements are not seen. Potential adverse effects of these agents include histamine release, hypotension or hypertension, tachycardia, and ventricular arrhythmias.

Concurrent use of isoflurane or halothane increases the potency of neuromuscular blocking agents. Animals that have undergone recent treatments with organophosphate insecticides also show an increased susceptibility to neuromuscular blocking agents. Other drugs, including corticosteroids, barbiturates, furosemide and other diuretics, anticancer drugs, epinephrine, tetracycline, and aminoglycoside antibiotics such as gentamicin, have been shown to affect the potency of neuromuscular blocking agents.

Muscle-paralyzing agents are normally given by slow intravenous injection. The dose required varies between patients and with the anesthetic protocol used. Most agents take effect within 2 minutes, and the duration of paralysis is approximately 10 to 30 minutes (although this varies considerably, depending on the agent used). If more prolonged paralysis is required, repeated doses can be given. Alternatively, some agents may be given by constant intravenous infusion.

Regardless of the agent used, only voluntary (skeletal) muscles are affected. These agents do not affect the involuntary muscles, including cardiac muscle and the smooth muscle of the intestine and bladder. Skeletal muscles are affected in a predictable order: facial and neck paralysis is seen first, followed by paralysis of the tail, limbs, and abdominal muscles. The intercostal muscles and diaphragm are affected last.

Anesthetic depth may be difficult to assess in animals that have been given muscle-paralyzing agents because of the inhibition or absence of normal reflex responses and the absence of jaw tone. Heart rate and blood pressure may give some indication of anesthetic depth. If salivation, tongue curling, or lacrimation is seen, the patient may not be deep enough for surgery.

Animals given muscle-paralyzing agents cannot blink and are predisposed to corneal drying. An ophthalmic lubricant must be used. The anesthetist must also monitor the patient for hypothermia, which is a common side effect resulting from the decreased muscle tone seen in patients given these agents. Hypothermia can slow the metabolism of the agents and delay recovery from anesthesia.

Nondepolarizing agents should be reversed with an anticholinesterase agent, even if the effects appear to be wearing off. Reversing agents have no effect on depolarizing agents. The most commonly used reversing agents are edrophonium (Tensilon), neostigmine, and pyridostigmine (Regonol). The patient should be maintained at a light anesthetic depth until the reversal agent has taken effect. After reversal of muscle-paralyzing agents, signs of returning muscle function include diaphragmatic movements, eye rotation, an active palpebral reflex, and increasing jaw tone. Sometimes, the effect of the reversing agent wears off before the muscle-paralyzing agent is eliminated, in which case respiratory support may be required.

Reversing agents may have undesirable side effects such as bradycardia and increased bronchial and salivary secretions and should be given only after pretreatment with atropine or glycopyrrolate.

KEY POINTS

1. Local anesthesia is the use of a chemical agent on sensory and motor neurons to produce a temporary loss of pain sensation and movement. Because of low patient toxicity, low cost, and minimal recovery time, local anesthesia may be preferred to general anesthesia in some patients. Disadvantages include lack of patient restraint, risk of overdose in smaller patients, and technical difficulties.
2. If sufficient quantity of local anesthetics reaches the sympathetic ganglia, a sympathetic blockade may result. This causes flushing, increased skin temperature, and, occasionally, hypotension and bradycardia.
3. Local anesthetics have many topical uses, including application to the conjunctiva or the epithelium of the respiratory or urogenital tracts.
4. Local anesthetics may be injected in proximity to a peripheral nerve, blocking sensation from the tissues served by the nerve. Surgical preparation of the area is necessary before injection of a local anesthetic. Epinephrine is commonly added to the lidocaine to delay absorption of the local anesthetic agent from the site, but epinephrine must not be used at peripheral locations where blood supply may be compromised.

Continued

KEY POINTS

5. Epidural anesthesia is achieved by injecting local anesthetic in the epidural space, between the dura and the vertebrae. In dogs and cats, the injection is performed between the last lumbar vertebra and the sacrum. This technique is useful for surgical procedures in patients that are debilitated and in patients that require profound analgesia of the caudal abdomen, limbs, or pelvis.

6. Intravenous injection of local anesthetics may be useful for distal limb surgery, including amputation.

7. Local anesthetics may be harmful if injected into a nerve. They may also cause temporary paresthesia, which may result in self-mutilation.

8. Adverse systemic effects of local anesthesia include sedation, hyperexcitability, respiratory depression, and sympathetic blockade. Toxicity may be avoided by limiting the amount of lidocaine administered to the patient (a maximum 10 mg/kg in dogs, when given subcutaneously) and avoiding intravenous injection of bupivacaine.

9. Controlled or assisted ventilation may be used to deliver oxygen and anesthetic to the patient. Either a mechanical ventilator or manual bagging may be used. These procedures are particularly useful in patients with poor respiratory function. Controlled or assisted ventilation helps prevent the development of hypercarbia, respiratory acidosis, and pulmonary atelectasis.

10. Manual ventilation can be achieved by gently squeezing the reservoir bag at a rate of 8 to 12 breaths per minute and a pressure of 15 to 20 cm H_2O. Inspiration time should be 1 to 1.5 seconds, and expiratory time should be 2 to 3 seconds. Manual ventilation is difficult if a nonprecision vaporizer is used.

11. Mechanical ventilators may be incorporated into either a rebreathing or nonrebreathing system. Depending on the type of ventilator used, the anesthetist may control the pressure or volume of gas to be delivered, the respiratory rate, and the length of inspiration and expiration.

12. If controlled ventilation is used, the anesthetist must use caution to avoid excessive expansion of the alveoli, continuous positive pressure, and excessive ventilation rates.

13. Neuromuscular blocking agents may be useful in some anesthetic procedures to allow relaxation of voluntary muscles. They should never be used as the sole anesthetic agent.

14. Neuromuscular blocking agents may be depolarizing or nondepolarizing in their action. Nondepolarizing agents may be reversed by the administration of neostigmine or edrophonium.

15. Neuromuscular blocking agents may cause systemic effects such as hypothermia and respiratory failure. Mechanical or manual ventilation should be available when these agents are used.

16. Many drugs, including isoflurane, halothane, aminoglycoside antibiotics, organophosphates and diuretics, may alter the potency of neuromuscular blocking agents.

REVIEW QUESTIONS

1. In the healthy awake animal, the main stimulus to breathe is the result of:
   a. Excess oxygen concentration in the blood
   b. Excess carbon dioxide concentration in the blood
   c. Insufficient oxygen in the blood
   d. Insufficient carbon dioxide in the blood

2. In the healthy awake animal, exhalation lasts _____ times as long as inhalation.
   a. ½
   b. 2
   c. 3
   d. 4

3. The normal tidal volume in an awake animal is _____ ml/kg.
   a. 5 to 10
   b. 10 to 15
   c. 16 to 20
   d. 20 to 25

4. In the anesthetized animal that is breathing room air, the anesthetist may expect to see:
   a. An increase in the $Paco_2$ and a decrease in the Pao_2
   b. A decrease in the $Paco_2$ and an increase in the Pao_2
   c. A decrease in the $Paco_2$ and a decrease in the Pao_2
   d. An increase in the $Paco_2$ and an increase in the Pao_2

5. When used in a line block, a local anesthetic agent will have a direct effect on the:
   a. Peripheral nervous system
   b. Central nervous system
   c. Peripheral and central nervous systems

6. Local anesthetic agents may affect:
   a. Sensory neurons only
   b. Motor neurons only
   c. Sensory and motor neurons only
   d. Sensory, motor, and autonomic neurons

7. Local anesthetic agents work because:
   a. They mechanically block nerve impulse transmission
   b. They interfere with the movement of sodium ions
   c. They block all impulses at the spinal cord level
   d. They affect neurotransmission within the brain

8. When a local anesthetic is injected around a major nerve, the procedure is referred to as a/an:
   a. Line block
   b. Epidural block
   c. Infiltration nerve block
   d. Intravenous anesthesia

9. Epinephrine may be mixed with a local anesthetic agent to prolong the effects of the drug.

True   False

10. When performing an epidural, one must be aware that the spinal cord in a cat may extend as far caudally as:

a. T13
b. L6
c. L7
d. S1
e. The coccygeal vertebrae

11. The maximum subcutaneous dose of lidocaine for a dog is _____ mg/kg.

a. 1
b. 4
c. 10
d. 15

12. When performing intravenous anesthesia, one should use lidocaine

a. With epinephrine
b. Without epinephrine
c. Either with or without epinephrine

13. The term *atelectasis* refers to:

a. Excess fluid in the respiratory system
b. The absence of breathing
c. Collapse of the alveoli
d. Bronchial constriction

14. What is the most common acid-base abnormality in anesthetized patients?

a. Respiratory alkalosis
b. Metabolic alkalosis
c. Respiratory acidosis
d. Metabolic acidosis

15. When the lungs of a patient that is connected to a circle system with a precision vaporizer are continuously ventilated manually, it is customary to:

a. Increase the vaporizer setting
b. Decrease the vaporizer setting
c. Disconnect the patient from the circle system before starting manual ventilation
d. The lungs of patients that are connected to a circle system should not be manually ventilated

16. Which of the following can be used to monitor anesthetic depth in a patient that has been given a neuromuscular blocking agent?

a. Heart rate
b. Jaw tone
c. Palpebral reflex
d. Pedal reflex

17. A neuromuscular blocking agent will not only paralyze skeletal muscle, but will also give some analgesia.
    True   False

18. When an animal is given a _____ drug, an initial surge of muscle activity may be seen before there is paralysis of the muscles.
    a. Depolarizing
    b. Nondepolarizing

19. The muscle type that is most affected by neuromuscular blocking agents is:
    a. Cardiac
    b. Smooth muscle
    c. Skeletal muscle
    d. All types are equally affected

20. Both depolarizing and nondepolarizing drugs can be reversed.
    True   False

For the following questions, more than one answer may be correct.

21. Problems that may result from excessive controlled ventilation may include:
    a. A decreased cardiac output
    b. Muscle twitching
    c. A state of respiratory alkalosis
    d. Ruptured alveoli

22. Local anesthetic agents such as lidocaine or proparacaine work well when applied:
    a. Topically on the epidermis
    b. Topically on mucous membranes
    c. Topically on the cornea
    d. Through injection

23. Factors that may interfere with the action of local anesthetic agents include:
    a. Fat
    b. Scar tissue
    c. Rapid heart rate
    d. Hemorrhage

24. Clinical signs of systemic toxicity from a local anesthetic agent may include:
    a. Sedation
    b. Convulsions
    c. Muscle twitching
    d. Respiratory depression

25. The effects that could result from an epidural anesthetic if the drug reached the thoracic and cervical spinal cord include:
    a. Sympathetic blockade
    b. Paralysis of intercostal muscles
    c. Paralysis of diaphragm
    d. Hypertension

ANSWERS FOR CHAPTER 7

1. b	**2.** b	**3.** b	**4.** a	**5.** a
6. d	**7.** b	**8.** c	**9.** True	**10.** d
11. c	**12.** b	**13.** c	**14.** c	**15.** b
16. a	**17.** False	**18.** a	**19.** c	**20.** False
21. a, c, d	**22.** b, c, d	**23.** a, b, d,	**24.** a, b, c, d	**25.** a, b, c

Selected Readings

Heath RB: Lumbosacral epidural management, *Vet Clin North Am Small Anim Pract* 22(2):417-419, 1992.

Ilkiw JE: Advantages of and guidelines for using neuromuscular blocking agents, *Vet Clin North Am Small Anim Pract* 22(2):347-350, 1992.

Ko JCH, Pablo LS, Heaton-Jones TG: Epidural injection of anesthetics in dogs and cats, *Vet Tech* 17(3):143-154, 1996.

Martinez EA: Newer neuromuscular blockers, *Vet Clin North Am Small Anim Pract* 29(3):811-817, 1999.

Pascoe PJ: Advantages and guidelines for using epidural drugs for analgesia, *Vet Clin North Am Small Anim Pract* 22(2):421-423, 1992.

CHAPTER 8

Analgesia

PERFORMANCE OBJECTIVES

After completion of this chapter, the reader will be able to:

- Define the terms *analgesia, referred pain, hyperesthesia, splinting, preemptive analgesia, windup, endorphin, ceiling effect, prostaglandin,* and *cyclooxygenase.*
- Differentiate between visceral and somatic pain.
- List the changes in behavior and vital signs that may be exhibited by animals with mild, moderate, and severe pain.
- Describe the routes by which analgesia can be provided.
- Describe nursing care that helps to relieve discomfort in hospitalized patients.
- Explain the mode of action of opioid drugs and of nonsteroidal analgesic drugs.
- List the adverse effects associated with the use of morphine and other opioids.
- Describe the risks and benefits of epidural morphine administration.
- Describe the procedure for applying a fentanyl patch.
- List the beneficial properties and potential toxic effects of nonsteroidal analgesics.
- Outline the benefits of combination analgesic therapy and list examples.
- Describe ways in which analgesia can be provided to outpatients.

PRINCIPLES OF ANALGESIA
What Is Analgesia?

The anesthetist who safely guides a patient through anesthesia must take on a new role in the postoperative period: the delivery of appropriate medication to control pain. In this chapter, the provision of pain control is discussed in its widest sense, including both the prevention and treatment of pain, whether due to surgery, trauma, acute medical conditions (such as otitis externa, mastitis, and pancreatitis) and chronic medical conditions (such as osteoarthritis or cancer).

The International Association for the Study of Pain has defined pain as *an unpleasant sensory or emotional experience associated with actual or potential tissue damage. Analgesia* is the absence of the awareness of pain, achieved through the use of drugs or other modes of therapy. The term *analgesia* usually applies to the relief of pain without loss of consciousness.

For both ethical and medical reasons, the veterinarian and veterinary technician must ensure that analgesia is provided for every patient that requires it. The technician must strive to recognize procedures that are likely to be painful, to use techniques that minimize pain, to monitor behavior and physiologic variables as potential indicators of pain, and to promptly bring animals requiring analgesia to the veterinarian's attention (Shaffron, 1998).

Why Treat Pain?

In the past, pain control was reserved for animals undergoing extensive orthopedic or thoracic surgery and was seldom provided for painful medical conditions or for elective operations such as castration and ovariohysterectomy. However, this attitude has changed, and it is now generally accepted that most animals benefit significantly if analgesia is routinely provided whenever pain is present. This includes the postoperative period after surgery.

The current emphasis on analgesia in veterinary patients has arisen for several reasons:

- Veterinarians and veterinary technicians are becoming more aware of animals' need for analgesia. Although veterinary patients cannot verbally communicate their perceptions of pain, all the available evidence indicates that pain perception in human beings and animals is similar. A good rule of thumb is that if a procedure is known to be painful in human beings, it should be regarded as such in animal patients.
- Animal owners are increasingly concerned that their pet does not experience unnecessary postoperative pain.
- General anesthetics currently used in small-animal practice do not provide significant postoperative pain control. Anesthetics that lack analgesic effect include halothane, isoflurane, propofol, and barbiturates. In addition, recent information has indicated that some of the agents that have traditionally been considered to be good analgesics (for example, meperidine, ketamine, butorphanol, medetomidine, and xylazine) are not effective enough or long lasting enough to be used as the sole analgesic for animals with severe postoperative pain, such as that experienced after orthopedic surgery.
- An animal that experiences postoperative pain is more likely to have a poor anesthetic recovery in the immediate postoperative period. General anesthetic agents that were in common use before the 1980s (including methoxyflurane and pentobarbital) were characterized by slow recoveries and prolonged sleep after anesthesia. These have been largely replaced by agents that allow arousal within minutes after completion of an operation (for example, propofol and isoflurane). If no analgesia is provided, these recoveries not only are rapid, but also may be painful.
- It is no longer accepted that animals benefit from pain. In the past, many health care providers thought that pain served a useful purpose by preventing activity that could cause further tissue injury. The concern has also been expressed that the use of analgesia will mask signs of illness and result in inappropriate activity. However, it is now accepted that pain rarely has any useful function and is more likely to be harmful to the animal. Animals with untreated pain may have increased fear and anxiety, decreased cardiovascular function, decreased appetite, slower wound healing, and greater risk of infection and disseminated intravascular coagulation (DIC). Studies in seriously ill children show that survival is higher when pain is treated.

This is not to suggest that every patient must receive high doses of analgesic drugs. Overtreatment of postoperative pain can contribute to prolonged anesthetic recovery and may have significant side effects. The need for analgesia must be considered in the light of the individual patient's condition and the potential for serious side effects. Fortunately, many drugs are now available for pain control, and it is usually possible to select an analgesic that is safe and effective for a given patient.

The goal of the anesthetist is to provide adequate analgesia and sedation to allow the patient to move, eat, and sleep without undue discomfort, particularly in the first 12 to 24 hours after surgery. Fortunately, most veterinary technicians are sensitive to their patients' needs for analgesia. A recent survey revealed that veterinary practices that have a veterinary technician on staff are more likely to use postoperative analgesics, compared with practices in which there is no technician (Dohoo, 1996).

GENERAL PRINCIPLES OF ANALGESIA
Physiology of Pain

In recent years, significant progress has been made in understanding the physiology of pain. Pain results when nerve cells in the skin or deep tissues (called *nociceptors*) detect a noxious stimulus. Examples of noxious stimuli include heat, ischemia (lack of blood supply), distention or stretching, mechanical injury (such as a scalpel incision), and chemicals released by inflammation or tissue damage (including prostaglandins, leukotrienes, bradykinin, proteolytic enzymes, histamine, potassium ions, and serotonin).

Pain receptors convert the chemical, thermal, or mechanical stimuli into nerve impulses. These impulses are transmitted by a chain consisting of at least three neurons: a sensory neuron located in the peripheral tissue, a neuron in the spinal cord that conveys the impulse to the brain, and a neuron in the brain itself that conveys the conscious sensation of pain.

There are two types of sensory neurons that transmit most pain signals from the peripheral tissues to the spinal cord and brain. *A delta fibers* transmit sharp, discrete pain signals that allow the patient to localize the source of the pain to an exact site. These neurons are large and myelinated, and they conduct signals rapidly. Smaller, nonmyelinated *C fibers* transmit dull, aching, or throbbing pain sensations that cannot be exactly localized. It is thought that *somatic pain* (that is, arising from skin, subcutaneous tissue, muscle, bones, or joints) is transmitted by both A delta and C fibers. Somatic pain is often easily localized and is characterized as stabbing, throbbing, or aching. *Visceral pain* (arising from internal organs) is primarily transmitted by C fibers only. Visceral pain is more difficult to localize and is characterized as cramping, burning, or gnawing. The information from both types of neurons is conveyed to the dorsal horn of the spinal cord, where transmission of pain signals is suppressed or augmented by the effect of neural hormones such as substance P and cholecystokinin. The information is then transmitted to the thalamus and the sensory cortex of the cerebrum, where the perception of pain occurs.

Pain can be classified in several ways. The intensity of pain may be mild, moderate, or severe, and the duration may be acute or chronic. Because surgical pain has an abrupt onset and relatively short duration, it is classified as *acute pain*. Acute pain can usually be satisfactorily treated with analgesic drugs. In contrast, *chronic pain* (for example, pain associated with cancer or osteoarthritis) has a slow onset, a duration of several months or years, and may be unresponsive to drug therapy. *Referred pain* is a term used to describe pain that is felt in a body part other than that in which the cause is situated (for example, human patients who have had a heart attack may feel referred pain in the upper arm rather than in the chest). *Hyperesthesia* is an increased sensitivity to a stimulus such as touch, heat, or cold. The stimulus may or may not be perceived as painful. *Neuropathic pain* is pain that arises from direct damage to peripheral nerves or the spinal cord. It is often poorly responsive to analgesics.

Monitoring Signs of Pain

Monitoring animals for signs of pain is a complex task. It is sometimes difficult to differentiate pain from anxiety or emotional distress, and it is the challenging task of the veterinary technician to assist in alleviating each of these. If in doubt, it is best to treat the patient as if the problem were pain induced and to monitor the animal for alleviation of distress.

It is well recognized that the amount of pain that the patient has in the postoperative period will vary depending upon the site, duration, and nature of the surgical procedure (Table 8-1). Significant pain is most likely to arise after orthopedic procedures (especially amputations or operations involving the cervical vertebrae, femur, or humerus). Surgery of the ears, eyes, mammary glands, or joints may also be associated with severe postoperative pain. Other surgical procedures may result in a lesser degree of pain that can be treated with lower doses or less potent analgesics.

TABLE 8-1

Severity of Pain Associated with Medical and Surgical Procedures

IRRITATING OR MILDLY PAINFUL	MILDLY TO MODERATELY PAINFUL	MODERATELY TO SEVERELY PAINFUL	SEVERELY PAINFUL
Urine scald	Endoscopy with biopsy	Localized burns	Extensive burns
Clipper burns	Dental extraction	Corneal ulcerations	Pancreatitis
Intravenous or urinary catheterization	Arterial catheterization	Enucleation	Total hip replacement
Distended bladder	Aural hematoma	Thoracic or lumbar disk surgery	Cervical disk surgery
Superficial lacerations	Stabilized radial or tibial fracture	Onychectomy	Forelimb or hind limb amputation
Eyelid procedures	Castration	Stabilized femoral or humeral fracture	Ear ablation
Dental prophylaxis	Ovariohysterectomy	Pelvic fracture	Thoracotomy (especially sternal split)
	Ear flush	Mastectomy	Laminectomy
	Cystotomy	Cranial abdominal surgery	
		Anal sacculectomy	

Modified from Carroll GL: *Small animal pain management*, Lakewood, Colo, 1998, AAHA Press.

The anesthetist must also recognize that there is considerable variation among patients in the amount of analgesic required to control pain. It has been documented in human patients that there is a fivefold variation in the amount of narcotic medication needed to control pain after a standardized surgical procedure. Pain sensation varies according to level of consciousness, previous experience, behavioral training, emotional state, species, gender, age, breed, and other factors. Observation of the patient is the only way to determine whether sufficient analgesia has been provided. Because pain control is most critical in the first 24 hours after trauma or surgery, the patient should be repeatedly evaluated throughout this period to ensure that pain and discomfort are controlled as much as possible. If a patient has been treated with an analgesic but still appears uncomfortable, the veterinarian should be informed, because it may be necessary to administer an additional dose of analgesic or to change the type of analgesic used.

It is sometimes difficult to judge when a patient no longer requires analgesic drugs. In human medicine, patients with severe postoperative pain are usually treated for 2 to 5 days with injectable analgesics before switching to oral analgesics. In the case of animals, 3 days of analgesia is often adequate, but after the drug is discontinued, the patient should be closely monitored for signs of discomfort that would indicate a need for further analgesia.

Detection of pain in a veterinary patient may be difficult for the following reasons:
- The observer is usually unfamiliar with the individual animal's normal behavior or activity level.
- Some animals show no obvious signs of pain (particularly when interacting with people or in new, unfamiliar surroundings) or may demonstrate only subtle changes in their behavior. It is particularly challenging to determine if depressed, sick animals are in pain. The ability to suppress behaviors that show pain probably arises because in the natural world, animals that show pain or distress are more likely to become prey than are healthy animals.
- Many hospitalized patients have been given sedatives, which may alter the behavioral response to pain (although not the perception of pain by the patient).

For these reasons, the technician must be alert to even minor changes in normal behavior that may indicate that pain is present (Table 8-2). In fact, some authorities on veterinary anesthesia suggest that postoperative analgesics are indicated for all patients undergoing surgical procedures, regardless of the presence or absence of overt signs of pain. Because there is no single reliable measure of pain, analgesia should be used if it seems likely to the observer that the animal is experiencing pain, regardless of its outward demeanor.

Animal caregivers who take the time to observe animals after painful surgical procedures will soon realize that there is considerable variation in the way that animals show pain. Some animals become agitated or restless and may vocalize (for example, whimpering, groaning, barking, growling, and crying), whereas others appear quiet, depressed, and inactive. Some dogs and cats frown or squint, and lay their ears back. Some animals may become aggressive and resist handling, whereas others may seek contact with their caregivers. Other signs of pain may include difficulty sleeping and lack of appetite. Often, the patient will show stiff body movements and a reluctance to move or may be hesitant to jump or play. Cats with severe pain are commonly silent, assume a hunched position in sternal recumbency, appear

TABLE 8-2

Behavioral Responses to Pain

BEHAVIORAL RESPONSE	DOGS	CATS
Vocalization	Groan, whine, whimper, growl	Groan, growl, purr
Facial expression	Fixed stare, glazed appearance, ears back	Furrowed brow, squinted eyes
Body posture	Hunched or laterally recumbent	Sternal recumbency
Guarding/self-mutilation	Protects wound, limps, licks and chews wound and surgical site	Protects wound, limps, licks and chews wound and surgical site
Activity	Restless or restricted movement, trembling	Restricted movement, may see stereotyped movements such as circling
Attitude	Increased aggression or fearfulness	Comfort-seeking or hiding, may be aggressive
Appetite	Decreased	Decreased
Urinary and bowel habits	Increased urination, failure in house training, urinary retention	Failure to use litter box
Grooming	Loss of sheen in hair coat	Failure to groom, unkempt appearance
Response to palpation	Protecting, biting, vocalizing, withdrawing	Protecting, biting, scratching, vocalizing, withdrawing, attempts to escape

Modified from Mathews KA: Nonsteroidal antiinflammatory analgesics in pain management in dogs and cats, *Can Vet J* 37(9):539-545, 1996.

to distance themselves from their environment, and fail to groom themselves. Similarly, some dogs may "stare into space," seemingly oblivious to their environment.

With close observation, it is sometimes possible to determine the location of the pain. Patients may lick, bite, or scratch the source of the pain sensation. For example, animals with ear pain commonly shake their heads and scratch the affected ear. Dental pain may cause salivation and a reluctance to eat or drink. Animals with neck pain usually hold their neck straight and rigidly maintain that position. Patients with thoracic pain often have shallow abdominal respiratory movements and tend to sit or lie in sternal recumbency, reluctant to move. Animals with abdominal pain may have tense abdominal muscles (*splinting*) and often stand with the elbows back and the back arched. These patients may be reluctant to sit or lie down (or if lying down, they are reluctant to get up). Animals with head pain often appear depressed, immobile, and hold the head down, or press their head against a wall.

Pain may also cause changes in physiologic variables, leading to increased blood pressure and heart rate,* increased respiration rate and decreased tidal volume (sometimes panting), salivation, dilated pupils, pale mucous membranes, and prolonged capillary refill. Many of these changes arise from increased activity of the sympathetic nervous system. Laboratory findings may include neutrophilia and lymphocytosis, hyperglycemia, and elevated levels of hormones such as cortisol or epinephrine. Patients that receive appropriate analgesia should show improvement in both behavioral signs and vital signs, including a reduction in heart rate and respiratory rate.

Recently, an attempt has been made to quantify the amount of pain experienced by an animal, on the basis of the animal's behavior and vital signs (Box 8-1). This assessment scale is only a guide, and individual patients may differ significantly from the normal pattern. Behavioral characteristics are a continuum, and a given patient may show some signs that indicate moderate pain and other signs that indicate severe pain.

Methods of Pain Control

The most basic step in alleviation of pain (as with other medical conditions) is to take away the primary cause. This is not always possible, as in the case of postsurgical pain. However, painful medical conditions such as anal sac abscesses and otitis externa can be successfully treated, although analgesia may be required during the treatment period until pain is no longer present. The second step in alleviation of pain is to treat the pain itself. There are several effective methods of pain control, not all of which involve the administration of drugs.

Endorphins

Given that pain may be harmful to an animal, it is not surprising that the body has an internal mechanism to control pain. Within the central nervous system (CNS), chemicals similar to morphine (for example, beta endorphin, leu-enkephalin, and dynorphin) are released by neurons when the body is traumatized or under stress. These chemicals bind to opioid receptors and provide some analgesia. Acupuncture and transcutaneous electric nerve stimulation may effectively treat pain by stimulating the release of these chemical mediators. Other nonpharmacologic methods of pain control that may be effective in some situations include massage therapy, application of cold (for acute injuries) or heat (for chronic injuries), physiotherapy, magnetic therapy, and homeopathic or herbal remedies such as Bach flower remedies. The effectiveness of some of these therapies has not been demonstrated in controlled studies.

Nursing care

Patient discomfort can also be reduced through conscientious nursing care, including keeping the animal clean and dry, affording ample opportunity for defecation and urination (including bladder expression or catheterization if necessary),

---

*Although heart rate may be helpful in determining if pain is present, it is not always a reliable indicator of pain. Tachycardia may be mild or absent in painful animals, especially those that have received opioids. Also, tachycardia may be present in nonpainful animals as a result of excitement or other causes.

BOX 8-1   Recognition and Treatment of Postoperative Pain

This is a guide for pain assessment in veterinary patients. Pain can be graded on a scale of 0 (no pain) to 9 (severe to excruciating pain).

0 **No pain.** Patient is running, playing, eating, jumping, and sitting or walking normally. Sleeping comfortably with dreaming. Normal, affectionate response to caregiver. Heart rate should be normal, but if elevated it is the result of excitement. Cats will rub their face on the attendant's hand or the cage, may roll over and purr. Cats and dogs will groom themselves. Appetite is normal. If behavior different from this is associated with apprehension or anxiety in the hospitalized patient, no treatment necessary.

1 **Probably no pain.** Patient appears to be normal, but condition is not as clear-cut as above. Heart rate should be normal, or slightly increased as a result of excitement. Cats may still purr. No treatment necessary.

2 **Mild discomfort.** Patient will still eat or sleep but may not dream. May limp slightly or resist palpation of a surgical wound, but shows no other signs of discomfort. Not depressed. There may be a slight increase in respiratory rate and heart rate. Dogs may continue to wag their tail and cats may still purr. Reassess within the hour, then give analgesic if condition appears worse.

3 **Mild pain or discomfort.** Patient will limp or guard a surgical incision. The abdomen may be slightly tucked up if abdominal surgery was performed. Looks a little depressed. Cannot get comfortable. May tremble or shake. Appears to be interested in food and may still eat a little but somewhat picky. Respiratory rate may be increased and a little shallow. Heart rate may be increased or normal, depending on whether an opioid was given previously. Cats may continue to purr and dogs may wag their tail, even when they are in pain; therefore, disregard these behavioral patterns as indicators of comfort.

   Needs analgesia. The analgesic selected will depend on whether it is a repeat in the patient with moderate to severe pain, or the patient has a problem resulting in mild to moderate pain. If the patient has been previously treated with an analgesic, continue with morphine IM or SC (dogs 0.3 to 0.5 mg/kg, cats 0.05 to 0.1 mg/kg), oxymorphone (0.05 to 0.1 mg/kg IV or IM), hydromorphone IV (0.1 mg/kg), or injectable NSAID if patient status allows. If patient has not been previously treated and this is a mild to moderate pain situation, oxymorphone or hydromorphone or morphine is unnecessary and may cause dysphoria. Instead, administer butorphanol (0.2 to 0.4 mg/kg), buprenorphine, or NSAID where appropriate.

4 **Mild to moderate pain.** The patient resists touching of the surgery site, injured area, painful abdomen, neck, or other area. If there is abdominal pain, guards or splints the abdominal muscles or stretches all four legs out. May lick or chew at the painful area. The patient may sit or lie in an abnormal position and is not curled up or relaxed. May remain recumbent, without moving, for several hours (because movement causes pain). May tremble or shake. May or may not appear interested in food. May start to eat and then stop after one or two bites. Respiratory rate may be increased or shallow. Heart rate may be increased or normal. Pupils may be dilated. May whimper (dogs) or cry (cats) occasionally, be slow to rise, and hang tail down. There may be no weight bearing or only a toe touch on an injured limb. Will be somewhat depressed. Cats may lie quietly and not move for prolonged periods.

   Needs analgesia. Administer butorphanol 0.4 mg/kg every 2 to 4 hours for soft tissue injury or surgery, or painful medical conditions. For orthopedic or soft tissue injury, administer an opioid every 3 to 6 hours: oxymorphone (0.05 mg/kg) or hydromorphone (0.1 mg/kg) or morphine IM or SC (dogs 0.3 mg/kg, cats 0.1 mg/kg). Consider NSAIDs for orthopedic procedures or soft tissue injury or surgery where there are no concerns for hemorrhage, renal insufficiency, or gastric ulceration. If the patient has already received an opioid, consider an NSAID as an adjunct to opioid.

BOX 8-1 *Recognition and Treatment of Postoperative Pain—cont'd*

5 **Moderate pain.** Patient reluctant to move, depressed, and inappetant. May vocalize, bite, or attempt to bite when the caregiver approaches the painful area. Trembling or shaking with head down, depressed. There is definite splinting of the abdomen if affected (as in peritonitis, pancreatitis, hepatitis, and incisional pain). Patient is unable to bear weight on an injured or operative limb. The ears may be pulled back. The heart and respiratory rates may be increased. Pupils may be dilated. The patient is not interested in food, will lie down but does not really sleep, and may stand in the "prayer position" (tail and pelvis in the air, front legs extended and head close to ground) if there is abdominal pain. Cats may lie quietly and not move.

Needs analgesia. Treatment is same as for 4.

6 **Moderate pain.** Same signs as 5, but patient may vocalize or whine frequently, without provocation and when attempting to move. Heart rate may be increased or may be within normal limits if an opioid was administered previously. Respiratory rate may be increased with an abdominal lift. Pupils may be dilated.

Needs analgesia. Treatment with oxymorphone (0.1 to 0.2 mg/kg), hydromorphone (0.1 to 0.2 mg/kg), or morphine IM or SC (dogs 0.4 mg/kg, cats 0.2 mg/kg) every 3 to 6 hours, or morphine or fentanyl in IV fluids (see p. 328). If butorphanol was given within the last 20 minutes and the condition is still painful, a higher dose of morphine or oxymorphone is usually required because of the antagonistic effects of butorphanol; or may give injectable NSAID, especially if orthopedic pain and patient status permits.

7 **Moderate to severe pain.** Includes signs from 5 and 6, and patient appears very depressed and is not concerned with its surroundings. The patient will urinate and defecate without attempting to move. Will cry out when moved or will spontaneously or continually whimper. Some animals do not vocalize. Heart and respiratory rates may be increased. Hypertension may be present; pupils may be dilated.

Needs analgesia. Patient requires a higher dose of morphine, fentanyl, oxymorphone, hydromorphone, or NSAID (if orthopedic pain) or combination of NSAID and opioid.

8 **Severe pain.** Signs same as in 7. Vocalizing may be more of a feature, or patient may be so consumed with pain that it does not notice your presence and lies quietly and is unresponsive. The patient may thrash around in the cage intermittently. If it is traumatic or neurologic pain, the patient may scream when approached (especially cats). Tachycardia and increased respiratory rate with increased abdominal effort and hypertension are usually present even if an opioid was previously given.

Needs analgesia. Treat with high-dose oxymorphone, hydromorphone, or morphine IM, SC, or in IV fluids to effect (dogs) or with fentanyl (dogs and cats). Add an injectable NSAID if orthopedic pain and patient status permits.

9 **Severe to excruciating pain.** As in 8 but patient is hyperesthetic. The patient will tremble involuntarily when any part of the body in proximity to wound or injury is touched. Neurologic pain (entrapped nerve or inflammation around the nerve) or extensive inflammation (peritonitis, pleuritis, myositis, or pancreatitis) usually present.

Needs analgesia. Requires high-dose oxymorphone, hydromorphone, or morphine IM, SC, or in IV fluids given to effect (dogs), or fentanyl (cats and dogs), plus NSAIDs where not contraindicated. Consider combining analgesics with epidurally placed opioids or local anesthetic block. Inciting cause must be found and if possible, removed.

providing comfortable bedding and quiet surroundings, and gently reassuring the patient. The patient should be positioned so that it does not lie on a surgery site or traumatized area. Some patients benefit from being turned every 2 to 3 hours. Unconscious animals may require the application of ophthalmic ointment to prevent corneal drying. Treatments and monitoring should be scheduled so that the patient is not disturbed unnecessarily.

PHARMACOLOGIC ANALGESIA

There are many situations in which nursing care is of limited benefit for treating pain and the use of analgesic drugs is indicated. Ideally, pain control in the surgical patient should be available at every stage of hospitalization and treatment: during the preanesthetic period, the surgical procedure itself, the immediate postoperative period, the remainder of the hospital stay, and, if necessary, after the patient's return home.

The veterinarian has many options in choosing the method of delivering analgesic drugs. The first choice is the agent to be used, which may be an opioid, a nonsteroidal antiinflammatory drug (NSAID), a local anesthetic, or a combination of these. The choice of analgesic is governed by the severity and type of pain and the animal's general condition. The veterinarian also selects the route of delivery, which may include injection (SC, IM, IV, intraarticular, epidural, local infiltration), oral administration, rectal suppository, or transdermal patch.

Preemptive Analgesia

It is often advantageous to administer analgesics before tissue damage occurs or the patient has an awareness of pain (for example, before or during surgery, rather than after surgery). This fundamental principle of analgesia is called *preemptive use*. One method of providing preemptive analgesia is to give the patient a drug such as butorphanol, medetomidine, or meperidine as a preanesthetic. Other examples of preemptive pain control include epidural morphine administration and the use of bupivacaine or lidocaine local and regional nerve blocks. Animals that receive preemptive analgesics are less likely to show signs of a painful recovery compared with an animal that has not received analgesics in the preanesthetic period.

Because the effect of meperidine or butorphanol is short in dogs (1 to 2 hours), it is unlikely that these drugs are still active in the body by the time the patient wakes up from anesthesia. Why then does the animal appear to have a less painful recovery then expected? It is thought that meperidine and other preanesthetic analgesics act during the surgical period itself to prevent the buildup of chemical mediators that intensify the pain response. In contrast, an animal that has not been treated with analgesics during the preanesthetic period will experience the buildup of these mediators within the spinal cord in response to surgical manipulation (a phenomenon called windup). Although the animal will not be aware of pain during the surgical period itself, it is likely to be painful when it regains consciousness in the immediate postoperative period and becomes aware of the effect of the pain mediators. This results in the need for greater amounts of postoperative analgesic in these patients, compared with those that received preemptive analgesics. It must be emphasized, however, that the use of preemptive analgesics only prevents sensitization of the CNS and does not replace or eliminate the need for postoperative analgesic drugs.

In addition to providing effective pain relief in the recovering patient, preemptive use of analgesics also allows the anesthetist to reduce the amount of general anesthetic needed during the operation itself. For example, a patient that has been given IM morphine immediately before an operation may require considerably less halothane for maintenance of anesthesia than an unmedicated patient. This anesthetic-sparing effect is also useful if a patient shows pain during an operation, in response to surgical stimulation. In this case, the anesthetist may decide to administer a powerful analgesic such as hydromorphone (0.05 to 0.2 mg/kg), oxymorphone (dogs and cats, 0.05 to 0.2 mg/kg IM), or morphine (dogs 0.25 to 0.5 mg/kg IM; cats 0.1 to 0.2 mg/kg IM), rather than increasing the depth of anesthesia. When given by the IM route, morphine requires almost 15 minutes to reach maximum analgesic effect.

The recommendation for preemptive use of analgesics applies best to opioid agents (such as butorphanol, meperidine, hydromorphone, and morphine) and local anesthetics (such as bupivacaine and lidocaine). In the case of NSAIDs, preemptive use may not be advisable because it may increase the incidence of adverse effects such as decreased blood flow to the kidney during anesthesia and hemorrhage at the surgery site. Some NSAIDs, such as carprofen, can be used preemptively under certain conditions (see the section on NSAIDs).

Preemptive pain relief may not be possible in some patients (for example, patients with severe trauma). In this case, analgesics should be given before the return of consciousness after anesthesia. It is inhumane and often ineffective to delay the administration of analgesics until the patient wakes up and vocalizes because of pain.

Mechanisms of Pain Relief

Analgesic drugs prevent pain perception by several mechanisms. NSAIDs such as aspirin or carprofen work at the tissue level to prevent the production of chemicals such as prostaglandins that mediate inflammation and pain. Some NSAIDs also have a direct effect on the brain. Local anesthetics such as lidocaine block transmission of pain impulses by sensory nerves. Opioids such as morphine and alpha-2 agonists such as medetomidine affect multiple sites in the brain and spinal cord to diminish the perception of pain.

Because there are many pathways and mechanisms that lead to the perception of pain, it is unlikely that any one agent can effectively treat all patients for all kinds of pain. The nature of pain varies depending on the surgical procedure and the patient, and the optimal analgesic treatment will therefore vary between cases. For any given animal, different analgesics may be used at different times. The anesthetist should have a good knowledge of several agents and techniques that can be used and should consult with the veterinarian on which drug or combination of drugs is most appropriate for a particular patient's situation.

Whatever the type of analgesia chosen, there is considerable variation among patients in the amount of analgesic they require and the duration of its effect. Whether a patient receives injectable butorphanol, epidural morphine, a fentanyl patch, or an NSAID such as ketoprofen, the aim is the same: the patient should be able to sleep comfortably and move freely when awake. If this aim is not achieved after administration of an analgesic, the patient should be reassessed and further treatment given as necessary. Because different classes of agents differ in their mechanisms of action, it is sometimes helpful to combine two drugs from different classes (such as an opioid and an NSAID, or an opioid and a local analgesic) to achieve more effective analgesia (see section on combination therapy).

CLASSES OF ANALGESIC DRUGS

Pharmacologic analgesia can be achieved through a variety of agents, including opioids, NSAIDs, alpha-2 agonists, ketamine, and local anesthetics.

Opioid Agents

Opioids appear to act on pain receptors in both the spinal cord and brain. Doses, routes, and side effects of opioids used for postoperative analgesia are given in Table 8-3.

TABLE 8-3			
Dosages of Opioids Used for Postoperative Analgesia*			
DRUG	SPECIES	DOSAGE	DURATION
Morphine	Dog	Loading dose is 0.1 mg/kg slowly IV every 3-5 minutes until desired effect achieved. Add same dose to IV fluids and administer over next 4 hours. Maintenance dose is 0.2-1 mg/kg IM or SC, or 0.05-0.3 mg/kg/hr constant IV infusion. Oral dose 1-3 mg/kg every 4-8 hours PO (2 mg/kg every 12 hours for sustained-release tablets)	2-4 hours for injection, 4-12 hours PO
	Cat	0.05-0.2 mg/kg SC	
Oxymorphone	Dog	0.03-0.2 mg/kg IM, SC, IV	3-4 hours
	Cat	0.03-0.05 mg/kg IM, SC	3-4 hours
Hydromorphone	Dog and cat	0.05-0.2 mg/kg IV, IM, SC	4 hours
Meperidine	Dog and cat	2-10 mg/kg IM, SC	Less than 1 hour
Butorphanol	Dog and cat	0.2-0.8 mg/kg IM, SC, IV	1-2 hours for injection in dogs, 4 hours in cats
		0.5-1 mg/kg PO	6-12 hours PO
Buprenorphine	Dog and cat	0.01-0.02 mg/kg IM or IV	6-12 hours
Fentanyl	Dog and cat	Loading dose is 20 µg/kg in dogs and 2 µg/kg in cats Infusion rate 0.6-0.7 µg/kg/min	30 minutes

Modified from *Veterinary teaching hospital undergraduate manual,* Guelph, Ontario, Canada, 1992, Ontario Veterinary College.
*Dosages are approximate and patient should be monitored for efficacy and duration.

As outlined in Chapter 1, opioids have many uses in veterinary anesthesia, including the following:

- Opioids are commonly included in injectable premedications, often in combination with an anticholinergic and a tranquilizer such as acepromazine or medetomidine. With preemptive use they diminish windup, although perhaps not as effectively as local anesthetics. The analgesic effect of these preanesthetic mixtures is generally gone by 2 to 4 hours after administration, and they are usually inadequate to prevent or control even moderate pain after surgery.
- At higher doses, opioids can be used in combination with tranquilizers to induce a state of potent sedation (neuroleptanalgesia) that offers considerable analgesia throughout the surgical period and for some time after surgery. (See the discussion on neuroleptanalgesia on pp. 41 and 137-138.)
- Opioids can be used on their own or in combination with other agents (for example, NSAIDs and local anesthetics) to provide postoperative pain control (see the following discussion on the use of opioids in the postoperative period by injectable, epidural, transdermal, and other routes).

Individual opioids vary in their potency, duration, and side effects. For the purpose of pain control, opioids can be divided into two groups. Pure agonists* such as morphine, hydromorphone, oxymorphone, and fentanyl produce significant sedation and excellent analgesia but may induce significant respiratory and cardiovascular side effects. They are used for moderate to severe pain. Other agonists, including meperidine, buprenorphine, and nalbuphine, and mixed agonist/antagonists such as butorphanol are less potent. Sedation is also less pronounced, as are adverse effects on the cardiovascular and respiratory system. Because of their weaker analgesic effect, these agents should be reserved for use as preanesthetics and for treatment of mild to moderate pain.

In addition to their analgesic properties, many opioids cause some degree of sedation and relieve anxiety. If used as sole agents and at high dosages, some may induce excitement, nausea, and vomiting in awake patients. Many are effective cough suppressants.

Opioids are metabolized in the liver. Animals with liver disease may have impaired drug metabolism, and these agents should be given at reduced dosages.

Opioid agents used for moderate to severe pain

The potent opioid analgesics most commonly used in veterinary medicine are morphine, oxymorphone, hydromorphone, and fentanyl.

Morphine (morphine sulfate, Duramorph, Astramorph/PF). Morphine was the original opioid agent used in human and veterinary medicine and is still extensively used in veterinary practice as a preanesthetic and analgesic. It is a pure agonist with affinity for both mu and kappa opioid receptors (see Chapter 1). Morphine can be used in both dogs and cats; however, the canine dosage may cause excitement in cats, and a lower dosage is warranted in this species. Restlessness is seen in some dogs shortly after morphine administration, especially in the absence of pain.

---

*See Chapter 1 for a discussion of opioid agonists and mixed agonist/antagonists.

Morphine is an inexpensive and effective option for treatment of moderate to severe pain in most patients. It is effective in treating both visceral and somatic pain and can be given by several routes, including slow IV (dogs only), IM, SC, intraarticular, epidural, or spinal injection. Morphine is also available in regular or sustained release tablets for oral use and in a rectal suppository form. Efficacy of oral morphine varies considerably among patients.

When morphine is given IV to dogs, care should be taken to avoid too rapid injection, which may cause release of histamine (characterized by a fall in blood pressure, flushing, and pruritus). One technique for use in dogs is to draw up a loading dose of 0.1 to 0.5 mg/kg, which is given slowly IV (over 5 minutes) and repeated until the patient appears free of pain. The same total dose is then added to the IV fluids and administered over the next 4 hours. Morphine can also be administered IV by constant rate infusion. In this technique, morphine contained in a syringe is slowly administered through an IV catheter by means of a syringe pump at a rate of 0.05 to 0.3 mg/kg/hr.

Administration of morphine (and oxymorphone or hydromorphone) by the IM route gives a slightly longer duration of action than IV administration and avoids the risk of hypotension. IM injection appears to be somewhat painful, and SC injections cause less patient discomfort (although SC injections have a slightly slower onset of effect). The incidence of excitement, dysphoria, and vomiting in cats is lower when morphine is given by the SC, rather than IM, route. Cats should not receive morphine by the IV route.

Although morphine provides potent analgesia and sedation, it is associated with several undesirable side effects, including gastrointestinal stimulation and vomiting, salivation, and defecation. The incidence of vomiting can be reduced by pretreatment with acepromazine (0.02 mg/kg IM, 15 to 20 minutes before the morphine is given). Morphine also has the potential to cause severe respiratory depression, although this is less common in animals than in human patients. Excitement (particularly in cats given doses greater than 0.1 mg/kg), bradycardia, panting, increased intraocular pressure, increased intracranial pressure, urinary retention, miosis (in dogs), mydriasis (in cats), and hypothermia are also encountered in some patients after morphine administration. Fortunately, these side effects are seldom a significant problem in painful patients treated with analgesic dosages. Morphine also reduces cardiac afterload and is sometimes used in dogs with congestive heart failure, especially if sedation is desirable.

Morphine has a strong tendency to cause physical dependence (addiction) in humans. It is therefore classified as a Schedule II drug in the United States and is designated as a narcotic in Canada.

Oxymorphone (Numorphan). Oxymorphone is a pure agonist opioid with a greater analgesic potency and sedative effect than morphine, fewer side effects, and a longer duration of analgesia (4 hours). Despite these advantages, use of oxymorphone in veterinary practice is somewhat limited by its high cost.

Oxymorphone has less tendency to induce vomiting than morphine does. Also, unlike morphine, it does not induce histamine release and therefore does not decrease blood pressure. For this reason, it is preferred to morphine in patients with trauma, which may be in shock or at increased risk of developing hypotension.

Oxymorphone may cause respiratory depression in some animals, especially in animals under inhalation anesthesia. Paradoxically, it also induces panting in many patients, which may make some procedures (such as thoracic radiography) difficult. Oxymorphone causes some animals to become hyperresponsive to sound, and affected animals are easily startled by sudden noises. Bradycardia is also a potential side effect of this drug but can be prevented by pretreatment with atropine or glycopyrrolate.

Oxymorphone can be administered by many routes, including IV, IM, SC, or epidurally. Oxymorphone may be given rapidly IV to dogs, but IV administration may cause excitement in cats. A tranquilizer such as medetomidine, acepromazine, or diazepam may be used concurrently to prevent excitement and supplement the sedative effect of oxymorphone. Oxymorphone mixed with sterile saline and administered by IV drip is a safe analgesic agent in very sick or debilitated animals. Oxymorphone can be mixed with acepromazine (0.05 to 0.1 mg/kg acepromazine, not to exceed 3 mg, and 0.2 mg/kg oxymorphone) and used to induce anesthesia. Oxymorphone and diazepam (IV, administered alternately with separate syringes) can also be used to induce anesthesia and has less risk of hypotension or decreased cardiac contractility than oxymorphone-acepromazine.

Oxymorphone is classified as a Schedule II drug in the United States and as a narcotic in Canada.

Hydromorphone (Dilaudid). Hydromorphone is an opioid agonist with slightly less potency than oxymorphone and with a similar duration of effect. Hydromorphone is much less expensive than oxymorphone. It can be given IV, IM, or SC to both cats and dogs at a dose of 0.05 to 0.2 mg/kg. Unlike morphine, it is not associated with histamine release and has less potential to cause excitement in cats. Otherwise, side effects are similar to those seen with morphine: respiratory depression, bradycardia, vomiting, panting, excessive sedation, and excitement (seen especially at doses greater than 0.2 mg/kg).

Like oxymorphone, hydromorphone can be used as a premedication (at 0.1 to 0.2 mg/kg IM, alone or in combination with a tranquilizer), as an analgesic (at 0.05 to 0.2 mg/kg IM or SC for dogs and cats, repeated every 4 to 6 hours), or as an induction agent for high-risk patients (0.05 to 0.2 mg/kg hydromorphone slow IV followed by 0.04 to 0.6 mg/kg diazepam IV). It is also given by the epidural route (0.03 to 0.1 mg) and has a similar effect to morphine.

Hydromorphone is classified as a Schedule II drug in the United States and as a narcotic in Canada.

Fentanyl (Duragesic). Among the most potent analgesics known, fentanyl has a rapid onset and short duration of effect in small animals (onset approximately 2 minutes, duration of effect approximately 30 minutes after IV injection). It is most commonly administered by continuous IV drip or by means of a skin patch (see following section). It also can be used as an induction agent with midazolam or diazepam, with separate syringes. When fentanyl is given IV, the loading dose is 20 µg/kg (0.02 mg/kg) in dogs and 2 µg/kg (0.002 mg/kg) in cats. Analgesia during surgery can be maintained in dogs, with an infusion rate of no greater than 0.6 to 0.7 µg/kg/min. It can also be given by IM, SC, or epidural injection.

Fentanyl can induce profound sedation, bradycardia, and respiratory depression in human patients, and like oxymorphone it may cause panting or increased sensitivity to sound. Side effects of fentanyl are further discussed in the section that follows on transdermal patches.

Fentanyl was formerly used in combination with droperidol in the injectable neuroleptanalgesic Innovar-vet; however, this combination is no longer commercially available. Fentanyl is sold in combination with fluanisone (Hypnorm) in some countries.

Fentanyl (including fentanyl patches) is a Schedule II drug in the United States and is classified as a narcotic in Canada.

Opioid agents used for mild to moderate pain

Meperidine/pethidine (Demerol). A synthetic opioid, meperidine has been extensively used in veterinary medicine as an analgesic and preanesthetic agent. Although meperidine is classified as a pure agonist opioid, its analgesic properties are less potent than the other pure agonists. Meperidine is usually administered by SC injection, because IM injection may be painful and rapid IV injection may cause severe hypotension, excitement, and seizurelike activity.

Meperidine has a wide safety margin and causes less respiratory depression and gastrointestinal stimulation than morphine. It decreases salivary and respiratory secretions, a property that may be helpful in preanesthesia. Like morphine, it may cause histamine release in some patients, and pretreatment with histamine blockers may be advisable before IV injection.

In the past, meperidine was commonly used on its own as a postoperative analgesic, at a dose rate of 2 to 5 mg/kg IM or SC. Unfortunately, its analgesic effect is weak and of short duration, particularly in cats. For this reason it is no longer considered to be suitable for postoperative analgesia in animals, and in recent years it has been superseded by other opioids, particularly butorphanol and buprenorphine.

Despite its weak analgesic properties in animals, meperidine is still a useful drug for veterinary anesthesia and analgesia. Meperidine is commonly used to formulate preanesthetic mixtures in combination with atropine and low doses of acepromazine (see Box 1-1). When administered with a tranquilizer (usually diazepam or acepromazine), meperidine also provides effective neuroleptanalgesia in puppies. Meperidine is also used in conjunction with injectable NSAIDs such as ketoprofen because it confers analgesia during the 30 to 60 minutes before the NSAID takes effect.

Meperidine is a Schedule II drug in the United States and is classified as a narcotic in Canada.

Butorphanol (Torbutrol, Torbugesic, Stadol). A synthetic opioid with both agonist and antagonist properties, butorphanol was first used in veterinary medicine as a cough suppressant. Butorphanol is widely used as a preanesthetic or sedative (at a dose of 0.5 mg/kg SC or IM or in mixtures with medetomidine or acepromazine) and is also an effective postoperative analgesic for mild to moderate pain.

Butorphanol is a mixed agonist-antagonist agent in that it stimulates kappa receptors and antagonizes or blocks mu receptors (see Chapter 1). As such, it is not as effective as the pure agonists (morphine, fentanyl, hydromorphone, and oxymorphone) for treating severe pain, especially orthopedic pain. Butorphanol is, however, an effective and safe treatment for mild to moderate visceral pain, especially cranial abdominal pain, in both dogs and cats. It is also extensively used in horses.

Butorphanol is available in several concentrations, including 0.5 mg/ml, 2 mg/ml, and 10 mg/ml. Injectable butorphanol may be given IV, IM, or SC. It is potentially toxic to the spinal cord, which limits its use for epidural injection. Tablets are available for long-term administration (at a dose of 0.4 to 1 mg/kg tid) and may be dispensed for postoperative pain.

The duration of analgesia provided by butorphanol may be short (as little as 1 hour in dogs after IM or SC injection). To avoid frequent redosing, butorphanol can be given as a constant rate infusion (in IV fluids or by syringe pump) at a dose of 0.1 to 0.2 mg/kg/hr, after a loading dose of 0.2 to 0.4 mg/kg.*

Butorphanol produces less sedation, dysphoria, and respiratory depression than most opioids. Although moderate doses of butorphanol may cause some respiratory depression, higher doses do not depress respiration further (a phenomenon known as the *ceiling effect*). Heart rate, blood pressure, and cardiac output may be decreased after the administration of butorphanol; however, the effect is less than that of morphine and pretreatment with atropine is not usually required. Panting, vomiting, bradycardia, and histamine release are seldom seen with this drug.

Butorphanol can be used as an antagonist to partially reverse respiratory depression and sedation induced by opioids such as morphine or fentanyl; the anesthetist must be aware that it will also partially reverse the analgesic effect of these drugs. The dose used for reversal is 0.2 to 0.4 mg/kg, administered IV to effect in increments of 0.01 to 0.05 mg/kg every 3 minutes. The antagonistic effect of butorphanol is less predictable and less potent than that of naloxone and can be overridden by subsequent administration of high doses (2 to 3 times the normal dose) of morphine.

Since 1997, butorphanol has been classified as a Schedule IV drug in the United States. In Canada it is classified as a controlled drug.

Buprenorphine (Buprenex, Temgesic). Buprenorphine is a partial agonist. It stimulates mu receptors, producing some analgesia, but is less effective than morphine and other pure agonists. Buprenorphine has a "bell-shaped" dose response curve, which means that high doses may have less analgesic effect than moderate doses.

Buprenorphine can be given by the IV, IM, or epidural route. It has a delayed onset of action (15 minutes IV and 40 minutes IM) but provides a longer duration of analgesia than other opioids (authorities suggest as little as 6 hours or as long as 12 hours after IM injection and 18 to 24 hours after epidural injection). Like butorphanol, buprenorphine does not provide adequate analgesia for severe pain (such as orthopedic pain), but it is useful for mild to moderate pain. It is commonly used to provide analgesia for rodents and other species used in research, as well as postoperative analgesia for dogs and cats.

Like butorphanol, buprenorphine can be used to reverse the sedation and respiratory depression induced by other opioids while maintaining some analgesic effect. Its effectiveness as a reversing agent is not as dramatic as butorphanol because of the delay in its onset of action.

---

*The calculation of the butorphanol dose can be done as follows: suppose a 10-kg patient is receiving 100 ml of IV fluid per hour, and the dose of butorphanol selected is 0.2 mg/kg/hr. The patient should receive 2 mg butorphanol per hour (10 kg × 0.2 mg/kg/hr). Because the patient receives 100 ml of IV fluids per hour, 2 mg of butorphanol (0.2 ml of a 10-mg/ml solution) can be added to 100 ml of fluids in a burette, or one can add 10 times this amount (20 mg or 2 ml of a 10-mg/ml solution) to a liter bag of fluids, mix thoroughly, and administer over the next 10 hours at a rate of 100 ml/hr.

Buprenorphine at high doses may induce respiratory depression, which is difficult to reverse with naloxone. Analeptic agents such as doxapram may be somewhat effective in correcting buprenorphine-induced respiratory depression. Intubation and assisted ventilation are necessary in some patients, because there is a potential for carbon dioxide retention and increased intracranial pressure.

Although buprenorphine has little sedative effect on its own, it can prolong sleep times with other agents.

Buprenorphine is a Schedule V drug in the United States and is unavailable in Canada. It is relatively expensive and is provided in ampules that are inconveniently large for small-animal patients. Buprenorphine can, however, be transferred to sterile vials for use on multiple patients.

Nalbuphine. Nalbuphine is a kappa agonist and mu antagonist like butorphanol, but its antagonist properties are greater. It is currently the only injectable opioid agent for veterinary use that is not classified as a controlled drug in the United States. It is a weak analgesic and sedative and can be used as an opioid reversing agent. Bradycardia, respiratory depression, and sedation are uncommon with this agent.

Use of opioid injections to treat postoperative pain

Opioids can be administered by a variety of routes for prevention or treatment of postoperative pain. In many practices, opioids are given by IM or SC injection, preferably before the animal regains consciousness from anesthesia. Injections may be repeated as necessary to prolong the analgesic effect (see Table 8-3 for information on dosage and duration).

From the standpoint of analgesia, one major disadvantage of opioid agents is their relatively short duration of effect when given SC or IM. Morphine offers 2 to 3 hours of analgesia for severe pain and 4 to 6 hours for moderate or mild pain; oxymorphone 1.5 to 5 hours; meperidine less than 1 hour; and butorphanol 1 to 2 hours in dogs and up to 4 hours in cats. Repeat injections can be used, but this tends to be expensive, requires hospitalization, and creates "peak-and-trough" blood levels instead of a constant, effective blood concentration.

A second disadvantage of opioid use is the potential for side effects such as respiratory depression, bradycardia, excitement (usually exhibited as apprehension, hypersalivation, and mydriasis), excessive sedation, panting, increased sensitivity to sound, urinary retention, nausea, and vomiting. These side effects are seldom severe when analgesic dosages are used. However, it is probably advisable to avoid opioid use or use with caution in high-risk patients such as those with hypotension, hepatic disease, preexisting respiratory difficulties, CNS disorders such as head injuries or increased intracranial pressure, or altered bowel motility.

Both disadvantages of opioids—their short duration and potential for side effects—may be partially overcome by giving these drugs by routes other than IM or SC injection. Alternative routes for opioid administration include IV infusion, epidural injection, transdermal patches, and intraarticular administration. When used by these alternative routes, opioids may produce effective, economic, and long-acting analgesia with minimal side effects. However, use of opioids by these routes constitutes off-label use in many animal species, and informed consent should be obtained from the animal's owner.

Intravenous infusion of opioids

Morphine, fentanyl, oxymorphone, hydromorphone, and butorphanol can be given IV by constant rate infusion. This is sometimes the only method of analgesic delivery that is effective in constant, unremitting pain. Animals are given an initial loading dose (for example, 0.1 mg/kg morphine IV every 3 to 5 minutes) until the desired effect is achieved. Animals should be closely monitored for signs of histamine release (pruritus, hypotension) when morphine is administered IV. The same dose is then given over 4 hours, through a constant flow of IV fluids. At its most elaborate, IV infusion consists of an automated infusion pump or syringe pump. Practices that lack this type of specialized equipment can deliver opioid analgesics continuously through the use of IV fluids by adding an opioid directly to the bag of fluids or the burette and rotating the bag several times to mix (see Table 8-3 for dosages). Patients must be frequently monitored for signs of inadequate pain control (in which case the rate of administration should be increased) or excessive sedation, dysphoria, respiratory depression, bradycardia, panting, and other signs that indicate excessive dosing. If these signs are present, the rate of administration should be decreased. The duration of pain control (for morphine) is 30 minutes past the discontinuation of the IV fluids. If morphine is inadequate to control pain, lidocaine also can be added to the fluids and infused at 5 to 20 µg/kg/min.

Intraarticular use of opioids

Opioids may be given by the intraarticular route, particularly after elbow or stifle surgery. In this technique, 0.1 to 0.3 mg/kg of morphine is diluted in 1 ml saline per 10 kg body weight and instilled into the joint with a sterile catheter, immediately after closure of the joint capsule. The morphine can also be combined with a local anesthetic such as bupivacaine (0.5% bupivacaine, 1 ml/4.5 kg). This technique provides 8 to 12 hours of postoperative analgesia.

Epidural use of opioids

With the instillation of a small dose of an opioid or other analgesic into the epidural space at the lumbosacral junction, it is possible to achieve excellent analgesia of the hind limbs, abdomen, caudal thorax, pelvis, and tail. Currently, morphine is the drug most commonly used for epidural analgesia. Oxymorphone is more expensive, butorphanol is less effective and may have some spinal toxicity, and local anesthetics such as lidocaine may impair movement, urination, defecation, and may cause a sympathetic blockade if the drug diffuses too far cranially (see Chapter 7). Occasionally, morphine and local anesthetics are used epidurally in combination.

Morphine given by the epidural route offers more profound analgesia and for a longer time than morphine given by IM or SC injection. The analgesia is not sufficient for a surgical procedure unless supplemented with general anesthesia; however, it is an excellent means of securing postoperative pain relief. Epidural morphine has direct, long-lasting effect on the pain receptors in the spinal cord, but because it does not reach high concentrations in the bloodstream, side effects such as sedation (dogs), excitement (cats), respiratory depression, and nausea are rare.

To achieve preemptive analgesia for postoperative pain, epidural morphine should be given after induction but before the surgical procedure. Epidural morphine is significantly less effective when administered in the postoperative period. Preservative-free morphine (Duramorph) is preferred, because the preservatives typically found in morphine preparations (formaldehyde and phenol) are potentially neurotoxic.

The technique for epidural morphine administration is similar to epidural administration of lidocaine (see Procedure 7-1). Normally, the animal is anesthetized or deeply sedated and positioned in sternal recumbency with the head slightly elevated and the hind limbs pulled forward to open the lumbosacral space. An epidural puncture is performed. Once it is determined that the needle is in the epidural space, morphine is injected over 30 seconds. Currently, the recommended dose for epidural morphine is 0.1 mg/kg in dogs and 0.05 to 0.1 mg/kg in cats. Ideally, a single dose vial of formalin-free morphine should be used, diluted with sterile saline to a volume of 0.3 ml/kg. The maximum volume that can be injected is 6 ml in a dog and 1.5 ml in a cat. Onset of analgesia is approximately 20 to 60 minutes after injection and lasts 6 to 24 hours. If more prolonged analgesia is required, an epidural catheter can be used to instill morphine into the epidural space over a longer period (hours to days).

Although epidural analgesia is regarded as a safe procedure, it should not be undertaken in animals with septicemia, local infections in the lumbosacral space, bleeding disorders, spinal trauma, or neurologic disease of the spinal cord. It is relatively difficult to administer epidural anesthetics to obese animals. Epidural hematomas and abscesses may result from improper needle placement or unsterile technique. Urinary retention may occur in the first 24 hours after surgery and the bladder should be monitored closely in all patients that have received epidural analgesics. Urinary catheterization may be necessary in some patients. Pruritus, delayed respiratory depression, sedation, vomiting, and nausea have been reported in human patients but are uncommon in dogs. These symptoms, if they occur, can be treated with naloxone hydrochloride (0.01 mg/kg). Animals that have received epidural morphine should be repositioned every 2 to 4 hours because normal sensation may be absent. Failure to reposition animals may result in pulmonary atelectasis or prolonged pressure on superficial nerves, leading to temporary or permanent loss of function.

Transdermal use of opioids

Transdermal patches containing fentanyl are another convenient option for long-term opioid administration. Fentanyl patches (Duragesic patches) have been used for several years in the treatment of severe pain in human patients. The analgesic effect of a fentanyl patch is thought to be comparable to IM oxymorphone, but the duration of analgesia is considerably longer.

A "patch" consists of a reservoir of 5 mg fentanyl enclosed in plastic. It can be applied to the clipped skin of a dog or cat and left in place for several days (Procedure 8-1). A 25-µg/hr patch is used in cats* and in dogs that weight less than 7 kg. A 50-µg/hr patch is used in dogs weighing 7 to 20 kg; a 75-µg/hr patch is used in dogs weighing 20 to 30 kg; and dogs that weigh more than 30 kg receive a 100-µg/hr

---

*For cats weighing 6 kg or more, the entire patch is exposed by removing the protective liner. For cats weighing less than 6 kg, only one half to two thirds of the patch should be exposed, and the rest should remain covered by the protective liner. Some authorities suggest that fentanyl patches should not be used in cats weighing less than 3.5 kg.

patch. Patches should not be cut or trimmed because this will cause erratic drug release and possible human exposure. In patients showing signs of inadequate pain control 24 hours after patch application, a second patch or another analgesic agent can be added.

Because fentanyl is relatively slowly absorbed through the skin, there is a delay of 4 to 12 hours in cats and 12 to 24 hours in dogs before therapeutic blood levels are achieved. To achieve preemptive analgesia, apply the patch at least 6 hours before the start of anesthesia in cats and at least 12 hours before the start of surgery in dogs. If application of the patch is delayed until after surgery, it is necessary to

| PROCEDURE 8-1 | Applying a Fentanyl Patch |

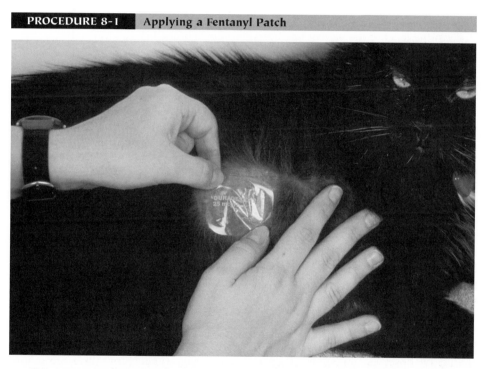

FIG. 8-1   Application of a fentanyl patch. (*Photo courtesy Dr. Margie Scherk.*)

1. Various locations can be used for patch application, including the lateral thorax, dorsal neck, and the ventral abdomen. Once applied, the patch should not contact sources of external heat.
2. The skin is clipped, taking care not to nick the skin (which may result in the fentanyl being absorbed too rapidly). If soiled, the skin can be cleansed with water (only) and dried.
3. The patch is removed from its protective backing and handled by the edges only. The adhesive side of the patch is held onto the skin for 1 to 2 minutes with hand pressure.
4. The patch should be handled by its edges, or gloves should be worn to avoid contact with the patch membrane.

Continued

| PROCEDURE 8-1 | Applying a Fentanyl Patch—cont'd |

5. The patch is applied to the shaved skin and held in place for 1 to 2 minutes. If the patch does not adhere to the skin, a Tegaderm patch or light dressing can be placed over the fentanyl patch. Tissue adhesive should not be used to attach the patch to the patient because it alters the absorption of the fentanyl. If necessary, the patch may be covered with bandage material to prevent removal by the patient (particularly dogs*).

6. The patch remains in place for several days, during which time the fentanyl is gradually absorbed. Blood levels remain at therapeutic levels for approximately 5 days in cats and 3 days in dogs, although there is considerable variation in duration and effectiveness between patients.

7. At the end of this time the patch should be peeled off and disposed by flushing down the toilet. If the patient has been discharged in the interim, it may be advisable to return to the clinic for patch removal and assessment.

8. If a longer duration of analgesia is required, a new patch can be applied at a separate, clipped site.

---

*Accidental ingestion of the patch produces no signs in dogs or cats if the patch reaches the stomach or intestines intact, because any fentanyl absorbed is metabolized rapidly by the liver. However, overdose may occur after oral absorption (for example, if a patch is chewed and punctured).

provide the patient with another opioid (for example, morphine, hydromorphone, or oxymorphone) or NSAID such as meloxicam, ketoprofen, or carprofen until the patch takes effect. Butorphanol or buprenorphine should not be used concurrently with a fentanyl patch because either may partially block the opioid receptors, reducing the analgesic effect.

Many types of patients benefit from a fentanyl patch, including postoperative patients (for example, after onychectomy, orthopedic procedures, or abdominal surgery) and those that have trauma, burns, cancer, or painful abdominal conditions such as pancreatitis.

Recent studies have shown considerable variation among animals in the concentration of fentanyl absorbed from a transdermal patch. One study showed that a 50-µg/hr patch in dogs delivered as little as 13.7 and as much as 49.8 µg/hr. Patients should be observed for signs of breakthrough pain (which may indicate a low plasma fentanyl concentration) and supplemented with morphine, oxymorphone, hydromorphone, or an NSAID as required.

Excessively high plasma fentanyl concentrations may develop in some patients. If this occurs, the most common signs are ataxia and sedation in dogs and dysphoria and disorientation in cats. Affected cats appear fearful or excited, are hypersensitive to sound, and may have widely dilated pupils. Panting is also a problem in some animals. Treatment, if necessary, consists of removing the patch or giving a narcotic antagonist (for example, naloxone or butorphanol).

There have been some reports of death caused by respiratory failure when human patients self-administered more than one patch at a time, but respiratory depression is apparently uncommon in veterinary patients with fentanyl patches. Respiratory depression may be seen in trauma patients, particularly animals with CNS signs. Other side effects reported in human patients include constipation, physical dependence, muscle rigidity, miosis, mood changes, bradycardia, and bronchoconstriction. Use of fentanyl patches is not recommended in human patients with respiratory disease, increased intracranial pressure, impaired consciousness, bradycardia, pulmonary disease, hepatic or renal dysfunction, or brain tumors, and these recommendations may also hold true for animals. Some patients may exhibit a mild transient dermatitis at the patch site after removal, and delayed hair regrowth at the patch site is common.

Transdermal patches may release excessive amounts of fentanyl if they are heated, and fentanyl overdoses have been reported in human beings who lie under electric blankets while wearing a patch. It is therefore suggested that fentanyl patches be avoided in animals with fevers and that patch contact with hot water bottles and other external sources of heat be avoided.

There is some concern regarding the potential for abuse or ingestion of the patch by a child. For this reason, the manufacturer does not support the use of fentanyl patches in animals. Some veterinarians address this concern by using the patch only on hospitalized animals or by carefully selecting and educating owners before discharging an animal that is wearing a patch.

Nonsteroidal Antiinflammatory Drugs

NSAIDs, also called nonsteroidal antiinflammatory analgesics or NSAAs, are a large group of agents that have been used for many years to control minor pain in human beings and animals. The NSAID group includes such common drugs as acetylsalicylic acid (aspirin) and acetaminophen (Tylenol) and newer agents such as carprofen (Rimadyl), meloxicam (Metacam, Mobicox), etodolac (EtoGesic), and ketoprofen (Anafen). Dose and toxicity information for individual NSAID agents are summarized in Table 8-4.

Traditionally, veterinarians have thought that NSAIDs are not potent enough to treat anything other than mild postoperative pain. However, newer and more powerful NSAIDs such as ketoprofen, meloxicam, and carprofen are increasingly used for postoperative analgesia after procedures as diverse as ovariohysterectomy and fracture repair. In some cases (for example, degloving injuries and some orthopedic procedures) analgesia provided by injectable NSAIDs may be equal or superior to that provided by opioids. NSAIDs are also useful for treatment of dental pain, panosteitis, osteoarthritis, meningitis, mastitis, and other painful medical conditions.

Mode of action

NSAIDs have several beneficial effects on animal patients, including the following:
- All NSAIDs appear to be effective analgesics for somatic (musculoskeletal) pain. Some NSAIDs such as aspirin have little efficacy against visceral (organ-related) pain, whereas others such as ketoprofen and carprofen are potent analgesics for both somatic and visceral pain. All NSAIDs require approximately 30 to 60 minutes to achieve full analgesic effect, regardless of the route of administration.
- Many NSAIDs have antiinflammatory properties. This, combined with their analgesic effect, is the basis for the widespread use of drugs such as aspirin and carprofen in the treatment of osteoarthritis, panosteitis, hypertrophic osteodystrophy, and muscular pain.
- Some NSAIDs are antipyretic (reduce fevers).

TABLE 8-4

Dose and Toxicity of Nonsteroidal Antiinflammatory Drugs (NSAIDs)*

AGENT	DOSE	COMMENTS
Aspirin (acetylsalicylic acid, ASA)	Dogs: 10-25 mg/kg PO, every 12 hours Cats: 10 mg/kg PO, every 48-72 hours	Gastric irritation. Enteric coated formulations decrease GI effects but unpredictable absorption. Increased bleeding time because of effect on platelets. Prolonged half-life in cats, neonates, and geriatrics.
Acetaminophen (Tylenol, Tempra)	Dogs: 5-10 mg/kg PO every 8 hours Cats: NONE!	Less potent than aspirin but less gastric irritation. Weak anti-inflammatory effect. Very toxic to cats (hepatic necrosis, methemoglobinemia), hepato toxic to dogs. No effect on platelets.
Ibuprofen (Advil, Motrin, Nuprin)	Dogs: 10 mg/kg PO every 24-48 hours but not recommended	Common cause of poisoning in small animals. Renal and gastric effects, severe gastric ulceration in some dogs. GI upset may occur at therapeutic doses. Narrow safety margin, especially for cats.
Flunixin (Banamine)	Dogs: 0.25-1 mg/kg IV, IM, or SC every 24 hours for three-dose maximum Cats: 0.25 mg/kg SC or IM, one dose only	Significant renal toxicity, especially in hypotensive patients. Risk of gastric ulceration. Use with ulcer prophylaxis, IV fluids, one dose only. Do not use with methoxyflurane. Chief use is for ophthalmic surgery.
Ketoprofen (Anafen, Ketofen, Orudis, Oruvail)	Dogs and cats: 2 mg/kg first dose, give IV, SC, or IM in dogs, SC in cats Maintenance dose 0.5-1 mg/kg PO every 24 hours, maximum 5 days	Potential for renal toxicity in hypotensive patients. Vomiting, abnormal stool, gastric irritation and ulceration may occur at therapeutic doses. Potential for increased bleeding times. Potent analgesic, especially for orthopedics.
Ketorolac (Toradol)	Dogs: 0.3 mg/kg every 8-12 hours, IV or IM, one to three treatments only Cats: 0.25 mg/kg every 8-12 hours, one or two treatments only	Can cause gastric ulceration and renal insufficiency in geriatric or hypotensive patients. Use with misoprostol, sucralfate. Potent analgesic, comparable to morphine.

Modified from Mathews KA: Nonsteroidal antiinflammatory analgesics in pain management in dogs and cats, *Can Vet J* 37(9):539-545, 1996.

GI, Gastrointestinal.

*Doses given are for healthy, young patients with normal renal function and no evidence of bleeding or gastrointestinal ulceration. For dose ranges, give lower doses IV and high doses IM or SC.

Continued

TABLE 8-4

Dose and Toxicity of Nonsteroidal Antiinflammatory Drugs (NSAIDs)—cont'd

AGENT	DOSE	COMMENTS
Piroxicam (Feldene)	Dogs: 0-3 mg/kg PO every 24 hours	May cause vomiting, diarrhea, gastric ulceration. Use with misoprostol. Useful for treatment of bladder tumors.
Carprofen (Rimadyl, Zenecarp)	Dogs: 2 mg/kg PO every 12 hours or 4 mg/kg every 24 hours; 2-4 mg/kg IV, SC, IM every 24 hours[†] Cats: same dose SC or 1 mg/kg PO, one treatment only	Less potential for gastric ulceration than some NSAIDs. Renal toxicity seen in dogs and GI ulceration in cats after chronic use. Hepatocellular toxicosis reported, especially Labrador retrievers.
Meloxicam (Metacam, Mobicox)	Dogs: 0.1 mg/kg PO every 24 hours Cats: 0.3 mg/kg initial dose, then 0.1 mg/kg every 24 hours	Vomiting, diarrhea, inappetence may occur. Less potential for gastric ulceration and renal toxicity than some NSAIDs. Cats: 5-day limit at this dose.
Tolfenamic acid (Tolfedine)	Dogs: 4 mg/kg PO every 24 hours for 3 days Cats: 2-4 mg/kg PO, up to 3 doses	Vomiting, diarrhea, inappetence may occur. Less potential for gastric ulceration and renal toxicity than some NSAIDs, but gastric erosions may occur after chronic use.
Meclofenamic acid (Arquel)	Dogs only: 1.1 mg/kg PO every 24 hours	Side effects include vomiting, diarrhea, and GI ulceration. Maximum duration 5 days.
Etodolac (EtoGesic)	Dogs only: 10-15 mg/kg PO every 24 hours	Difficult to accurately dose small dogs. Adverse reactions include vomiting, lethargy, diarrhea, and hypoproteinemia. Elevated doses may cause GI ulceration and anemia because of fecal blood loss.
Naproxen (Naprosyn)	Dogs only: 3 mg/kg PO every 24-48 hours	Induced gastric ulceration; less toxic approved drugs are available.

[†]Injectable carprofen is not yet available in the United States.

The clinical effects of NSAIDs stem chiefly from their inhibition of *prostaglandin* synthesis. Prostaglandins (often abbreviated PG) are a group of extremely potent chemicals that are normally present in all body tissues and are involved in the mediation of pain and inflammation after tissue injury. Most NSAIDs prevent pain and inflammation by inactivating the enzyme cyclooxygenase (COX), which catalyzes one of the steps in the production of prostaglandins. There are actually two types of cyclooxygenase (COX-1 and COX-2). The relative effect of an NSAID on these enzymes will determine both the analgesic potency and the severity and type of adverse effects after the administration of that particular drug (see the separate section on side effects).

Although some NSAIDs are active against prostaglandins in peripheral tissues only, others (for example, acetaminophen and ketorolac) exert their effects mainly on prostaglandin synthesis in brain tissue and are therefore said to be "central acting." Some agents (ketoprofen, meloxicam) appear to exert their effects both centrally and in the peripheral tissues.

As a group, NSAIDs are well absorbed orally, and many are available in tablet or liquid form. Recently, potent injectable NSAIDs have also become available. Injectable NSAIDs can be given at the end of surgery to provide 24 hours of pain relief. Some NSAIDs, for example carprofen, can also be used before surgery in selected patients to achieve preemptive analgesia. If long-term analgesia is required, injections can be repeated in some cases, or tablets can be dispensed.

All NSAIDs are eliminated by metabolism and conjugation within the liver, followed by renal or biliary elimination. The NSAID group of drugs is unusual in that there is significant variation in duration of effect between species. For example, the plasma half-life of aspirin is 1 hour in the horse, 8 hours in the dog, and 38 hours in the cat. The prolonged half-life of aspirin in the cat is a result of the low levels of the enzyme glucuronyl transferase (one of the enzymes that metabolizes salicylate NSAIDs such as aspirin) in that species. There is also significant variation between species in the toxicity of particular NSAIDs. For example, acetaminophen (Tylenol) is extremely toxic in cats but is a useful agent in dogs. Similarly, ibuprofen (Advil, Motrin, Nuprin) is considered to be safe for use in humans but has significant toxicity in dogs and cats. Because of this variation, the safety of any NSAID in one species does not imply that it can be used with impunity in all species (see Table 8-4 for dosages and cautions for specific agents). *In particular, it cannot be assumed that dosages and administration schedules that are appropriate for dogs can be safely used in cats.*

NSAIDs have some advantages over opioids: they are not subject to the storage, handling, and record-keeping regulations that govern narcotics, they have little abuse potential, and they are effective when given orally. Unlike opioids, NSAIDs have a negligible effect on the cardiovascular and respiratory systems. NSAIDs also do not depress the CNS and therefore lack the sedative effect of opioids. When used in healthy young to middle-aged dogs and cats according to label directions, they provide effective and safe relief for mild to moderate pain. For some applications, their analgesic effect appears to be superior to that of butorphanol or meperidine.

Adverse effects

Unfortunately, NSAIDs as a group have significant potential for toxicity in small-animal patients. Most people who work in veterinary hospitals are aware of the toxicity of acetaminophen (Tylenol) in cats. A single 320-mg capsule may cause acute hepatotoxicosis within 4 hours of ingestion because of the formation of toxic metabolites within the liver. Many NSAIDs are safe for use in healthy dogs and cats but can have serious toxic effects on animals that are dehydrated or hypotensive.

Many of the adverse effects of NSAIDs are attributable to the fact that they reduce not only the production of the prostaglandins that produce pain, inflammation, and fever, but also the production of beneficial prostaglandins. Pharmaceutical companies have attempted to formulate NSAIDs that will prevent the production of harmful prostaglandins while preserving the production of beneficial prostaglandins. This can be achieved if the NSAID inhibits the enzyme COX-2 (which is active in damaged or inflamed tissues and synthesizes the prostaglandins that cause pain) but does not affect COX-1 (which synthesizes the prostaglandins that help maintain normal physiologic functions such as protection of the gastric mucosa and modulation of blood flow to the kidney). In theory, it is possible to produce NSAIDs that have more than 1000-fold specificity for COX-2 over COX-1 and are therefore extremely safe for use. However, the drugs currently available do not have this degree of specificity. Confusingly, an agent that has pronounced specificity for COX-2 in one species does not necessarily show the same specificity in another species.

One example of a beneficial prostaglandin that is adversely affected by many NSAIDs is prostacyclin, which is normally present within the stomach mucosa and helps reduce gastric acid secretion and promote mucus production. When prostacyclin levels are reduced by the administration of an NSAID, gastric acid secretion increases and mucus production decreases, which sometimes leads to the production of stomach ulcers. Up to 50% of dogs treated with aspirin have mild stomach ulceration within a few days of treatment, which may result in vomiting, gastrointestinal bleeding, and inappetence but more often is not clinically apparent. Occasionally, animals with gastrointestinal ulceration resulting from NSAID use may undergo a sudden episode of life-threatening hemorrhage. In dogs, ulcerogenic potential appears to be high for ketoprofen, naproxen, ibuprofen, flunixin, prioxicam, and meclofenamic acid, and use of these agents for prolonged periods (over 5 days) is associated with a high incidence of adverse effects. Meloxicam, carprofen, and etodolac have less ulcerogenic activity in dogs and are preferred for long-term use, as in dogs with osteoarthritis.

In an effort to avoid gastrointestinal problems in human beings and animals receiving NSAIDs, pharmaceutical companies have prepared enteric-coated or buffered formulations. Enteric coating does not appear to reliably reduce the toxicity of these drugs; however, buffered formulations may have reduced toxicity. It is also helpful to administer oral NSAIDs with a meal to dilute the drug that is present in the stomach. In susceptible patients, it may be advisable to use gastrointestinal protectants such as sucralfate suspension (Sulcrate, at a dose of 0.25 to 0.5 g PO tid a day in cats, 0.5 to 1 g PO tid in dogs) in conjunction with an NSAID to prevent or treat gastrointestinal effects. Sucralfate forms a proteinaceous complex that adheres to damaged gastric mucosa, preventing further injury. Sucralfate should be administered on an empty stomach, at the same time as the NSAID. Another helpful gastrointestinal protectant is the synthetic prostaglandin misoprostol (Cytotec), which is given orally at a dose of 2 to 4 mg/kg tid.* Histamine-blocking agents such as famotidine (Pepcid) or ranitidine are also helpful in treatment of stomach ulcers but should not be given at the same time as sucralfate.

Another potential side effect of NSAID administration is renal toxicity. A beneficial prostaglandin, PGE_2, normally maintains adequate blood flow within the kidney. In anesthetized animals and other animals that are prone to hypotension (such as trauma patients), PGE_2 plays a vital role in maintaining renal blood flow.

---

*Misoprostol should not be given at the same time as sucralfate (ideally it should be administered 1 hour before or 2 hours after). It should not be given to pregnant animals.

By blocking synthesis of PGE_2, NSAIDs have the potential to decrease renal blood flow in these patients, leading to renal hypoxia. Dogs are apparently very susceptible to development of renal failure when blood pressure decreases and there are several reports of acute renal failure after the administration of NSAIDs during anesthesia. To avoid the risk of renal damage in anesthetized patients, the use of NSAIDs should be postponed until after anesthesia, and preemptive or intraoperative use is not advised unless the patient is receiving intraoperative IV fluids and arterial blood pressure monitoring is available. Fortunately, NSAID-induced renal insufficiency is usually reversible (in young, healthy patients) with the administration of IV fluids. It is much more difficult to reverse in geriatric patients with preexisting renal failure. It is a prudent practice to screen geriatric patients for renal disease before anesthesia (by determining values for blood urea nitrogen, creatinine, and/or urine specific gravity) and to avoid NSAIDs in patients with decreased renal function.

Another potential side effect of NSAID administration is impaired platelet aggregation, which can lead to prolonged bleeding times. This effect may be beneficial in some circumstances (for example, by lowering the risk of stroke in human patients who regularly take aspirin). However, there is a potential for increased bleeding in patients that are given NSAIDs before or during surgery. As with the potential for renal toxicity, this concern can be minimized by postponing the use of NSAID agents until after surgery is completed. If preemptive use of an NSAID is indicated, carprofen can be used (in the dog), because it has been shown to have less renal toxicity and platelet-inhibiting effect than some other NSAID agents.

Liver damage appears to be associated with the use of NSAID agents in some patients. Carprofen has been extensively studied in this regard, and although the incidence of liver disease is small, this is a recognized adverse effect of this drug. Hepatocellular toxicosis appears to be most common in Labrador retrievers and may be evident as soon as 2 weeks after initiation of treatment. Monitoring bile acid levels appears to be a sensitive method of detecting early signs of toxicity.

NSAIDs may antagonize the action of several drugs commonly prescribed for cardiac disease and hypertension, including angiotensin-converting enzyme (ACE) inhibitors (such as Fortekor and Enalapril), and some diuretics.

As with most drugs, there is great variation between individual patients in the potency, duration, and side effects produced by NSAIDs. When used for postoperative pain control, NSAIDs should only be used in well-hydrated young to middle-aged dogs or cats, with normal renal and hemostatic function. NSAIDs should be used with care or avoided entirely in dehydrated patients and in animals with liver or kidney dysfunction. Because of the potential for gastrointestinal ulceration, these agents should be avoided in patients with gastrointestinal disorders and in patients that are receiving corticosteroids (which also contribute to ulcer formation). Animals that have low blood pressure, congestive heart failure, or hemostatic disorders such as thrombocytopenia are generally high-risk candidates for NSAID therapy. Patients with trauma should not receive NSAIDs unless they are in stable condition with no indication of hemorrhage, they are receiving IV fluids, and no surgery is anticipated in the next 48 hours. For some patients (for example, geriatric patients and patients with renal disease) NSAIDs should only be used in conjunction with IV fluids and blood pressure monitoring. Opioids appear to be a safer therapeutic option in these patients.

Other Analgesic Agents

Although opioids and NSAIDs are the mainstays of postoperative pain control, other agents may be useful in some circumstances. These include local anesthetics, alpha-2 adrenergic agonists (for example, xylazine and medetomidine) and ketamine.

Local anesthetics

Local anesthetic agents have long been used to allow surgical procedures in conscious animals, but their use in preventing or treating postoperative pain is relatively recent. Local anesthetic can be sprayed or injected at the site of an injury or a surgical site or infiltrated around nerve supplying the affected area. They can also be used to desensitize an entire region, as with epidural administration or IV infusion. Local anesthetics have many advantages, including complete anesthesia of the affected area, low toxicity (when given at the appropriate dosage), and rapid onset of action. Unfortunately, the duration of action is relatively short, and the danger of CNS and cardiac toxicity prevents repeated use. The use of local anesthetics for pain control is discussed in detail in Chapter 7.

Alpha-2 adrenergic agonists

Although alpha-2 adrenergic agonists such as xylazine and medetomidine provide some analgesia, their use for pain control in small animals is limited by three factors: (1) the short duration of their analgesic effect (in the case of xylazine, 30 to 60 minutes and for medetomidine, 30 to 90 minutes), (2) the profound sedative effect of these agents, and (3) the potential for serious side effects (respiratory depression, vomiting, bradycardia, heart block, and hypotension, which may be exacerbated by opioids). It is difficult to determine the quality or duration of analgesia in some patients because the sedative effect of these drugs remains even after the analgesic effect has worn off. In dogs and cats, these agents should only be used for young to middle-aged, healthy patients. However, when used in low doses (for example, xylazine at 0.1 mg/kg IV, IM, SC; and medetomidine at 0.005 to 0.01 mg/kg IV, IM, SC), these agents appear to potentiate the effect of opioids and may contribute to the quality of analgesia in the postoperative period. Butorphanol and medetomidine in combination appear to provide effective analgesia and sedation for minor clinical procedures.

Recently, alpha-2 adrenergic agonists have been shown to give significant analgesia when administered by the epidural route (alone or in combination with opioids and other agents). Medetomidine (0.005 mg/kg) can be added to morphine to prolong the duration of epidural analgesia.

The analgesic effect of xylazine and medetomidine is antagonized by yohimbine and atipamezole.

Ketamine

Ketamine is thought to be a good analgesic for superficial pain (particularly involving the skin and SC tissue) but a poor analgesic for bone, muscle, or visceral pain (such as pain originating in the abdominal and thoracic organs). The analgesic effect of ketamine is enhanced by concurrent administration of opioids such as butorphanol.

Ketamine can be used as an analgesic in the following two ways:

- Ketamine (5 mg/kg IM or SC) is sometimes used as a preanesthetic in cats, in combination with acepromazine, and as an anticholinergic.

- Ketamine at a dose rate of 0.5 to 2 mg/kg IV, 2 to 4 mg/kg IM, or 10 mg/kg by mouth has been suggested as a means of controlling pain in dogs and cats, if opioids are unavailable or ineffective. It is particularly useful in patients with trauma because of the minimal adverse cardiovascular and respiratory effects at this dose. Duration of effect is 30 minutes. Catalepsy and unconsciousness are not seen at the lower dosages.

Ketamine should not be used in patients with hypertrophic cardiomyopathy or in cats with compromised renal function. Side effects of ketamine are dose related and seldom seen at analgesic dosages, but may include tachycardia, increased blood pressure, increased intraocular and intracranial pressure, seizures and postoperative delirium, and salivation.

Tranquilizers

Although acepromazine, diazepam, and other tranquilizers are not considered to be analgesics, they may potentiate the effect of opioids in some patients (possibly because pain appears to be intensified in anxious patients). Animals that have received adequate analgesia but are restless may become calmer after administration of acepromazine (0.01 to 0.05 mg/kg SC, IM, or IV) or diazepam (0.2 mg/kg IV). Tranquilizers are also useful in cats that show excitement after opioid administration. Because tranquilizers have no analgesic effect, they should not be used as a substitute for opioids or other analgesic agents. Acepromazine should be used with caution in patients with blood loss, dehydration, or low blood pressure.

Combination Therapy

Because there are several mechanisms by which pain is produced, it is often helpful to use more than one type of analgesic to relieve pain. Combination therapy (also known as multimodal or balanced analgesia) may be more successful than treatment with any single agent, probably because pain perception is affected at several points along the pain pathway. For example, it has been shown in human patients that the use of piroxicam (an NSAID) and buprenorphine (an opioid) together provides analgesia that is superior to either agent alone. The concurrent use of NSAIDs with opioids may allow a 20% to 50% reduction in the opioid dose.

One familiar example of combination therapy is a mixture of acetaminophen and codeine (Tylenol 3, Tylenol 4), which is an effective oral treatment for moderate to severe pain in the dog. When given orally at a dose rate of 10 mg/kg acetaminophen and 0.5 to 1 mg/kg codeine every 6 to 12 hours, the combination is safe in healthy dogs for up to 5 days. If necessary, the codeine can be supplemented up to 4 mg/kg. Constipation and sedation are common side effects of this drug combination, and the diet should be supplemented with a fiber source such as bran or psyllium. Tylenol/codeine should never be given to cats and should also be avoided in dogs with hepatic disease.

Opioids and NSAIDs may be given to a patient simultaneously or at different times. For example, a fentanyl patch may be applied to a cat and a dose of meloxicam given at the same time to provide analgesia during the lag time when the patch has not yet taken effect. Alternatively, a dog undergoing an orthopedic operation can be premedicated with morphine (0.2 to 0.3 mg/kg IM) followed by administration of an injectable NSAID (such as meloxicam or carprofen) at the end of operation and followed up with an NSAID given orally for 3 days. This type of "balanced analgesia" allows the use of relatively modest doses of analgesics with a low risk of side effects yet achieves effective pain relief in many patients.

Home Analgesia

There are several options for pain relief in dogs and cats discharged from the hospital. Fentanyl patches can be used sequentially for a period of up to several months in patients with chronic pain (for example, cancer). Meloxicam, carprofen, and etodolac are commonly prescribed for long-term therapy of osteoarthritis and other chronic painful conditions Oral morphine is available as a sustained-release tablet that is effective when given to dogs or cats twice daily, beginning with a low dose and gradually increasing the dose as needed. Tylenol with codeine (dogs only) and butorphanol are also available in tablet form and are suitable for treatment of mild to moderate chronic pain.

KEY POINTS

1. The veterinarian and veterinary technician have an obligation to provide analgesia for patients with painful medical disorders and for patients that undergo surgical procedures.
2. Pain has little if any beneficial effect and may decrease cardiovascular function, appetite, wound healing, resistance to infection, and patient survival.
3. Pain is perceived when nociceptors are stimulated by mechanical injury, ischemia, heat, or chemicals such as prostaglandins. Pain is transmitted by a chain of at least three neurons, through spinal cord pathways to the brain.
4. Pain may be classified according to the location of origin (somatic or visceral pain) or duration (acute or chronic pain).
5. Animals vary in their behavioral response to pain, and even close observation may not be adequate to determine if a given patient is experiencing pain.
6. To some extent, pain may be quantified by observing behavior and physiologic variables such as heart rate, respiration rate, pupil dilation, and hormone levels.
7. Patient discomfort should be addressed through nursing care, including the provision of comfortable bedding and allowing opportunity for urination and defecation.
8. Various classes of drugs can be used as analgesics. Classes vary in their site of action, potency, duration of effect, and side effects. If necessary, pain should be managed by simultaneously administering more than one type of drug to a given patient.
9. Analgesics may be delivered by many routes, including injection (IV, SC, IM, epidural, intraarticular, nerve infiltration) transdermal patch, oral, and rectal administration.
10. Analgesic administration is most effective when used preemptively (that is, before the animal has an awareness of pain). This may not be possible in the case of NSAIDs, which can interfere with blood clotting and may decrease renal perfusion during anesthesia.

Continued

KEY POINTS—cont'd

11. Opioids may be used to provide analgesia during the preoperative, operative, or postoperative periods. Some opioids (for example, most pure agonists) are potent enough to treat severe pain, whereas others (for example, agonist/antagonists and meperidine) are more suited to treatment of mild to moderate pain.

12. Side effects of opioid administration may include respiratory depression, bradycardia, and hypotension after IV administration, vomiting and defecation, urinary retention, increased intracranial and intraocular pressure, increased sensitivity to noise, and panting. Side effects other than sedation are generally uncommon when analgesic doses are used.

13. The duration of effect of opioids may be extended if they are administered by the epidural, transdermal, or intraarticular routes.

14. NSAIDs have analgesic, antiinflammatory, and antipyretic properties. Their effects are mainly a result of inactivation of the enzyme cyclooxygenase, which catalyzes the production of prostaglandins.

15. NSAIDs may impair platelet function, cause gastrointestinal ulceration, and decrease renal perfusion during anesthesia. Agents that preferentially inhibit the enzyme COX-2 have fewer adverse effects than other NSAIDs. It is safest to reserve NSAID analgesia for young patients with normal renal, gastrointestinal, and hemostatic function. Patients receiving NSAIDs may benefit from IV fluids during surgery and the use of sucralfate and other drugs.

16. Local anesthetics such as lidocaine and bupivacaine may be used to prevent postoperative pain in patients undergoing surgical or dental procedures.

17. Alpha-2 adrenergic agonists and tranquilizers may be used to supplement the analgesic effect of opioids but should not be used on their own to provide analgesia.

18. NSAIDs or opioid drugs can be dispensed for pain control in outpatients.

REVIEW QUESTIONS

1. Which of the following anesthetic agents provides some analgesia in the postoperative period?
   a. Isoflurane
   b. Propofol
   c. Thiopental
   d. Ketamine

2. Visceral pain arises from damage to:
   a. Muscle
   b. Skin
   c. Nerves
   d. Internal organs

3. Pain receptors are called:
   a. C fibers
   b. Nociceptors
   c. Prostaglandins
   d. Endorphins
4. If you wait until an animal shows signs of pain before treating with an analgesic, a higher dose will be required.
   True   False
5. Animals do not readily show pain compared with human beings because:
   a. They do not feel as much pain
   b. Animals lack neurologic pathways for pain transmission
   c. Animals that appear stressed are more likely to become prey for other animals
   d. Animals release sufficient endorphins to alleviate pain
6. The dosage for injectable morphine is greater for the dog than for the cat.
   True   False

7. Compared with morphine, meperidine has a _____ duration of effect.
   a. Shorter
   b. Similar
   c. Longer
8. Which of the following is an agonist/antagonist opioid?
   a. Oxymorphone
   b. Meperidine
   c. Butorphanol
   d. Fentanyl

9. When applying a fentanyl patch to a cat, one can expect a _____ onset of effect.
   a. Quick (less than 1 hour)
   b. Moderate (1 to 4 hours)
   c. Delayed (more than 4 hours)
10. Increased amounts of fentanyl may be released from a patch if the patient has a fever or if heat is applied to the area where the patch is located.
    True   False
11. All of the following are characteristics of NSAIDs except:
    a. Decrease musculoskeletal pain
    b. Antipyretic
    c. Inhibit prostaglandin synthesis
    d. Reversed by naloxone or buprenorphine
12. Which of the following NSAIDs provides safe and effective analgesia for cats with moderate orthopedic pain in the immediate postoperative period?
    a. Ketoprofen
    b. Ibuprofen
    c. Acetaminophen
    d. Aspirin

Continued

13. NSAIDs may interfere with the action of drugs used for treatment of cardiac disease.

    True   False

14. An NSAID agent that is COX-2 selective is likely to be more toxic than an agent that is not COX-2 selective.

    True   False

15. Ketamine is most useful in treating pain in what part of the body?

    a. Bone
    b. Gastrointestinal system
    c. Chest
    d. Bladder
    e. Skin

16. Which of the following can be used as a reversing agent for morphine?

    a. Oxymorphone
    b. Meperidine
    c. Butorphanol
    d. Fentanyl

17. As analgesics, medetomidine and xylazine have a prolonged effect.

    True   False

18. The potential side effects of opioids include all of the following except:

    a. Bradycardia
    b. Gastrointestinal bleeding
    c. Panting
    d. Increased sensitivity to noise

19. The potential side effects of NSAIDs include all of the following except:

    a. Platelet inhibition
    b. Decreased renal perfusion
    c. Respiratory depression
    d. Gastrointestinal ulceration
    e. Liver disease

20. Tranquilizers such as acepromazine should be used instead of analgesics when treating painful, excited animals.

    True   False

ANSWERS FOR CHAPTER 8

1. d	2. d	3. b	4. True	5. c
6. True	7. a	8. c	9. c	10. True
11. d	12. a	13. True	14. False	15. e
16. c	17. False	18. b	19. c	20. False

Selected Readings

Carroll GL: How to manage perioperative pain, *Vet Med* April:353-357, 1996.

Carroll GL: *Small animal pain management,* Lakewood, Colo, 1998, AAHA Press.

Dohoo SE, Dohoo IR: Factors influencing the postoperative use of analgesics in dogs and cats by Canadian veterinarians, *Can Vet J* 37:552-556, 1996.

Dohoo SE, Dohoo IR: Attitudes and concerns of Canadian animal health technologists toward postoperative pain management in dogs and cats, *Can Vet J* 39(8):491-496, 1998.

Gaynor J, Muir W: *Handbook of veterinary pain management,* St Louis, 2002, Mosby.

Hardier EM: Recognition and management of pain in small animals, *Small Anim Med Dig* 2(2):89-96, 1996.

Heller PW, Gaynor J: Acute post-surgical pain in dogs and cats, *Compendium* 20(2):140-153, 1998.

Ko JCD, Eaton-Jones TG: Epidural anesthesia in dogs and cats, *Vet Tech* 17(3):143-154, 1996.

Mathews KA: Nonsteroidal antiinflammatory analgesics in pain management in dogs and cats, *Can Vet J* 37(9):539-545, 1996.

Pettifer G, Dyson D: Hydromorphone: cost-effective alternative to the use of oxymorphone, *Can Vet J* 41:135-136, 2000.

Quant JE, Railings CR: Reducing postoperative pain for dogs: local anesthetic and analgesic techniques, *Compendium* 18(2):101-111, 1996.

Scherk-Nixon M: A study of the use of a transdermal fentanyl patch in cats, *J Am Anim Hosp Assoc* 32(1):19-24, 1996.

Shaffron N: Pain in critically ill small animals: ethical aspects, *Vet Tech* 19(5):349-353, 1998.

Socman JE: Pain management. In McCurnin DM, editor: *Clinical textbook for veterinary technicians,* ed 4, Philadelphia, 1997, WB Saunders.

Taylor PM: Newer analgesics: nonsteroidal anti-inflammatory drugs, opioids, and combinations, *Vet Clin North Am Small Anim Pract* 29(3):719-736, 1999.

Tranquilli WJ, Grimm KA, Lamont LA: *Pain management for the small animal practitioner,* Jackson, Wyo, 2000, Teton New Media.

CHAPTER 9

Anesthesia of Rodents and Rabbits

Paul Flecknell

PERFORMANCE OBJECTIVES

After completion of this chapter, the reader will be able to:

- Summarize the common problems that may arise when anesthetizing rodents and rabbits.
- List the preanesthetic and anesthetic agents suitable for use in these species.
- Describe the technique of endotracheal intubation in rabbits.
- Describe the problems that can arise when monitoring anesthesia in rodents and rabbits.
- State aspects of intraoperative care that are of particular importance when anesthetizing rodents and rabbits.
- Describe how to cope with common anesthetic emergencies in rodents and rabbits.
- Describe the most common problems associated with postanesthetic care of rodents and rabbits.
- List the analgesics that can be used in rodents and rabbits.

A nesthesia of small mammals (rabbits, guinea pigs, rats, mice, gerbils, and hamsters) is a specialized branch of veterinary anesthesia, but the general principles of good anesthetic practice provide basic guidance. The main difficulties encountered when anesthetizing these animals are due to:

- Lack of familiarity with the species
- Lack of suitable equipment
- A failure to appreciate the poor health status of some patients
- The difficulties of providing supportive care

Once these problems are appreciated, anesthesia of small mammals and other exotic species should be as successful as anesthesia of dogs and cats.

PATIENT EVALUATION

To anesthetize small mammals safely and effectively, it is important to perform a clinical examination and obtain a case history. Although the information required is similar to that needed for more familiar species, many of these small animals are owned by children, and accurate information may not always be obtainable. Even when an adult or older child is caring for the animal, it may be difficult to be certain that the animal is eating and drinking normally, because many of these species are fed ad lib.

It should be recalled that the life span of these small mammals is considerably shorter than that of dogs and cats. Geriatric animals present a greater risk when anesthetized; a hamster, for example, will be nearing the end of its natural life when aged only 18 to 24 months. Some basic biologic data are given in Table 9-1.

For a physical examination to be performed, any animal must be safely and humanely handled and restrained. Handling is easier if small rodents are brought to the veterinary clinic in a small container, although they should not be left in a cardboard box for a prolonged period because they can easily gnaw through the container and escape. Rabbits can usually be transported in a small transport box, and cat-sized carriers are suitable. Because rabbits are a prey species and cats are one of their predators, it is not surprising that placing a rabbit in a transport box that has been previously used for cats can be extremely stressful and should be avoided.

Before the animal is handled, it should be observed undisturbed so that its normal behavior and respiratory pattern and rate can be noted.

Handling and Restraint
Mouse

Mice are best picked up a by the base of the tail and lifted clear of their transport box. They can then be allowed to rest on the operator's forearm and their external appearance assessed. To restrain them for administration of injectable anesthetics or other drugs, allow mice to rest on a rough surface (for example, a towel or the bars of their cage). They can then be grasped by the skin overlying the shoulders

TABLE 9-1

Biologic Data for Small Mammals

	GERBIL	GUINEA PIG	HAMSTER	MOUSE	RABBIT	RAT
Adult body weight (g)	85-150	700-1200	85-150	25-40	2000-6000	300-500
Respiratory rate (bpm)	90	50-140	80-135	80-200	40-60	70-115
Heart rate (bpm)	260-300	150-250	250-500	350-600	135-325	250-350
Average adult blood volume (ml) (65-70 ml/kg)	9	60	9	2.5	250	30
PCV (%)	41-52	37-48	36-55	36-49	36-48	38-50
Blood glucose (mmol/l)	3-7	4.5-6	3-8	3.5-9	4-8	3-8
Total protein (g/dl)	4.3-12.5	4.6-6.2	5.9-6.5	3.5-7.2	5.4-7.5	5.6-7/6
BUN (mg/dl)	17-27	9-32	10-25	12-28	17.0-23.5	6-23
ALT (IU)	—	25-59	12-36	74-232	35-38	17.5-30
Life span (yr)	3-5	4-8	1.5-2	2-2.5	5-10	2-3.5

ALT, Alanine aminotransferase; BUN, blood urea nitrogen; IU, international units; PCV, packed cell volume.

and lifted clear. The tail can be gripped between the operator's fingers as shown in Fig. 9-1. Subcutaneous administration of medication is made into the skin overlying the shoulders and can be carried out single-handedly. An assistant should administer intraperitoneal and intramuscular injections while the operator restrains the animal as shown in Figs. 9-2 and 9-3. Restraining the mouse by its scruff can interfere with respiration. This causes no problems in healthy animals, but care should be taken if the animal is showing signs of respiratory disease. Young mice can be extremely active and may jump out of their transport box as soon as the lid is removed; handling these agile young animals requires fast reactions.

Rat

Most pet rats are friendly and easy to handle. They should be picked up around the shoulders and lifted clear of the transport box. They can then be allowed to rest on the handler's forearm and be gently restrained by the tail or around the shoulders. If the animal resents handling (which it may if it is in pain; for example, if it has arthritis), it can be picked up by the base of the tail as mice are. It can then be placed on a rough surface and grasped around the shoulders. When holding a rat in this way, the operator can avoid being bitten by positioning the thumb under the mandible as shown in Fig. 9-4. It is important not to grasp the animal's chest too firmly because this can interfere with respiratory movements, causing the animal to panic and struggle. Although subcutaneous injections can be given into the scruff

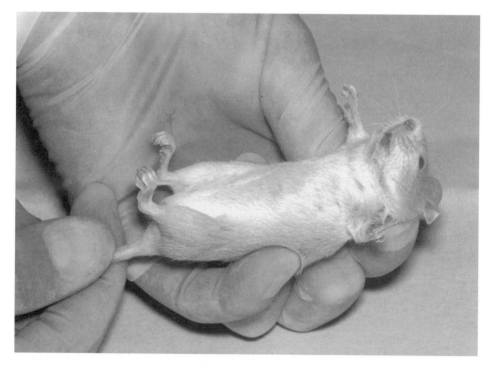

FIG. 9-1 Mice can be restrained by the skin overlying the shoulders, with the tail held between the operator's fingers.

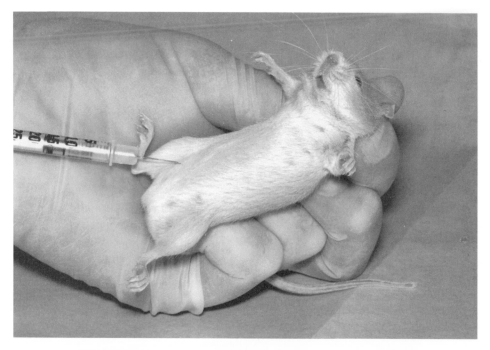

FIG. 9-2   Intraperitoneal injection is made into one posterior quadrant of the abdomen, along the line of the hindlimb.

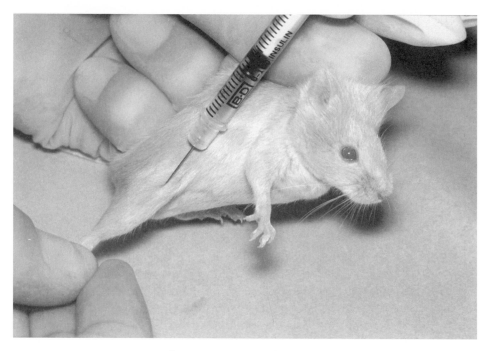

FIG. 9-3   Intramuscular injection is made into the quadriceps muscle.

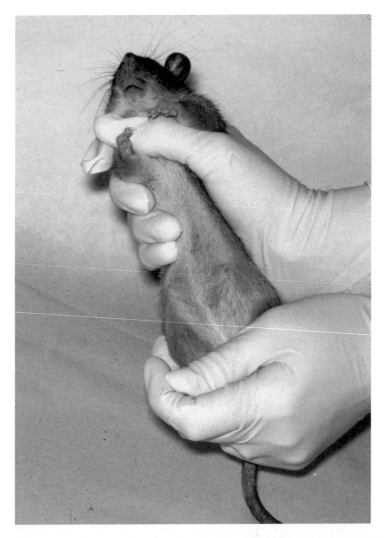

FIG. 9-4   Restraint of a rat. Note the thumb is positioned below the mandible to prevent biting. The chest is held gently to avoid interfering with respiration.

while also restraining the animal, it is usually easier to obtain the assistance of a colleague. Intramuscular and intraperitoneal injections are given in the same way as in the mouse, but an assistant is needed for these procedures (Figs. 9-5 and 9-6).

Hamster

Hamsters vary considerably in their temperament, and care should be taken when handling them. This species is normally active at night and asleep during the day, and if necessary they should be gently awakened before being handled. Most animals can be cupped in the operator's hands, as shown in Fig. 9-7, and an external examination carried out. If it is necessary to immobilize the animal, it should be covered by the operator's hand (Fig. 9-8) with the skin overlying the shoulders and back

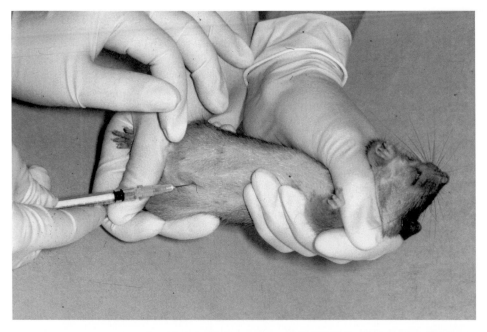

FIG. 9-5 Intraperitoneal injection in the rat. An assistant extends one hindlimb and injects into one posterior quadrant of the abdomen.

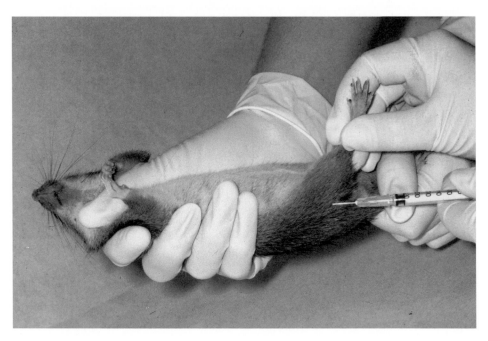

FIG. 9-6 Intramuscular injection in the rat. An assistant extends and immobilizes one hindleg and injects into the quadriceps muscle.

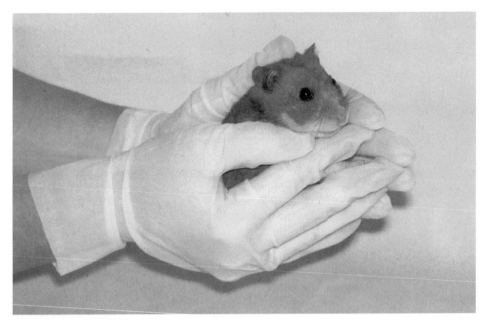

FIG. 9-7   Restraint of a hamster for clinical examination by cupping in the operator's hands.

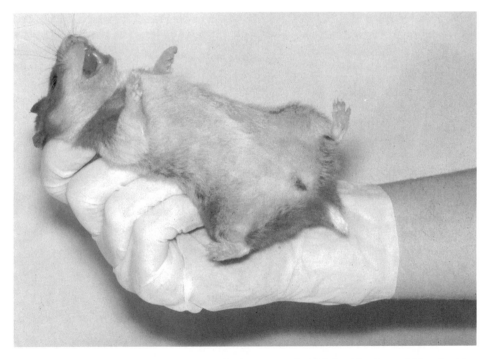

FIG. 9-8   For more secure restraint, the hamster should first be immobilized with the operator's hand and the skin overlying the back and shoulders grasped firmly.

grasped firmly (Fig. 9-9). It is important to grasp sufficient skin; otherwise, the animal can turn in the operator's grasp and may bite. An assistant can make intramuscular, intraperitoneal, or subcutaneous injections into the same sites as in the rat and mouse. Hamsters should not be allowed to run unrestrained on the consulting room table because they appear to lack depth perception and may fall to the floor and injure themselves.

Gerbil

Gerbils are very active and can easily escape from their transport container unless quickly immobilized. Preventing escape is best achieved by the operator covering the animal with a hand and grasping around the animal's shoulders with the thumb positioned under the mandible to prevent biting. With the animal immobilized in this way, an assistant can administer subcutaneous injections into the flank or intramuscular or intraperitoneal injections in the same site as for other small rodents. Gerbils can also be immobilized by grasping the base of the tail, but the skin of the tail is delicate and easily damaged.

Guinea pig

On initial examination, a guinea pig may be completely immobile, but when attempts are made to restrain it, the animal can become very agitated and run around its transport box at high speed. It should be immobilized by grasping it swiftly and firmly around the shoulders. It can then be lifted clear of the transport container,

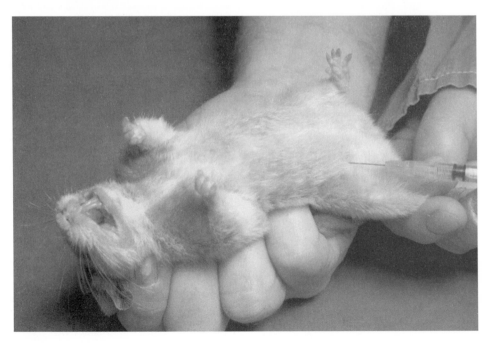

FIG. 9-9   The hamster can then be held securely for injections to be carried out by an assistant.

and the operator's other hand can be used to support its hindquarters (Fig. 9-10). With the animal restrained in this way an assistant can administer subcutaneous injections into the flank and intramuscular and intraperitoneal injections into the same site as with other rodents. If drugs are to be given by the subcutaneous route, an alternative approach is placing the restrainer's hands on either side of the guinea pig's body to immobilize the animal on the examination table. An assistant can then inject into the skin overlying the shoulders.

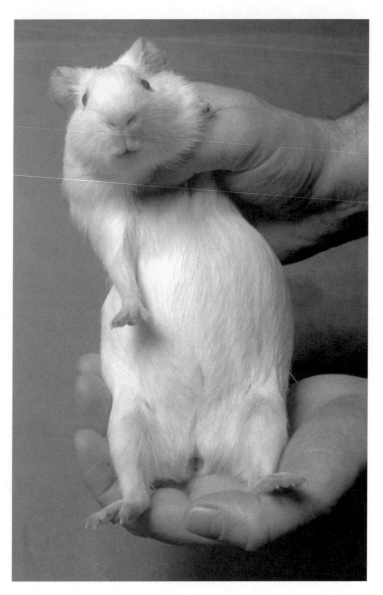

FIG. 9-10 Guinea pigs should be grasped around the shoulders and the hindquarters supported.

Rabbit

Rabbits vary considerably in body weight, ranging from dwarf breeds weighing as little as 400 g up to giant breeds that can weigh 10 kg. Most domestic rabbits weigh between 2 and 5 kg and are relatively easy to restrain, but care must be taken because they are easily frightened. When attempting to escape, they may kick out with their back legs. This can injure the person attempting to handle them and may also result in serious injury to the rabbit (for example, fracture of the lumbar verte-brae). It is therefore important to provide support to the animal's back at all times and never to leave the animal unrestrained on the consulting room table.

Rabbits should be grasped by the skin overlying the shoulders and lifted clear of the transport container. As the rabbit is lifted, the operator's other hand should be positioned under the animal's abdomen to support its body weight as shown in Fig. 9-11. The rabbit can then be placed on the examination table. The animal should not be released until its feet are in firm contact with the table surface. It can then be restrained by gently holding the skin over the shoulders. Rabbits should never be picked up by the ears because these are delicate structures.

An assistant can make intramuscular injections into the quadriceps or into the lumbar muscles while the operator restrains the animal by placing hands and arms along either side of its body. Intravenous injection is most easily carried out into the marginal ear veins. The skin of the ears is sensitive, and animals will often jerk in response to venipuncture. To avoid a jerk and to prevent discomfort, the skin over-

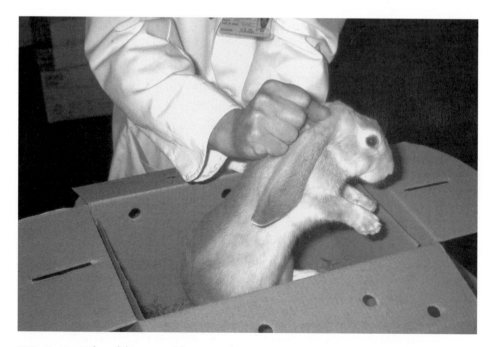

FIG. 9-11   When lifting a rabbit out of its transport box or cage, the skin overlying the shoulders should be grasped firmly and the abdomen supported. The operator's forearms are used to provide support to the animal's back.

lying the vein can be desensitized using a local anesthetic cream (for example, EMLA, AstraZeneca). The cream is applied thickly over the vein and covered with a waterproof dressing (for example, plastic food wrap) and a protective adhesive bandage. The cream is left in place for approximately 45 minutes and then removed and the ear wiped clean. This provides full skin thickness anesthesia for at least an hour. This technique is particularly useful when placing "over the needle" catheters. As an alternative to the ear veins, the cephalic veins on the forelegs can also be used. These vessels are fragile, and it is easy to produce a hematoma, even when venipuncture has been carried out successfully on the initial attempt.

If an assistant is unavailable, rabbits can be securely restrained by wrapping them in a towel or lab coat, as shown in Fig. 9-12. Provided it is wrapped securely, the animal will remain immobile, and it is usually possible to carry out venipuncture successfully with the marginal ear veins.

Physical Examination of Small Mammals

As mentioned earlier, the animal should first be observed undisturbed in its transport box if possible and can then be restrained as previously described for more detailed examination. The animal's respiratory rate and pattern can be assessed and its heart rate recorded either by palpating the heartbeat or by using a stethoscope. Although normal rates are given in Table 9-1, these will rarely be observed in patients because most will show a marked increase in heart and respiratory rates due to the stress of examination. Rabbits, for example, frequently have respiratory rates in excess of 250 breaths per minute during routine clinical examination. The

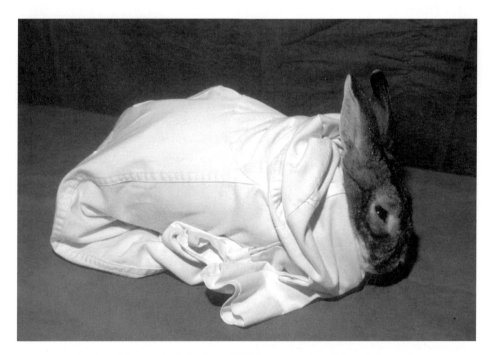

FIG. 9-12   Restraint of a rabbit by wrapping it in a lab coat.

type of examination that can be carried out is limited by the size of the species being examined, but in rabbits it is possible to auscultate and percuss the chest as in cats. In all species, the following are of particular importance:

- Discharges from the eyes and nose may indicate the presence of respiratory disease. Rats are commonly seen with a black or reddish brown discharge around their eyes or nose. This is a buildup of porphyrin secretions, which when wiped with a damp swab, will appear bright red. This can lead owners to report that their animal has been bleeding from its eyes or nose. These secretions are a nonspecific response to stress or illnesses such as chronic respiratory disease.
- Labored or noisy respiration is also indicative of respiratory disease.
- Soiling of the perineum can indicate gastrointestinal disturbances.
- An unkempt or "starey" appearance of the coat is a general sign of ill health in small mammals.
- Loss of skin tone in response to dehydration is more difficult to detect in small mammals than in the dog and cat. If loss of elasticity is noted, it usually indicates that more than 10% of body weight has been lost as fluid. When small mammals are markedly dehydrated, the eyes become sunken. This is commonly seen in rabbits and small mammals that are anesthetized for treatment of dental disease. Because the disease may have been present for some time, the animal may have had a prolonged period of reduced food and water intake. It is essential that these animals receive supportive fluid therapy before anesthesia.
- Palpation of the regions overlying the back and pelvis is helpful in assessing body condition. If the prominences of the vertebrae and of the pelvis are easily palpable, it is likely that the animal has lost a considerable amount of body fat.
- It is difficult to examine the mucous membranes in small rodents, but in the rabbit both the gingiva and conjunctiva can be inspected easily. They should have a normal reddish coloration, and the capillary refill time should be under 1 second. As with the dog and cat, abnormal coloration of the mucous membranes may indicate underlying disease.

Diagnostic Tests

Preanesthetic blood tests are rarely undertaken in small rodents but may be of value in some circumstances (for example, in rabbits with suspected hepatic lipidosis). Urine samples are easily obtained from small rodents because these species frequently urinate when handled. Diabetes mellitus is relatively common in Chinese hamsters and is also seen occasionally in rabbits and guinea pigs. In these latter species it is frequently asymptomatic.

Radiography may be required before some surgical procedures. For example, radiography of the skull is helpful in assessing underlying dental problems before flushing the tear ducts to correct blockage. Radiography is also indicated before removal of suspected uterine adenocarcinoma in rabbits to identify secondary tumors in the lungs.

PREANESTHETIC PATIENT CARE
Withholding Food Before Anesthesia

Small rodents and rabbits do not vomit, and there is generally no reason to withhold food or water before anesthesia. Withholding food from small rodents for prolonged periods can be detrimental because it can predispose to hypoglycemia. Withholding

TABLE 9-2

Volumes of Fluid for Administration for Adult Small Mammals*

ROUTE	GERBIL	GUINEA PIG	HAMSTER	MOUSE	RABBIT	RAT
Intraperitoneal	2-3 ml	20 ml	3 ml	2 ml	50 ml	5 ml
Subcutaneous	1-2 ml	10-20 ml	3 ml	1-2 ml	30-50 ml	5 ml

*All fluids should be warmed to body temperature before administration.

food from rabbits and guinea pigs can also trigger digestive disturbances that can result in enterotoxemia, which may be fatal. One exception to the no-fasting rule is if the planned operation involves the stomach, in which case a 3- to 4-hour fasting period will reduce the volume of digesta.

Successful recovery from an operation and anesthesia in these species is critically dependent on reestablishing a normal feeding pattern. It is therefore strongly recommended that food be available up until 1 to 2 hours before anesthesia and provided again as soon as the animal has recovered. The anesthetist should be aware that many of these animals are nocturnal and will not feed during the day. Postoperative pain and discomfort can also decrease appetite in the period after the operation.

Correction of Preexisting Problems

If animals are in poor condition, every attempt should be made to commence supportive therapy before anesthesia. One common problem is dehydration. Unfortunately the small body size of these animals makes administration of fluids difficult. In the rabbit, the marginal ear veins and cephalic veins can be used, but in rodents the small size of the veins does not allow intravenous catheterization. One alternative is to administer fluids by the subcutaneous or intraperitoneal route, although subcutaneous administration is unlikely to be effective if dehydration is severe. The intraosseous route can also be used and can be a valuable means of providing prolonged fluid therapy in rabbits, guinea pigs, and rats.

Calculation of fluid volume and administration rates is done according to body weight. Small mammals require higher maintenance rates than dogs and cats (100 ml/kg every 24 hours). All of the commonly used fluids used in small animal practice can be administered to rodents and rabbits. Suggested volumes for administration are listed in Table 9-2.

PREANESTHETIC AGENTS

Although the general principles governing the use of preanesthetic agents apply in small mammals, these agents are less frequently used than in dogs and cats. This is primarily due to the methods of anesthesia that are used in small mammals. Because many anesthetic protocols include a combination of anesthetic agents to be given by subcutaneous, intraperitoneal, or intramuscular injection, there is often little advantage in giving a sedative agent before this. If anesthesia is to be induced with an anesthetic chamber, prior sedation is rarely needed except in rabbits. However, preanesthetic agents should be used in the following circumstances:

- Preanesthetics can be used to reduce salivation associated with some anesthetics (for example, ketamine) and to reduce bronchial secretions, particularly in animals with preexisting respiratory disease. Atropine is frequently used for this purpose, but in rabbits it is often relatively ineffective, because many animals have high levels of atropinesterase. It is therefore advisable to use glycopyrrolate in rabbits.
- Opioid analgesics may be given 30 to 45 minutes before induction of anesthesia. This reduces the concentration of volatile anesthetic needed to maintain anesthesia and provides preemptive analgesia.
- Sedatives or tranquilizers should be given to rabbits before induction of anesthesia with volatile agents (see detailed discussion later in this section).

All of the agents that are commonly used for preanesthetic medication in dogs and cats can be used in small mammals. Their properties and side effects are very similar, but some vary in their actions. Suggested dose rates and effects are listed in Table 9-3.

Anticholinergics

Both atropine and glycopyrrolate can be used in small mammals with the same indications as in dogs and cats. As mentioned earlier, glycopyrrolate is preferred to atropine for use in rabbits because the effect of atropine is less predictable in this species.

Phenothiazines

Phenothiazines such as acepromazine can be used to sedate small mammals. When used in rodents, acepromazine will sedate the animal but will not immobilize it. In rabbits, acepromazine has excellent sedative effects and will often provide sufficient restraint for procedures such as radiography.

Benzodiazepines

Both diazepam and midazolam have marked sedative effects in rodents and rabbits, unlike their effects in dogs and cats. They can be administered by intraperitoneal, intramuscular, or intravenous injection and are often used in combination with other agents to produce balanced anesthesia. The sedative properties, although pronounced, are not usually sufficient to immobilize an animal for minor procedures such as radiography.

Alpha-2 Adrenoreceptor Agonists

Both xylazine and medetomidine can be used to produce sedation with some analgesia in small mammals. At higher dose rates the effects can be sufficient to immobilize some animals. This effect is most reliable in the rabbit, and medetomidine can be used to provide sedation and restraint for radiography in this species. One side effect of medetomidine, vomiting (which is often seen in dogs and cats), does not occur in small mammals because these animals do not vomit. The other side effects of these agents, such as hyperglycemia, diuresis, and respiratory and cardiovascular system depression, do occur. A major advantage of these sedatives is that their action can be reversed by administration of specific antagonists. Both yohimbine and atipamezole have been used for this purpose in small mammals. Atipamezole is preferable because it has fewer side effects. It can be given through the subcutaneous, intraperitoneal, intramuscular, or intravenous routes. Absorption after subcutaneous injection is rapid, generally acting within 5 to 10 minutes. Dose rates

TABLE 9-3

Preanesthetic Agents for Use in Small Mammals

DRUG	SPECIES	DOSE RATE	EFFECT
Acepromazine	Rat, guinea pig	2.5 mg/kg IP or SC	Sedation, but still active
	Mouse, hamster, gerbil	3-5 mg/kg IP or SC	
	Rabbit	1 mg/kg SC or IM	Sedation, often immobilized
Acepromazine and butorphanol	Rabbit	0.5 mg/kg + 1.0 mg/kg IM or SC	Sedation, often immobilized, some analgesia
Atropine	Mouse, hamster, gerbil, rat, guinea pig	40 µg/kg SC or IM	Reduced bronchial and salivary secretions, inhibition of vagal responses, ineffective in many rabbits
Diazepam	Mouse, hamster, gerbil, guinea pig	5 mg/kg IP	Sedation
	Rat	2.5 mg/kg IP	
	Rabbit	1-2 mg/kg IM	
Glycopyrrolate	Rabbit	0.01 mg/kg IV or 0.1 mg/kg SC or IM	Reduced bronchial and salivary secretions, inhibition of vagal responses
Innovar Vet (fentanyl/ droperidol)	Rabbit	0.22 ml/kg IM	Sedation and analgesia, often sufficiently immobilized for minor surgical procedures
	Mouse	0.5 ml/kg IM	
	Hamster	1.5 ml/kg IM	
	Guinea pig	0.4 ml/kg IM	
Hypnorm (fentanyl/ fluanisone)	Mouse, hamster, gerbil, rat, guinea pig	0.5 ml/kg SC or IP	Sedation and analgesia, often sufficiently immobilized for minor surgical procedures
	Rabbit	0.3-0.5 ml/kg SC or IM	
Medetomidine	Mouse, hamster, rat	30-100 µg/kg SC or IP	Sedation and some analgesia, immobilized at higher dose rates
	Rabbit	100-500 µg SC or IP	
Midazolam	Mouse, hamster, gerbil, guinea pig	5 mg/kg IP	Sedation
	Rat	2.5 mg/kg IP	
	Rabbit	1-2 mg/kg IM	
Xylazine	Mouse, hamster, rat	5 mg/kg SC or IM	Sedation and some analgesia, immobilized at higher dose rates
	Rabbit	2.5 mg/kg SC or IM	

IP, Intraperitoneal.

of 0.5 to 1.0 mg/kg are required, depending on the dose of medetomidine that has been administered

Opioids

The use of these agents in the preanesthetic period to provide preemptive analgesia is discussed on p. 363. More commonly, opioids are used in small mammals in combination with sedative agents to provide chemical restraint and analgesia for minor procedures such as suturing superficial wounds and draining abscesses. In North America a commercially prepared mixture of fentanyl and droperidol (Innovar Vet) was formerly available for this purpose, and a similar mixture of fentanyl and fluanisone (Hypnorm) is still available in Europe. A mixture of acepromazine and butorphanol is useful when getting blood samples from rabbits because it provides some sedation and analgesia and dilates the ear veins.

GENERAL ANESTHESIA
Induction Techniques and Agents

Although techniques similar to those used for anesthetic induction in dogs and cats can be used in small mammals, practical considerations limit the use of the intravenous route except in rabbits. A wide range of different anesthetic agents can be used in these species and suggested dose rates are given in Table 9-4. Formulas for anesthetic mixtures used in small mammals are given in Box 9-1.

In rabbits, the subcutaneous or intramuscular routes are often used, although intravenous injection of short-acting agents is also possible in some animals. For small mammals, intraperitoneal injection is a simple and relatively painless injection route for induction agents. The intraperitoneal route appears to be less painful than intramuscular injection, although the technique is less familiar. The technique is similar in most small rodents, in which an assistant extends the right hindlimb and injects the anesthetic into the middle of the right posterior quadrant of the abdomen. This technique avoids the bladder, which lies in the midline just in front of the pelvis. Use of the right side of the abdomen also avoids the cecum, which is large and thin-walled in rodents.

Although the technique for intraperitoneal injection is simple to carry out, administration of anesthetics by this route has important practical implications. If an anesthetic is given intravenously, the dose that is administered can be titrated to provide the required effect in that particular animal. It is therefore relatively simple to adjust the dose to account for individual, breed, and strain variation, and overdosing or underdosing is easy to avoid. When anesthetics are given intraperitoneally (or by subcutaneous or intramuscular injection), a calculated dose is given, and there is no opportunity to adjust it to suit the requirements of the particular animal. As large variations in response to anesthetics have been noted in small rodents, so it is advisable to select an anesthetic regimen that has a wide safety margin (preferably one that is completely or partially reversible) if injection routes other than IV are used.

A further problem associated with use of the intraperitoneal or intramuscular route is that relatively high dose rates are required compared with those that are needed when drugs are given intravenously. One consequence is that recovery times tend to be prolonged, which is particularly undesirable in small mammals because of the high risk of hypothermia.

TABLE 9-4

Anesthetic and Related Drugs for Use in Small Mammals*

ANESTHETIC AND RELATED AGENTS	GERBIL	GUINEA PIG	HAMSTER	MOUSE	RABBIT	RAT
Atipamezole	1 mg/kg SC, IM, IP, IV	1 mg/kg SC, IM, IP, IV	1 mg/kg SC, IM, IP, IV	1 mg/kg SC, IM, IP, IV	1 mg/kg SC, IM, IP, IV	1 mg/kg SC, IM, IP, IV
Doxapram	5-10 mg/kg IV or IP	5-10 mg/kg IV or IP	5-10 mg/kg IV or IP	5-10 mg/kg IV or IP	5-10 mg/kg IV or IM	5-10 mg/kg IV or IP
Fentanyl/fluanisone and diazepam†	0.3 ml/kg IM + 5 mg/kg IP	1.0 ml/kg IM + 2.5 mg/kg IP	1 ml/kg IM + 5 mg/kg IP	0.3 ml/kg IM + 5 mg/kg IP	0.3 ml/kg IM + 2 mg/kg IP or IV	0.3 ml/kg IM + 2.5 mg/kg IP
Fentanyl/fluanisone and midazolam‡	8 ml/kg IP	8 ml/kg IP	4 ml/kg IP	10 ml/kg IP	0.3 ml/kg IM + 2 mg/kg IP or IV	2.7 ml/kg IP
Ketamine and medetomidine	—	40 mg/kg + 0.5 mg/kg IP	100 mg/kg + 0.25 mg/kg IP	75 mg/kg + 1 mg/kg IP	15 mg/kg + 0.25 mg/kg IM	75 mg/kg + 0.5 mg/kg IP
Ketamine and xylazine	50 mg/kg + 2 mg/kg IP	40 mg/kg + 5 mg/kg IP	200 mg/kg + 10 mg/kg IP	80 mg/kg + 10 mg/kg IP	35 mg/kg + 5 mg/kg IM	75 mg/kg + 10 mg/kg IP
Pentobarbitone	60-80 mg/kg IP	37 mg/kg IP	50-90 mg/kg IP	40-50 mg/kg IP	30-45 mg/kg IV	40-50 mg/kg IP
Tiletamine and zolazepam (immobilizes, does not usually produce anesthesia)	60 mg/kg IM	40-60 mg/kg IM	50-80 mg/kg IM	80-100 mg/kg IM	5-25 mg/kg IM	20-40 mg/kg IM

IP, Intraperitoneal.
*Note that there may be considerable variation between strains, and these dose rates should be taken as a general guide only.
†These drugs cannot be mixed together and must be given separately.
‡Doses are milliliters of a combination of fentanyl/fluanisone and midazolam, prepared as 2 ml water for injection plus 1 ml of 5 mg/ml midazolam and 1 ml of "Hypnorm" (Janssen, fentanyl/fluanisone).

BOX 9-1 *Formulas for Anesthetic Mixtures for Small Mammals*

- Many of these solutions can be stored for a few days if made up carefully and placed in a sterile multidose ampule. There is some risk of instability with prolonged storage, and this practice is not recommended by the manufacturers.
- If necessary, solutions can be diluted with sterile water for injection or sterile saline to provide an appropriate volume for accurate administration. The appropriate volume for mice is 0.1 ml/10 g (therefore an adult mouse would need 0.2 to 0.4 ml IP or SC). The appropriate volume for a rat is 0.2 ml/100 g (therefore an adult rat would need 0.5 to 0.8 ml IP or SC).
- See Tables 9-3 and 9-4 for dosages used in each species.

EXAMPLES

1. To make up a 2-ml mixture of ketamine (75 mg/kg) and medetomidine (0.5 mg/kg) for rats, mix together the following:

Ketamine (100 mg/ml)	0.75 ml
Medetomidine (1.0 mg/ml)	0.5 ml
Sterile saline (0.9%)	0.75 ml

Administer at 0.2 ml/100 g IP.

2. To make up a 5-ml mixture of ketamine (75 mg/kg) and medetomidine (1.0 mg/kg) for mice, mix together the following:

Ketamine (100 mg/ml)	0.38 ml
Medetomidine (1.0 mg/ml)	0.5 ml
Sterile saline (0.9%)	4.12 ml

Administer at 0.1 ml/10 g IP.

IP, Intraperitoneal.

Cyclohexamine agents

When used alone, ketamine has limited effect in small mammals, even at high doses. In rodents it barely immobilizes the animal and does not provide sufficient analgesia even for superficial surgical procedures such as suturing of skin wounds. In rabbits, use of ketamine alone provides restraint, but the degree of analgesia is insufficient for surgery. Ketamine/acepromazine and ketamine/diazepam or midazolam produces surgical anesthesia in some rabbits, but these combinations generally produce only light anesthesia in small rodents. Ketamine is most effective when combined with an alpha-2 agonist such as medetomidine or xylazine, because these agents have analgesic activity. Ketamine with medetomidine or xylazine produces surgical anesthesia in most rodents and rabbits, but the effects of these agents are less uniform in guinea pigs, and some animals may not be at a sufficient depth of anesthesia for an operation to be carried out humanely. Because ketamine has limited effects when used alone in small mammals, reversal of xylazine or medetomidine will considerably reduce the length of the recovery period. However, because the analgesic effects are also reversed, another analgesic should be administered to provide postoperative pain relief.

Tiletamine in combination with zolazepam (Zoletil, Telazol) produces light to medium planes of anesthesia in small rodents. It offers little advantage in comparison with ketamine combined with diazepam or midazolam, and it produces less analgesia than ketamine in combination with xylazine or medetomidine.

Neuroleptanalgesics

As mentioned earlier, the combinations of fentanyl/droperidol and fentanyl/fluanisone provide restraint and analgesia in small mammals. Fentanyl and fluanisone also can be combined with a benzodiazepine to provide surgical anesthesia. The addition of midazolam or diazepam provides muscle relaxation and increases the depth of anesthesia. Recovery can be enhanced by reversal of fentanyl with a mixed agonist/antagonist opioid such as butorphanol or nalbuphine. This reverses the respiratory depression and some of the sedation caused by the fentanyl component of the anesthetic mixture but continues to provide postoperative analgesia. Although antagonists of benzodiazepine (for example, flumazenil) can be administered to speed recovery, their duration of action is short, and resedation may occur.

The effects of fentanyl and droperidol together with benzodiazepines are less predictable, and this mixture is best avoided in small mammals.

Barbiturates

Although pentobarbital has been widely used for anesthesia of small mammals, it has a very narrow safety margin and produces severe cardiovascular and respiratory depression. Recovery from pentobarbital is prolonged and can be associated with involuntary excitement. For these reasons its use is best avoided. Thiopental and methohexital can be given by intravenous injection in rabbits to produce a short period of anesthesia, and they have effects similar to those seen in dogs and cats.

Propofol

Propofol produces short periods of surgical anesthesia in small rodents, but because it must be given by intravenous injection, it is rarely used in these species. Propofol can be used in rabbits to provide a short period of light anesthesia, sufficient for induction of anesthesia followed by endotracheal intubation and maintenance of anesthesia with gas anesthetics. If high doses of propofol are given to rabbits in an attempt to produce a surgical plane of anesthesia, respiratory arrest often occurs.

Inhalation anesthetics

Induction of anesthesia with inhalation agents is probably the safest and most effective means of providing anesthesia in small rodents. Although mask induction is possible, it is usually most convenient to induce anesthesia in an anesthetic chamber. Suitable chambers can be purchased commercially or can be constructed from clear plastic containers. The size of the chamber should be such that it can be filled rapidly with anesthetic vapor from the anesthetic machine. This will ensure that induction of anesthesia is rapid and smooth with a brief period of involuntary excitement. Anesthetic vapors are denser than air, so the chamber should be filled from the bottom and excess anesthetic gases removed from the top. A suitable design is shown in Fig. 9-13.

Halothane, isoflurane, desflurane, and sevoflurane can all be used safely in small rodents. The concentrations required for induction and maintenance are similar to those used in dogs and cats. Provided the anesthetic chamber is filled rapidly, induc-

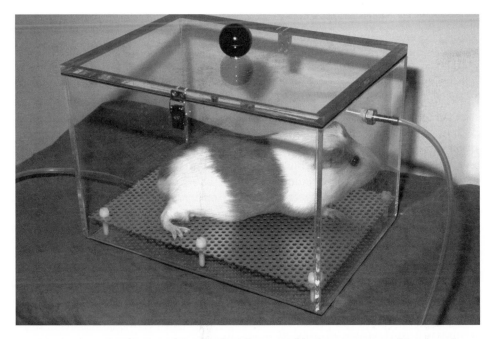

FIG. 9-13 Anesthetic induction chamber suitable for use in small mammals.

tion is generally complete in 2 to 3 minutes. Recovery is also rapid, with rodents recovering their righting reflex within 5 to 10 minutes after 20 to 30 minutes of anesthesia. After a further 10 to 15 minutes they will appear to be fully recovered. As in dogs and cats, induction of anesthesia and recovery are more rapid with isoflurane in comparison with halothane and even more rapid with desflurane and sevoflurane.

Inhalation anesthetics should be delivered with a precision vaporizer. Induction of anesthesia in a chamber in which liquid anesthetic is placed on a gauze pad is extremely dangerous because high concentrations (>20%) of anesthetic vapor are produced.

After induction of anesthesia, the animal can be removed from the chamber and brief (<30 seconds) procedures carried out. For longer procedures it is usually more convenient to maintain anesthesia by placing a face mask on the animal. Suitable masks can either be purchased commercially or constructed from plastic syringes. As with dogs and cats it is important that waste anesthetic gases are scavenged effectively, and this is most easily achieved by using a commercial apparatus designed for this purpose.

The use of gas anesthetics in rabbits can be difficult because animals frequently hold their breath when exposed to these agents. Breath holding can be prolonged and is sometimes associated with marked bradycardia. If a mask is used, animals appear to resent the procedure and may struggle violently. If placed in an anesthetic chamber, they attempt to avoid inhaling the anesthetic and may make violent attempts to escape. It is therefore preferable to administer preanesthetic medication (for example, acepromazine, diazepam, or medetomidine) before inducing anesthesia with a face mask or chamber. After this medication has taken effect, a mask can be used to administer 100% oxygen for 1 to 2 minutes before introducing the inducing agent. The animal may still hold its breath but is unlikely to struggle. If breath holding occurs, the mask should be briefly removed and replaced when the animal commences breathing again. An alternative approach is to administer a short-acting induction agent such as propofol and maintain anesthesia with an inhalation agent.

Summary of Recommended Techniques

Because of the ease of control of depth of anesthesia, the simple and convenient method of induction, and the rapid recovery, inhalation agents are often the anesthesia method of choice in small mammals. If injectable anesthetics are preferred, ketamine in combination with xylazine or medetomidine, or fentanyl and fluanisone and benzodiazepines are the combinations of choice. If an injectable anesthetic combination has been administered and the desired depth of anesthesia is not reached, it is possible to administer an additional drug to deepen anesthesia. However, it is often preferable to deepen anesthesia with a low concentration of an inhalation agent or alternatively to provide local analgesia by infiltrating the surgical site with local anesthetic. These techniques are also useful when dealing with high-risk patients. In these circumstances a low dose of an injectable anesthetic combination can be given to provide a light plane of anesthesia, and inhalation anesthetics or local anesthetics can be used to provide surgical anesthesia.

Intubation and Maintenance of Anesthesia

The apparatus used to anesthetize small rodents and rabbits is similar to that used in dogs and cats, but the size of the patient limits some of the equipment that can be used. Generally, anesthetic gases are delivered with a face mask; however, in rabbits endotracheal intubation is a relatively simple technique to perform and is recommended as a routine procedure. Endotracheal intubation can be carried out by visualizing the larynx with a laryngoscope and blade created for this purpose (such as a Wisconsin blade) or a canine otoscope. Alternatively, a blind technique can be used. These procedures are outlined in detail in Procedure 9-1.

PROCEDURE 9-1   **Rabbit Endotracheal Intubation**

1. Have ready an appropriate size tube, local anesthetic spray, a laryngoscope or otoscope, and an cer (Fig. 9-14). Check that the batteries in the otoscope or laryngoscope are functioning.
2. Measure from the nares to the thoracic inlet and trim the length of the endotracheal tube if necessary.
3. Anesthetize the animal, ensuring that it has lost the chewing reflex elicited when the mouth is opened. Place the animal on its back and administer oxygen through a face mask for 2 minutes.
4. Open the mouth and pull the tongue forward into the gap between the incisors and premolars. The incisors are sharp, so take care not to damage the tongue. Insert the blade of the laryngoscope or the otoscope speculum into the gap between teeth on the opposite side of the mouth and advance until the end of the soft palate or the larynx is visible. In some animals the epiglottis will be positioned behind the soft palate, hiding the larynx from view. To expose the larynx, use the introducer to reposition the epiglottis and soft palate (Fig. 9-15).

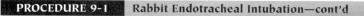

PROCEDURE 9-1   Rabbit Endotracheal Intubation—cont'd

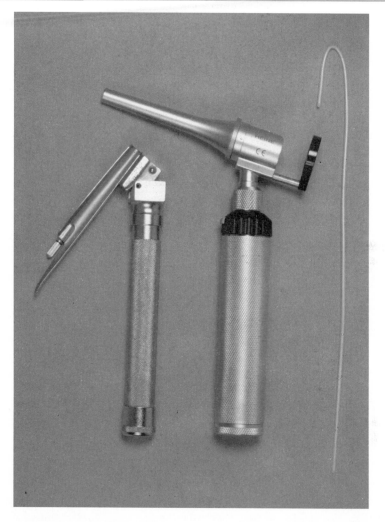

FIG. 9-14 Apparatus for endotracheal intubation in the rabbit. A laryngoscope *(left)* or otoscope *(center)* is used to visualize the larynx, and an introducer *(right)* is used to guide the endotracheal tube into the airway.

5. The larynx is sprayed with local anesthetic.
6. The introducer is advanced though the larynx into the trachea. If an otoscope is used, the introducer is threaded through the speculum, the otoscope is removed, and the endotracheal tube is threaded onto the introducer. If a laryngoscope is used, the tube and introducer are advanced into the mouth together and into the larynx and trachea. The introducer is used to guide the endotracheal tube into the trachea and is then withdrawn. Although introducers are commercially available, a dog or cat urinary catheter can be used to stiffen and straighten the endotracheal tube and act as a guide.

Continued

PROCEDURE 9-1   Rabbit Endotracheal Intubation—cont'd

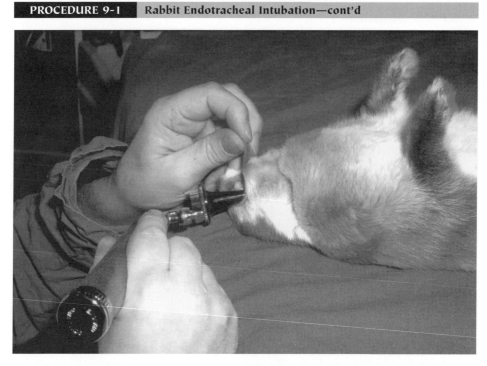

FIG. 9-15   Endotracheal intubation with an otoscope to visualize the larynx of a rabbit (in dorsal recumbency).

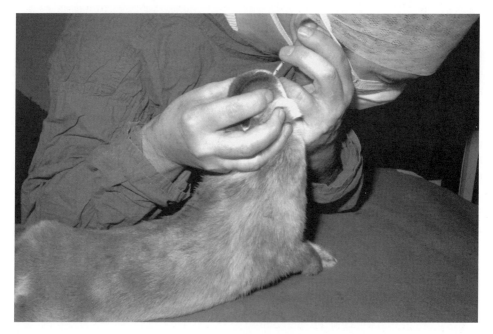

FIG. 9-16   Rabbit positioned for endotracheal intubation with a "blind" technique.

7. When a blind intubation technique is used, the rabbit is placed on its chest and oxygen is supplied through a face mask for 2 minutes. The rabbit is held around the base of the skull and positioned so its head and neck are elevated (Fig. 9-16). The endotracheal tube is introduced into the gap between the incisors and premolars and slid on into the pharynx. As it reaches the larynx, some increase in resistance is felt. The tube can then be advanced into the larynx and trachea; this is usually accompanied by a slight cough. In some cases the tube passes into the esophagus and will need to be withdrawn and repositioned. The position of the tube can be monitored by listening at the end of the tube. If breath sounds can be heard, the tube is in the pharynx or the trachea.

8. Successful placement of the tube can be confirmed by observing condensation in the tube on each expiration, by observing movement of a small piece of tissue paper or a tuft of fur placed at the end of the tube, or by using a capnograph to detect carbon dioxide. After attaching the tube to an anesthetic circuit, auscultate the chest and ensure that both sides are inflated when the reservoir bag is compressed or the expiratory limb of the circuit occluded.

Uncuffed endotracheal tubes are preferred. A typical 3-kg rabbit requires a tube with a 3- to 3.5-mm diameter. Very small rabbits (<800 g) need tubes with a diameter of less than 2.5 mm, which can be purchased from specialist suppliers. As an alternative to intubation, a nasal catheter can be passed and positioned in the back of the pharynx. This allows oxygen supplementation during oral surgery but does not enable ventilation to be assisted effectively.

An anesthetic machine with an out-of-circuit precision vaporizer should be used. Open, nonrebreathing systems are preferred to closed circuit systems because they offer less resistance and have less equipment dead space. Examples of suitable nonrebreathing systems include the Bain circuit and Ayres T piece. With smaller rabbits, it is advisable to use low–dead space pediatric connectors to attach the endotracheal tube to the breathing circuit. Low–dead space T pieces designed for use in human beings are also useful for rabbits (Fig. 9-17). Fresh gas flow rates are calculated in the same way as for dogs and cats (see Box 4-1).

Monitoring
Depth of anesthesia

Before a surgical or other painful procedure is started, it is essential to ensure that the animal is at an appropriate depth of anesthesia. The most reliable method in rodents is to assess the pedal withdrawal (discussed in Chapter 2) or tail pinch reflex. To assess the tail pinch, the operator firmly pinches the tip of the tail with fingernails. It is important to pinch hard enough to produce a painful stimulus, but not so hard as to damage the tail. If the animal is too lightly anesthetized for surgery, it will flick its tail and may vocalize. The tail pinch response is usually lost at light to medium planes of anesthesia, and this is followed by a loss of the pedal withdrawal response at medium to deep planes of anesthesia. Most surgical

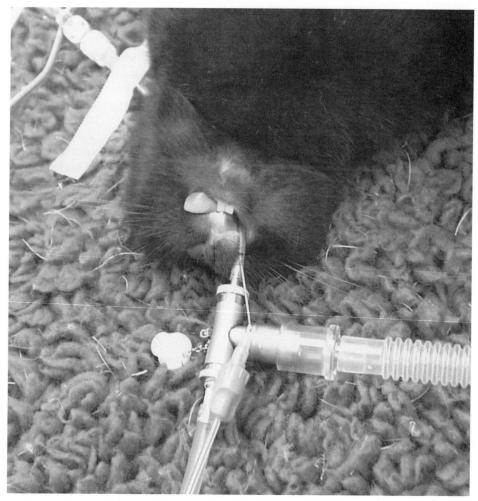

A

FIG. 9-17 Low–dead space pediatric T piece and endotracheal connector suitable for anesthetic delivery in a rabbit.

procedures can be carried out when the pedal withdrawal reflex is absent or barely detectable. In rabbits and guinea pigs, the ear pinch reflex can also be used to measure anesthetic depth.

Ocular reflexes are not as useful in small mammals as in the dog and cat. With most anesthetic regimens, the position of the eye remains fixed in rodents, and the palpebral (blink) reflex may still be present at surgical planes of anesthesia. In rabbits, there is considerable variation in loss of ocular reflexes; however, at deep planes of anesthesia the eye may rotate and protrude. Because cardiac arrest may occur shortly after the animal reaches such a deep plane of anesthesia, this appearance indicates that supportive measures should be initiated immediately and administration of anesthetic should be reduced or terminated.

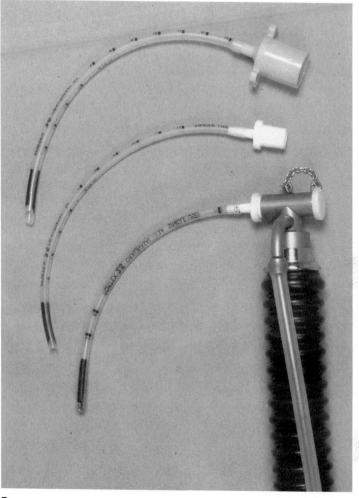

B

FIG. 9-17, cont'd Endotracheal tube connectors. *Top,* Standard connector; *middle,* pediatric connector; *bottom,* pediatric connector and T piece.

Heart rate and rhythm

The small size of rodents and rabbits and their rapid heart rate can make it difficult to monitor heart rate and rhythm, and it is not usually possible to palpate a peripheral pulse. Auscultation of the chest wall is possible in rabbits and guinea pigs, but difficult in smaller rodents. An esophageal stethoscope can be used in rabbits, and the heartbeat can be detected by palpating the chest wall in all species. However, because the heart rate often exceeds 250 beats per minute (bpm) in many of these animals, it is not possible to accurately assess the heart rate. Problems can also arise when an electrocardiogram (ECG) is used, because many instruments have an upper heart rate limit of 250 or 300 bpm and may also be unable to detect the low amplitude signals generated in small rodents.

Capillary refill time

The small size of rodents usually prevents use of capillary refill time as an assessment of peripheral perfusion, although it is possible to assess this in rabbits. The color of the mucous membranes can give some indication of problems associated with blood loss, cyanosis, and poor peripheral perfusion. In addition to inspection of the gingiva, the color of light reflected in the eyes can be used to detect cyanosis or pallor caused by blood loss in albino animals.

Blood loss

Because these animals are small, total blood volume is small—approximately 70 ml/kg of body weight. A 100-g hamster will have a total blood volume of only 7 ml. As in dogs and cats, loss of more than 15% (approximately 1 ml in this example) can lead to signs of circulatory failure. It is therefore critically important to monitor blood loss by carefully weighing swabs and assessing other losses at the surgical site.

Respiratory rate and depth

The pattern and depth of respiration can be monitored by observing the chest movements, although this becomes difficult once surgical drapes have been placed. Because of the small size of these animals, there is usually no reservoir bag in the anesthetic circuit, and respiration cannot be monitored by bag movement. It is helpful to use an electronic monitor, but as with the ECG, the small size of the animal and rapid respiratory rate can make some monitors ineffective.

Although both the pattern and rate of respiration change during anesthesia, this varies greatly depending on the anesthetic regimen used. Becoming familiar with one or two regularly used regimens allows changes to be interpreted more reliably. In general, once anesthesia has been induced, respiratory rate decreases markedly, especially because most of these animals will show tachypnea before induction. Typical respiratory rates during anesthesia are 50 to 100 breaths per minutes for small rodents and 30 to 60 breaths per minute for rabbits. A reduction to less than 50% of the estimated normal respiratory rate (see Table 9-1) should give cause for concern. As in dogs and cats, it is more common to see gradual changes in rate, rather than a sudden reduction. For this reason, it is helpful to keep a written anesthetic record when assessing the state of the animal during anesthesia.

Pulse oximetry

Pulse oximeters can be used to monitor both the adequacy of oxygenation and the heart rate, but not all instruments function well in small rodents. The high heart rates may exceed the upper limits of the monitor, and the low signal strength may not be detectable. A monitor with an upper limit of at least 350 bpm is needed, and it is useful to have a variety of different probe designs. A reliable signal can usually be obtained by placing the probe across the hind foot in small rodents or across a toe in larger rabbits, but the tail, tongue, and ear are also useful in some animals (Fig. 9-18).

Capnography

Side-stream capnographs can be used to monitor respiratory function in small animals, although the volume of gas sampled may be very large in relation to the

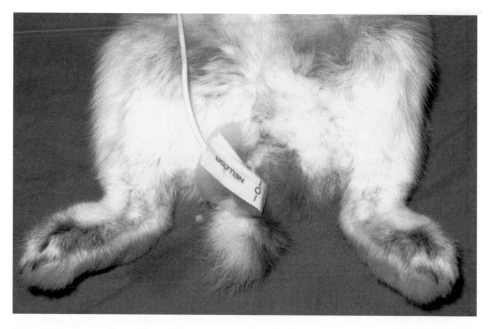

FIG. 9-18 Use of a pulse oximeter in a rabbit, with the probe positioned across the base of the tail.

animal's tidal volume. Mainstream capnographs introduce too much equipment dead space into the anesthetic breathing circuit and are not recommended in these species.

Thermoregulation

It is critically important to monitor and maintain body temperature during anesthesia and in the postoperative period. Because of their small body size, rodents and rabbits have an increased ratio of surface area to body weight, which may lead to rapid cooling during anesthesia. Heat loss can be much more rapid than in dogs and cats. For example, the rectal temperature in a mouse can fall 5° to 6° C (9° to 11° F) in 5 to 10 minutes after induction of anesthesia. The following procedures help avoid hypothermia:

- Monitor rectal temperatures using an electronic thermometer rather than a glass clinical thermometer. Glass clinical thermometers can only indicate a minimum temperature of 35° C, and the animal may be colder than this when the first measurement is made.
- Adopt good standards of asepsis, but keep the area of fur that is shaved at the surgical site to a minimum and use the minimum quantity of skin disinfectant.
- Place the animal on a warming pad as soon as it has lost consciousness and provide additional insulation if needed.
- Always warm fluids to body temperature before administration.
- Continue measures to prevent heat loss in the recovery period (see the following section).

POSTOPERATIVE CARE

The provision of appropriate postoperative care is critical to the successful outcome of anesthesia and surgery in small mammals. Supportive measures to maintain body temperature must be continued, and a quiet, warm, secure environment should be provided. Because heat loss can occur relatively rapidly, an appropriate recovery environment should be set up before starting anesthesia and an operation. The animal can then be transferred to the recovery area immediately after completion of the operation. While the animal is immobile and unconscious, an environmental temperature of approximately 35° C (95° F) should be maintained. This can be lowered to 26° to 28° C (79° to 81° F) as the animal recovers. Warm and comfortable bedding must be provided. Synthetic sheepskin is ideal, but if this is unavailable, shredded paper or tissues can be used. Sawdust is unsuitable because it tends to crust around the nose, eyes, and mouth. Good quality hay should be provided to guinea pigs and rabbits once they have recovered their righting reflex. This type of bedding allows the animal to surround itself with insulating material, which provides both warmth and a sense of security and encourages early feeding. Other species of small mammal should also be encouraged to eat soon after recovery and should be given their preferred foods.

Animals should also be provided with water, but care must be taken that they do not spill water bowls, because the animal will lose heat rapidly if it becomes wet. The animal may also fail to drink from an unfamiliar water container, and when a case history is obtained before anesthesia it is important to find out what type of container the animal is accustomed to using. In most circumstances, it is advisable to administer warmed (37° C or 98.6° F) subcutaneous or intraperitoneal dextrose/saline (4% dextrose, 0.15% saline) at the end of the operation to provide some fluid supplementation in the immediate postoperative period.

Postoperative analgesia is discussed on p. 380.

ANESTHETIC EMERGENCIES
Respiratory Depression

Changes in the depth and pattern of respiration usually precede respiratory arrest. Careful monitoring of respiratory function will usually allow corrective measures to be taken before an emergency arises. If the animal has been intubated, respiration can be assisted by delivering 100% oxygen from the anesthetic machine. As with larger species, it is important to check that the endotracheal tube is properly positioned and has not become disconnected from the breathing circuit or obstructed. If the animal has not been intubated, respiration can be assisted by extending the head and neck and gently compressing the chest. Attempts to assist ventilation with a face mask are usually unsuccessful. In small rodents, a soft piece of rubber tubing can be placed over the nose and mouth and the lungs inflated by gently blowing down the tube (Fig. 9-19). Respiration can also be stimulated by administration of doxapram, but this drug has a relatively short duration of action (approximately 10 minutes) and repeated doses may be needed. Efforts should be made to determine the cause of the respiratory depression and to initiate corrective measures.

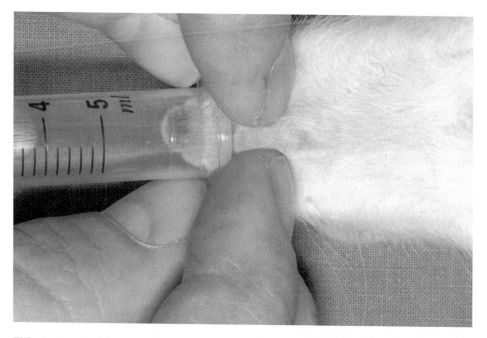

FIG. 9-19   Assisting ventilation in a rat by blowing down the barrel of a syringe placed over the mouth and nose.

Circulatory Failure

Treatment of circulatory failure and cardiac arrest is similar to that in dogs and cats, but the small size of these animals causes some practical problems. Fluid therapy is difficult because of the small size of the superficial vessels, although it is possible to place over-the-needle catheters in the tail vein of rats and the medial tarsal vein in guinea pigs. In rabbits, intravenous access is much easier, and catheters can be placed in the marginal ear veins or cephalic veins. The jugular vein is relatively mobile in the rabbit and is more difficult to locate and catheterize than in the dog and cat.

Loss of blood can be treated by transfusion from a donor animal. Fortunately, problems of incompatibility are rare on initial transfusion; however, it is likely to be more difficult to locate a suitable donor than when dealing with dogs and cats. As an alternative, a plasma volume expander such as Dextran or Hetastarch can be administered. All of the commonly available products can be administered safely to small mammals, providing appropriate allowance is made for their smaller circulating volumes. In smaller species in which intravenous access is not practical, intraperitoneal or subcutaneous administration of warmed electrolyte solutions can slowly replace fluid deficits or blood loss but will be of minimal benefit if rapid hemorrhage is occurring. As discussed earlier, preventing problems by minimizing hemorrhage through meticulous surgical technique is important.

If cardiac arrest occurs, external cardiac massage and emergency drugs such as epinephrine can be used to try to resuscitate the animal (see Chapter 6). One significant problem is the practical difficulty of rapidly calculating drug dose rates when an emergency occurs. It is much simpler to utilize a list of dose rates and volumes, expressed as the dose volumes for a typical adult animal of each species. This will help avoid errors and speed therapy (Table 9-5).

ANALGESIA

As discussed in Chapter 8, the use of analgesics in veterinary practice has become more widespread in recent years. Although most dogs and cats now receive at least some postsurgical analgesia, these drugs are often not used in small mammals. This is probably due to a number of factors, including poor ability to recognize pain in these small animals and a lack of knowledge of the safety and efficacy of analgesic agents. However, it is critically important to provide postoperative analgesia to these patients, because most small mammals will fail to eat or drink if they are experiencing postoperative pain.

Pain Assessment in Small Mammals

Pain assessment in dogs and cats is not always easy, but most veterinarians and veterinary technicians are relatively familiar with the normal behavior of these species. The normal behavior and general appearance of small rodents and rabbits are often less well appreciated, and as a result the signs associated with pain may be overlooked. In addition, several species of small mammals are nocturnal and may not be active when observed during normal working hours. They may also remain immobile in the presence of an observer if they perceive the observer as a threat. It is therefore not always easy to use behavior and changes in posture to assess pain. However, it is important to overcome these difficulties so that pain can be prevented or controlled effectively in these small animals.

TABLE 9-5

*Dose Rates for Emergency Drugs with Typical Dilutions and Volumes Needed for an Adult Animal**

DRUG	CONCENTRATION IN COMMERCIAL PREPARATION	DILUTION INSTRUCTIONS	VOLUME OF DILUTED DRUG FOR A TYPICAL ADULT ANIMAL
Doxapram	20 mg/ml	1 in 10	Mouse, 0.1 ml; hamster and gerbil, 0.25 ml, SC or IV
		Not required	Rat, 0.1 ml; guinea pig, 0.25 ml, SC or IV
Epinephrine	1:1000	1 in 10	Mouse, 0.03 ml; hamster and gerbil, 0.1 ml; rat, 0.3 ml; guinea pig, 0.7 ml, IV or intracardiac
Lidocaine	20 mg/ml	1 in 10	Mouse, 0.03 ml; hamster and gerbil, 0.1 ml; rat, 0.3 ml, guinea pig, 0.7 ml, IV or intracardiac
Sodium bicarbonate	1 mEq/ml	Not required	Mouse, 0.03 ml; hamster and gerbil, 0.1 ml; rat, 0.3 ml; guinea pig, 0.7 ml, IV

*For rabbits, dose rates are similar to those for dogs and cats.

As in dogs and cats, an initial assessment of the animal should be made without disturbing the animal. The animal's appearance and posture may be abnormal, and it may appear hunched. Its coat may be unkempt and ruffled because of a lack of grooming and the presence of piloerection. Rats may have a blackish discharge around their eyes and nose because of a buildup of secretions from their harderian glands. It is uncertain whether this buildup of material is due to reduced grooming or whether it is a response to stress, but it is a valuable indicator that the animal is not healthy and may be in pain. While it is being observed, the animal may demonstrate normal inquisitive behavior and explore its environment, but as mentioned earlier, if it remains motionless, this may be because it feels threatened rather than because it is in pain. If the animal has positioned itself in the back of its cage or pen or has hidden in bedding, this can also be a sign of fear but may also be due to pain.

When encouraged to move, the animal may have an abnormal gait or posture and may show uncharacteristic signs of aggression. Rats, mice, and gerbils will usually rear when investigating what has disturbed them, and the absence of this behavior may be due to pain. When handled, rather than attempting to evade capture, animals in pain may be apathetic or may be aggressive and bite the handler. When it is examined, the animal may respond to manipulation or palpation of a painful area by vocalizing or trying to bite. Confusingly, some small mammals such as guinea pigs will also vocalize loudly when not in pain and may respond to any manipulation by tensing their muscles and remaining immobile. Similar immobility can also be seen in rabbits.

Rabbits with abdominal pain may grind their teeth, and all small mammals may stop eating and drinking when experiencing pain. This can be difficult to detect if food is provided ad lib, but the subsequent loss in body weight can easily be monitored. This is one of the easiest ways of following an animal's progress after surgery or during treatment of any disease condition. The inappetence caused by pain is a serious problem in small mammals, because failure to drink can rapidly lead to significant dehydration and lack of food intake can predispose to the development of hypoglycemia in small rodents. In rabbits, guinea pigs, and chinchillas, disturbances in food intake can lead to the development of life-threatening gastrointestinal disturbances.

As experience is gained in observing the normal behavior patterns of small mammals, abnormalities will be detected with greater confidence. Although relatively specific signs of pain such as guarding of an injured area may be seen, many of the signs are relatively nonspecific and can also occur in response to nonpainful conditions. It is therefore important to consider the appearance of the animal in relation to its case history and other clinical findings. Although it is highly desirable to try to assess pain in each individual patient so that appropriate analgesia therapy can be administered, it is not unreasonable to accept that some analgesic treatment will be needed after every surgical procedure.

Analgesic Agents

None of the analgesics that are currently marketed for use in dogs and cats provide any product information regarding their use in small mammals. It is worth noting, however, that all of these products were originally tested for safety and efficacy in small rodents. This information provides reassurance that the drugs can be used safely to provide effective pain relief in these species. There is less information available on the use of analgesia in rabbits and guinea pigs, but extensive clinical experience indicates that most analgesics can be used safely in these animals. Suggested dose rates are listed in Table 9-6. The options for pain management are similar to those available in dogs and cats, but the small size of the animal may limit the use of techniques such as epidural administration of drugs or use of fentanyl patches.

Opioids

All of the morphine-like drugs that can be used in dogs and cats can also be used in small mammals but often have a shorter duration of action in these species. Meperidine lasts for only 30 to 60 minutes in rodents, for example. Buprenorphine, which has a duration of action of approximately 6 to 12 hours in small mammals, is often preferred. Some authorities question whether partial agonists such as buprenorphine are potent enough to control severe pain; however, clinical experience suggests that this analgesic is effective after most surgical procedures in small rodents and rabbits. Buprenorphine may cause behavioral abnormalities in small rodents (such as eating sawdust bedding in rats). However, this side effect appears rare, and most animals appear to benefit from the use of buprenorphine after surgery. If other opioid analgesics are to be used, repeated administration is likely to be needed to provide effective pain relief. One useful means of avoiding the need for frequent injections of drug is to combine administration of an opioid with the use of a nonsteroidal antiinflammatory drug (NSAID) (see the following section).

Nonsteroidal antiinflammatory drugs

NSAIDS (particularly the more potent NSAIDs such as carprofen, ketoprofen, and meloxicam) can provide very effective pain relief in small mammals. Considerable basic information is available from pharmaceutical companies concerning the safety and efficacy of these analgesics in small rodents. Although there have been no reports of adverse reactions to these drugs in small mammals, it seems advisable to adopt the same precautions as those in dogs and cats. Prolonged use (more than a few days) should be avoided when possible, although clinical experience suggests that meloxicam can be used for extended periods in rabbits to control dental pain. Because of the risks of renal toxicity should hypotension occur during anesthesia, only carprofen should be administered preoperatively. A significant advantage of the use of NSAIDs is that they appear to have a prolonged duration of action in small mammals. A single dose of carprofen, ketoprofen, or meloxicam may provide analgesia for 12 to 24 hours. Meloxicam has the additional advantage of being available in some countries as a palatable liquid preparation. This makes it easier for owners to continue analgesia administration if needed.

Local anesthetics

Local anesthetics can be used to provide postoperative analgesia. As in dogs and cats, they can be infiltrated around surgical wounds or administered as specific nerve blocks. Although the safety of these agents in small mammals is similar to that in dogs and cats, it is relatively easy to inadvertently overdose rodents because of their small size. Care must be taken to calculate the dose accurately (maximum recommended doses in rodents: lidocaine 10 mg/kg, bupivacaine 4 mg/kg; maximum

TABLE 9-6

Analgesic Agents for Use in Small Mammals*

ANALGESIC	GERBIL	GUINEA PIG	HAMSTER	MOUSE	RABBIT	RAT
Buprenorphine	0.1 mg/kg SC	0.05 mg/kg SC	0.1 mg/kg SC	0.1 mg/kg SC	0.01-0.05 mg/kg SC	0.05 mg/kg SC
Butorphanol	?	2 mg/kg	?	1-5 mg/kg SC	0.1-0.5 mg/kg SC	2 mg/kg SC
Carprofen	?	2.5 mg/kg SC daily	?	5 mg/kg bid SC or per os	1.5 mg/kg per os daily, 4 mg/kg SC daily	5 mg/kg bid SC or per os
Flunixin	?	?	?	2.5 mg/kg SC bid	1.1 mg/kg SC bid	2.5 mg/kg SC bid
Ketoprofen	?	?	?	?	3 mg/kg IM	5 mg/kg IM
Meloxicam	?	?	?	?	0.2 mg/kg SC daily	1.0 mg/kg SC or per os daily
Meperidine (Pethidine)	?	10-20 mg/kg SC or IM 2-3 hourly	?	10-20 mg/kg SC or IM 2-3 hourly	10 mg/kg SC or IM 2-3 hourly	10-20 mg/kg SC or IM 2-3 hourly
Morphine	?	2.5 mg/kg SC or IM 4 hourly	?	2.5 mg/kg SC or IM 4 hourly	2-5 mg/kg SC or IM 4 hourly	2.5 mg/kg SC or IM 4 hourly
Oxymorphone	?	?	?	?	0.1-0.2 mg/kg IM, IV	0.2-0.3 mg/kg SC

Data modified from Flecknell PA, Waterman-Pearson AE, editors: *Pain management in animals*, London, 2001, Harcourt International.
*Note that these are only suggestions based on clinical experience and the limited published data that are available. Dose rates should be adjusted depending on the clinical response of the animal. A "?" indicates that there is insufficient information to make a firm recommendation of an appropriate dose.

recommended dose in rabbits: same as for cats, see Chapter 7). It is important to note that the duration of action of some local anesthetics may be shorter in rodents than in larger species, such as dogs. As mentioned earlier, the application of topical agents such as EMLA cream provides analgesia for venipuncture or placement of intravenous catheters.

Chronic pain

Small mammals may have a range of chronic conditions that can cause pain. Rats may have arthritis; guinea pigs, chinchillas, and rabbits may have dental disease; and neoplasia is common in many species. NSAIDs can often be used successfully to control the pain associated with these conditions, although it is necessary to carefully monitor the patient for side effects, especially during long-term use of these agents.

Administration of Analgesics

Intravenous administration of analgesics is difficult in rodents but relatively straight-forward in rabbits. Because of the small muscle mass in rodents, subcutaneous administration is preferred. Oral dosing can be difficult and may require firm physical restraint that can exacerbate pain from surgical wounds. Provided the animal is eating, analgesics can be added to highly palatable food items (for example, doughnuts for rats and mice). Analgesics for rats or mice can also be incorporated into fruit or meat-flavored jelly. Commercial flavored jelly should be prepared with half of the recommended quantity of water, and after the mixture is allowed to cool, a measured quantity of analgesic is added. After the jelly has set, it can be cut into cubes of an appropriate weight. The remaining jelly should be labeled and stored in a refrigerator, taking note of any legal requirements concerning storage of controlled drugs. Commercial gelatin mixed with beef extract may also be used.

As in dogs and cats, preemptive administration of analgesics may provide more effective pain relief than postoperative use and may reduce the amount of anesthetic required for the surgical procedure. If volatile anesthetics are being used, opioids can be administered safely before the operation and the concentration of anesthetic delivered reduced as necessary to maintain a safe level of anesthesia. For example, when buprenorphine is administered preoperatively to rodents, the concentration of isoflurane needed to provide surgical anesthesia can be reduced by approximately 25% to 50%. If injectable agents are used, preemptive analgesia is more difficult, because injectable anesthetics are often given as a single dose by the intraperitoneal or subcutaneous routes and cannot be titrated according to their effect in the individual animal. Because the commonly used opioids will potentiate the actions of injectable anesthetic agents, their preoperative administration could lead to inadvertent anesthetic overdose. Because of the limited information available concerning the degree of interaction between injectable anesthetics and opioids, it is safer in this case to administer opioid analgesics at the end of the operation in small rodents, as the depth of anesthesia is becoming lighter.

Not all NSAIDs can be safely used preoperatively because of potential adverse effects such as renal hypotension and prolonged bleeding times. Carprofen is one NSAID that can apparently be safely used for preemptive analgesia.

Although the use of analgesic drugs remains the most important technique for reducing postoperative pain, pain medication must be integrated into a total scheme for perioperative care. Animals must be provided with a postoperative recovery area appropriate to their particular needs. For example, it is stressful for a small mammal to recover in the same room as their predators (for example, cats), and the resulting change in their behavior pattern could mask signs of pain.

REVIEW QUESTIONS

1. Glycopyrrolate should be used in rabbits, instead of atropine, because:
   a. Atropine is highly toxic in rabbits.
   b. Many rabbits have high levels of atropinesterase, so atropine is relatively ineffective.
   c. Rabbits are unable to metabolize atropine.
   d. Atropine causes marked bradycardia in rabbits.
2. Pulse oximeters can be used in small mammals, but they may not be reliable because:
   a. The heart rate of the animal may exceed the upper range of the instrument.
   b. The hemoglobin absorption characteristics are different in rodents and dogs and cats.
   c. Pulse oximeters do not function on animals that have dark fur.
   d. Small rodents have a rapid respiratory rate.
3. The position of the eye cannot be used to assess the depth of anesthesia in rodents because:
   a. The eye is too small to assess its position accurately.
   b. The position of the eye does not change during anesthesia.
   c. The eye rotates downwards at very light planes of anesthesia.
   d. The eyelids remain closed throughout anesthesia.
4. An advantage of using medetomidine combined with ketamine for anesthesia of rodents and rabbits is that:
   a. It is readily absorbed from body fat.
   b. It can be given by mouth to produce anesthesia.
   c. It promotes gut motility and so reduces the occurrence of postoperative inappetence.
   d. It can be partially reversed using atipamezole, allowing faster recovery.
5. An adult mouse weighing 40 g will have a blood volume of approximately:
   a. 10 ml
   b. 3 ml
   c. 50 ml
   d. 0.2 ml

6. When fluids such as lactated Ringer's solution are given to small mammals they should be:
   a. Used at about 4° C so that they are rapidly absorbed
   b. Administered orally, because it is not possible to use any other route
   c. Warmed to body temperature before administration, to avoid causing hypothermia
   d. Only given postoperatively, to avoid overloading the circulation
7. Anesthetic breathing circuits for use in small rabbits should:
   a. Only be constructed of plastic components because rabbits are allergic to latex
   b. Have low equipment dead space
   c. Have high equipment dead space
   d. Always include soda lime to prevent rebreathing
8. When small rodents are anesthetized with injectable anesthetics:
   a. It is not necessary to administer oxygen because most anesthetics stimulate respiration.
   b. Oxygen should be administered because most anesthetics depress respiration.
   c. Carbon dioxide should be included in the fresh gas mixture to stimulate respiration.
   d. Nitrous oxide should always be used; otherwise, the depth of anesthesia will be insufficient for surgery.
9. Postoperative analgesic should be given to rodents and rabbits to alleviate pain, but:
   a. NSAIDs cannot be used because they cause gastric ulceration at normal therapeutic doses in these species.
   b. Opioids (narcotics) cause severe respiratory depression and so must never be used.
   c. Opioids must be given with care if a neuroleptanalgesic mixture has been used for anesthesia.
   d. Local anesthetics cannot be used because they produce cardiac arrest even at low doses in these species.
10. If postoperative pain is not alleviated in rabbits, then:
    a. Animals will not eat or drink normally.
    b. Animals recover much faster from anesthesia.
    c. Rabbits will spend a great deal of time grooming themselves.
    d. Porphyrin staining will appear around their eyes.

ANSWERS FOR CHAPTER 9

1. b	2. a	3. b	4. d	5. b
6. c	7. b	8. b	9. c	10. a

Selected Readings

Flecknell PA: *Laboratory animal anesthesia,* London, 1996, Academic Press.
Flecknell PA, Waterman-Pearson AE, editors: *Pain management in animals,* London, 2001, Harcourt International.
Kohn DF, Wixson SK, White WJ, et al, editors: *Anesthesia and analgesia in laboratory animals,* San Diego, 1997, Academic Press.

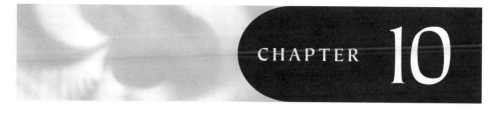

CHAPTER 10

Large Animal Anesthesia

Charles McGrath, Meghan Richey

PERFORMANCE OBJECTIVES

After completion of this chapter, the reader will be able to:
- Explain the importance of proper large animal handling and restraint.
- Describe a combination protocol for standing chemical restraint in the horse that includes sedation, analgesia, expected onset time, expected duration of effect, dosages, and routes of administration.
- Describe the expected corneal, palpebral, and anal sphincter reflexes of the equine patient in an anesthetic plane of field anesthesia.
- Describe the administration of a basic xylazine/ketamine combination in a horse, including dosage, route, and order of administration.
- List the different requirements of an anesthetic machine for an animal that weighs less than 150 kg versus a machine for an animal that weighs more than 150 kg.
- Describe three sites for arterial catheter placement in the horse for blood pressure measurement.
- Outline the reason for rapid intravenous (IV) fluid loading in a horse during anesthesia and describe the process.
- Describe how to set up a continuous dobutamine infusion for a 500-kg horse with a dose of 0.5 to 2.0 µg/kg/min.
- List two causes of regurgitation in anesthetized cattle and explain two means of prevention.
- Define "triple-drip," including the drugs used and the way in which this is administered to cattle.

GENERAL CONSIDERATIONS
Biologic Variation

For a better understanding of our patients and their different responses to anesthesia, an understanding of the general term *biologic variation* is required. From a pharmacologic perspective, patients may appear to have a consistent response to anesthetic drugs; however, subtle biologic differences existing among patients may cause variations in this response. For example, biologic variation may be caused by differences in basal metabolic rates, which vary with body size. Within a species, larger animals generally have a lower metabolic rate and require a lower dose on a milligram per kilogram basis. This is most obvious in the dog, in which body sizes vary from 1 kg to nearly 100 kg. This difference in metabolic rates is also seen between horses and ponies.

Each animal is a unique biologic entity. Within an apparently normal, healthy population of animals of the same species and approximate size, the response to anesthesia may vary significantly. It is unclear if this variation is a function of each individual animal's genetic makeup or if environmental factors play a role, or both. With many anesthetics (for example, inhalants), doses may be adjusted to compensate for individual variation. This approach is referred to as *dosing to effect* and is the typical method used to administer inhalant and some intravenous (IV) anesthetics such as propofol and thiopental. On the other hand, some anesthetics must be calculated and the whole dose administered IV.

Finally, a major component of biologic variation involves the difference in response to the same anesthetic agent among different species. A well-recognized example is the variation in response to xylazine (and other alpha-2 agonists) among various large animal species. In general, ruminants tend to be very sensitive to xylazine, horses are intermediate in their response, and swine are relatively resistant to the sedative effects of this agent. In contrast, most species exhibit an amazingly consistent response to inhalant anesthetics. For example, the minimum alveolar concentration (MAC) of isoflurane is approximately 1.3% in a variety of species ranging from horses to dogs to small rodents.

Handling and Restraint

Handling and restraint of large animal patients is an extremely important part of large animal anesthesia. A detailed discussion of this topic is well beyond the scope of this chapter; however, all technicians involved in large animal anesthesia should be thoroughly familiar with various techniques and equipment, including halters, ropes, cattle chutes, and other devices routinely used to handle various large animal species. Clearly, proper handling and restraint prevent injury to the patient and to veterinary personnel and clients.

For each of the following species, general considerations and problems unique to that species are presented. Additionally, common sedation and chemical restraint options, field anesthesia, injectable anesthetic induction and maintenance, and anesthetic monitoring considerations and expectations are discussed.

HORSES
Sedation and Standing Chemical Restraint

In situations in which good physical restraint is inadequate to perform a procedure, sedation and standing chemical restraint remain the best options for diagnostic and minor surgical procedures in the horse. For diagnostic procedures or minor surgery, sedation or standing chemical restraint has a significant advantage over general anesthesia in that the horse remains standing throughout the procedure. The potential for injuries that may occur during induction or recovery periods is eliminated. In addition, sedation and standing chemical restraint are less time-consuming than general anesthesia.

The drugs used to produce standing chemical restraint are most commonly given IV. Venipuncture in the standing horse is usually performed using the jugular vein. Some horses may be resistant to this procedure. In addition to good physical restraint, covering the ipsilateral eye to block the horse's rearward view and pinching the skin adjacent to the planned site of needle insertion may limit the response to venipuncture. Most drugs do not produce severe tissue reaction if extravasation occurs. However, using the right jugular vein is recommended so that if a tissue reaction does occur, it is limited to the side opposite the esophagus. Because the carotid artery is near the jugular vein, inadvertent intraarterial injection can occur, resulting in seizures within a few seconds of injection. Every effort should be made to avoid carotid arterial injection, including performing the venipuncture without the syringe attached. Once the needle is placed within the vessel, cessation of blood flow from the needle hub, when digital venous occlusion is removed, will serve as confirmation that the needle is in the jugular vein.

The drugs given for sedation include acepromazine, xylazine, detomidine, or romifidine. Sometimes two of these are used in combination to achieve a faster onset and/or longer duration of action. Regardless of the drug or drug combination, it is important to remember that some of these horses may be aroused from sedation by surgical or other stimulation. Acepromazine given at a dose of 0.05 mg/kg IV or IM will usually produce mild sedation within 15 to 20 minutes that will persist for about 90 minutes. Xylazine (0.5 to 1.1 mg/kg IV) produces sedation within 3 minutes of injection and persists for about 30 minutes. As an added benefit, xylazine also produces analgesia by activation of alpha-2 receptors in the central nervous system. Bradycardia in the form of second-degree atrioventricular block is seen fairly commonly within a few minutes of xylazine administration. Acepromazine (0.02 to 0.03 mg/kg IV) and xylazine (0.2 to 0.5 mg/kg IV) may be combined in an attempt to achieve a faster onset time (xylazine) and a longer duration (acepromazine).

The use of detomidine (Dormosedan) has increased dramatically since its introduction in 1989, partly because of its longer duration of action than xylazine and an onset time considerably faster than acepromazine (5 to 6 minutes). As an alpha-2 agonist, detomidine, like xylazine, produces sedation and analgesia. A third alpha-2 agonist, romifidine (Sedivet) is available in Canada for equine sedation. Some veterinarians prefer to use a mixture of xylazine (0.2 mg/kg IV) and detomidine (4 µg/kg IV) to improve sedation and analgesia during equine dental procedures.

Regardless of the alpha-2 agonist used, typical effects include sedation, analgesia, and skeletal muscle relaxation. Skeletal muscle relaxation may manifest itself as drooping of the eyelids and lips, as well as a head-down position. It should be remembered, however, that although horses appear sedate they may be aroused from sedation produced by alpha-2 agonists or acepromazine.

If sedation with acepromazine or an alpha-2 agonist is deemed to be inadequate, neuroleptanalgesic (NLA) agents are recommended to better ensure immobility. NLAs are a combination of a neuroleptic drug (tranquilizer) with an analgesic drug such as an opioid (see Chapter 1). NLAs are typically the most effective choice for standing chemical restraint. As with sedation or standing chemical restraint with acepromazine or xylazine, a horse that has been given an NLA remains standing throughout the procedure.

Several NLA combinations have been used in the past and many are still in current use. With most combinations, horses have a tendency to remain in a "sawhorse" stance. With some combinations, especially detomidine and butorphanol, they may tend to head-press if positioned directly in front of an immovable partition.

Field Anesthesia

In contrast to standing chemical restraint, the objective of field anesthesia is to create a state of light general anesthesia and recumbency with injectable anesthetics. Typically, field anesthesia is performed "on the farm" but may also be done for shorter surgical or diagnostic procedures at the clinic. As with all other animal patients, safety for the patient and personnel in the area must be addressed. At least one experienced handler is essential to minimize the risk of injury to the horse, handler, or other personnel.

The handler's role includes surveying the immediate area to be used for anesthesia for visible hazards. The area should be as flat as feasible given the terrain, and all obstacles such as rocks, boards, and farm implements should be removed. Contingency plans for possible escape of the horse should also be considered before inducing the patient. With few exceptions, owners should be excluded from the induction and recovery process.

During anesthesia induction, the handler holds the lead rope during the injection process and as recumbency ensues. A cotton lead rope is recommended to prevent rope burn or degloving injuries. The rope should never be wrapped around the hand, wrist, or shoulder. As the horse collapses to the ground, the handler, by using the lead rope, supports the head so that it does not forcibly strike the ground. As the recovery process commences, the lead rope may be used to assist the horse as it stands up again. Sometimes an unassisted recovery is preferred, but the lead rope should be kept attached or close at hand so that the horse's movements can be better controlled if it is unsteady on its feet. During recumbency, a towel should be placed under the "down" eye and over the "up" eye to minimize the risk of corneal abrasion. The towel can be lifted from the up eye periodically to check ocular signs as a part of assessing anesthetic depth.

When field anesthesia is induced, the plane of general anesthesia that is achieved is typically much lighter than that desired for the horse or small animal patient under inhalant anesthetics in a more controlled environment. Horses will usually exhibit a brisk corneal reflex, palpebral reflex, and anal sphincter reflex during field anesthesia. Spontaneous eyelid movement and nystagmus (a slow oscillatory movement of the eyeball) may also be present. Again, the principal objective is to keep the horse in recumbency at a plane of anesthesia that is just deep enough to allow the surgical procedure to be performed. In some instances, such as the actual period of testicular traction during castration, the horse may actually appear only lightly sedated but should remain recumbent.

Several injectable anesthetic combinations have been used in horses over the last three decades. Currently, the most common protocols are based on a combination of xylazine and ketamine. The basic xylazine/ketamine technique uses intravenous xylazine to produce a very sedate horse with the typical nose-to-knees sedative posture. When this posture is achieved, ketamine is given as an IV push. In this case, the entire predetermined ketamine dose is given, rather than giving the ketamine to effect, as it is for small animal induction. The recommended doses used for this technique are xylazine (1.1 mg/kg IV) followed 3 minutes later by ketamine (2.2 mg/kg IV) to effect recumbency. Xylazine must *always* be administered before ketamine. For the average-size horse, the xylazine and ketamine dose volumes are 5 ml and 10 ml, respectively. Use of a 5-ml syringe for xylazine and a 10-ml syringe for ketamine may help reduce the possibility of a reversed order of administration.

There are several variant combinations of the basic xylazine/ketamine induction technique in which another drug is added to permit some dosage reduction of xylazine, improve the smoothness of induction quality, enhance muscle relaxation, increase analgesia, or extend the duration of recumbency. The other drugs that are added in these combinations include guaifenesin, diazepam, and butorphanol.

Guaifenesin, also known as glyceryl guaiacolate and for that reason called *GG*, has skeletal muscle relaxant properties at the intravenous doses recommended here and is a useful adjunct to xylazine/ketamine anesthesia. Guaifenesin is prepared in either a 5% or 10% strength in a 5% dextrose solution. Because 5% dextrose is essentially iso-osmolar, the addition of guaifenesin to that solution dramatically increases the osmolality. Using guaifenesin solutions more concentrated than 15% has been associated with intravascular hemolysis in the horse. The usual IV dose of guaifenesin is 50 to 100 mg/kg, which is approximately 250 ml or 500 ml of 10% and 5% solutions, respectively. Because this volume is moderately large, this dose is given by IV infusion with an IV administration set and IV fluid container. Sequentially, the horse is given the usual or reduced dose of xylazine (0.4 to 1.1 mg/kg IV), and within about 2 to 3 minutes the infusion of guaifenesin is begun. When the approximate predetermined dose of guaifenesin has been given, ataxia will be clearly evident. At that time ketamine (2.2 mg/kg) is given by IV push with the injection port of the IV administration set. Again, the sequence in which the drugs are given (xylazine, guaifenesin, then ketamine) is important (Box 10-1).

Diazepam is also frequently used in equine practice. In addition to being an effective anticonvulsant, it causes mild sedation and a moderate degree of skeletal muscle relaxation. In the horse, diazepam is combined with the basic xylazine/ketamine induction technique. Diazepam, like most benzodiazepines, has few if any cardiorespiratory effects and a relatively small dose volume. Again, xylazine (0.4 to 1.1 mg/kg IV) is given first. Ketamine (2.2 mg/kg) and diazepam (0.11 mg/kg) are then given by IV push. Ketamine and diazepam may be mixed in the same syringe. A few ketamine and diazepam dosage variations have been reported, but the doses given here (representing equal volumes of ketamine and diazepam) are commonly used.

Butorphanol can be added to the xylazine/ketamine protocol to improve analgesia and to potentially increase the surgical time by a few minutes. Butorphanol (0.01 to 0.02 mg/kg IV) is added after xylazine (1.1 mg/kg IV) has been given. Another period of 2 to 3 minutes is allowed to elapse, and then ketamine (2.2 mg/kg) is given by IV push to achieve recumbency. Again, following the correct sequence of drug

---

BOX 10-1   *How to Administer Triple Drip to Horses**

Place an indwelling IV administration set and administer *in the following sequence:*
1. Xylazine 0.4 to 1.1 mg/kg IV and wait about 2 to 3 minutes
2. Guaifenesin 50 to 100 mg/kg (250 ml or 500 ml of 10% and 5% solutions, respectively) given through IV administration set until ataxia is apparent
3. Ketamine 2.2 mg/kg IV in injection port in IV administration set

---

*Dosages may vary depending on the source.

administration is important. Diazepam may also be administered with this protocol as outlined in the previous paragraph.

Other combinations exist, each with its own advantages and limitations. One limitation mentioned earlier in this section is that the horse will likely appear to be under a light depth of anesthesia, compared with small animal patients under gas anesthesia. A second limitation is the fairly short time available to perform an operation while the horse is recumbent. Repeated IV injections of one or more drugs may be administered to keep the horse in a recumbent position and at an adequate plane of anesthesia for surgery. However, increasing length of recumbency is correlated with an increased occurrence of postanesthetic myopathy and significant injuries on recovery. Therefore most equine surgical centers prefer to use inhalant anesthetics rather than injectable anesthetics alone for operations anticipated to last more than 20 to 30 minutes.

Inhalant Anesthesia

As in small animal practice, an anesthetic machine (Fig. 10-1) is required to administer inhalant anesthetics and oxygen to equine patients. For foals and smaller ponies (body weights less than 150 kg), the typical small animal machine equipped with a 5-L reservoir bag is suitable. However, for animals larger than 150 kg, the small diameter hoses and valve orifices of the small animal machine create too much resistance to breathing. In addition, the volume of the typical carbon dioxide absorber canister is too small. Therefore a larger anesthetic machine is needed. Notice that the vaporizer(s), oxygen flowmeter, pop-off valve, and scavenger system are the same as those found on small animal machines. The major difference is the diameter of the hoses and the valve orifices, as well as the size of the reservoir bag (15 to 30 L) and carbon dioxide absorber. Functionally, large animal and small animal anesthetic machines are identical.

As in small animal practices, there are several inhalant anesthetics from which to choose. Currently, the most commonly used agents are halothane, isoflurane, and sevoflurane. Selection of the inhalant is often made on the basis of familiarity and cost. In the horse, which must regain a standing position during recovery, the quality of anesthetic recovery is also a major selection criterion. Most individuals who provide equine anesthesia care agree that recovery quality from sevoflurane is better than halothane, which is better than isoflurane. Although isoflurane is the most commonly used inhalant in small animals, it tends to be the least commonly used inhalant in the horse because other agents are associated with smoother anesthetic recoveries.

To minimize introduction of food particles from the oral cavity into the trachea, thoroughly rinse the oral cavity with water before anesthetic induction (Fig. 10-2). Rinsing the oral cavity after the horse has been induced would place the horse at extreme risk of aspiration.

Before inhalation anesthesia, IV induction is performed with drugs and techniques similar to those described above for field anesthesia. In addition, the trachea is intubated via the oral cavity. In contrast to dogs, the larynx of the horse is difficult to see, because the mouth will not open more than a few inches and the dental arcades are fairly narrow. Therefore intubation in the horse and foal is usually done by using a blind technique.

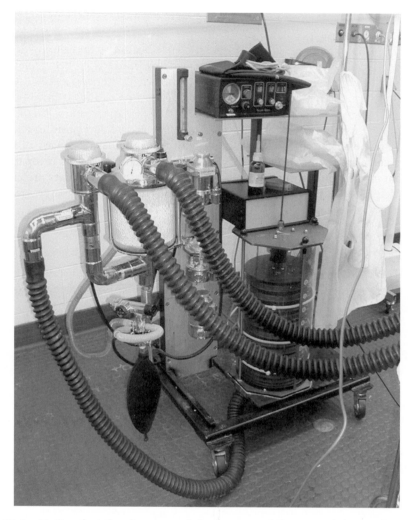

FIG. 10-1 Notice that the diameter of the hoses and the size of the unidirectional valves and carbon dioxide absorber on this large animal anesthetic machine are much bigger than on small animal machines. The bellows of the mechanical ventilator *(lower right of photo)* take the place of the reservoir bag that would normally be attached at the far left of photo. The smaller bag at lower left is a collection bag for the scavenger and is not the reservoir bag. The three vaporizers are mounted one above the other (from top to bottom, sevoflurane, isoflurane, and halothane).

After induction, a mouth speculum or a padded 4- to 5-inch length of 2-inch polyvinyl chloride (PVC) pipe is placed between the incisor teeth. A 24- to 30-mm inside diameter (ID) endotracheal tube is inserted past the molars to the oropharyngeal region (Figs. 10-3 and 10-4). At the next inspiratory attempt, the tube is advanced into the trachea. The insertion should be made with a very gentle technique. Verification of proper tube placement is made by breath sounds emanating

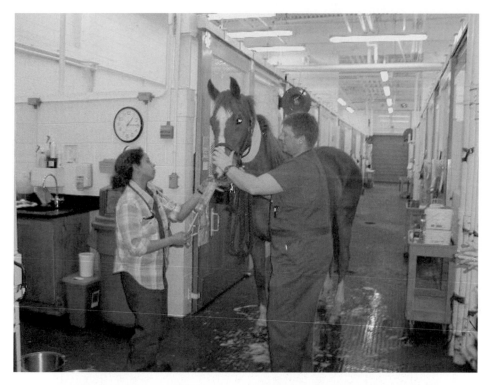

FIG. 10-2   A large-dose syringe is being used to flush the food and bedding particles from the mouth of this horse before anesthetic induction. This will minimize the risk of foreign particles being forced into the trachea during intubation.

from the tube. Accidental esophageal intubation can be confirmed by visualizing tube movement on the left side of the neck or by noticing extreme difficulty in advancing the tube.

Monitoring and Supportive Care

In most field anesthesia settings, routine monitoring of eye signs and other indicators of anesthetic depth along with evaluation of pulse quality and respiration are adequate. With longer anesthetic procedures in patients whose health may be less than optimal, more sophisticated monitoring and supportive care are necessary.

Positioning and protective padding

Positioning the horse after anesthetic induction usually requires use of an overhead monorail hoist that can lift the horse by the legs and place it on a padded surgical table (Fig. 10-5). Padding placed under the horse's body should be at least 6 inches thick. Vinyl-covered closed cell foam pads are commonly used for this purpose, but air-filled pads can also be used. The choice of padding depends on availability and the preferences of the specific equine clinic. In addition to padding underneath, horses positioned in dorsal recumbency will require some form of padding and support on each side to prevent them from rolling to the side (Fig. 10-6). It is

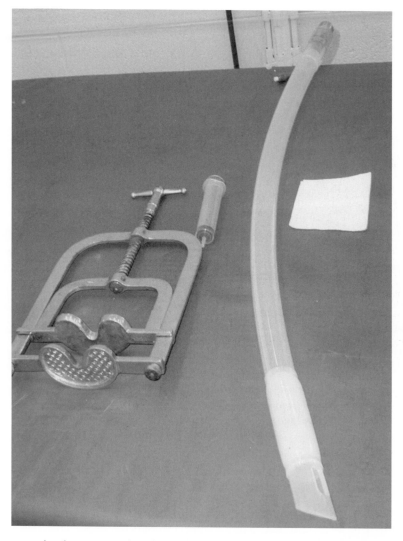

FIG. 10-3 This large animal endotracheal tube is a 26-mm inside diameter (ID). Compare the size to the 60-ml syringe and 4 × 4 gauze sponge. An equine mouth speculum as shown here can be used to keep the mouth open while the endotracheal tube is inserted.

important that this padding not compromise chest movement and breathing. For horses placed in lateral recumbency, a pad is placed on the surgery table and the horse is gently lowered onto the pad. Typically the "downside" front and hindlimbs are pulled forward, and additional support padding of sufficient thickness (often 8 to 12 inches) is placed between the down and up legs to keep the uppermost pair of legs approximately parallel to the floor surface.

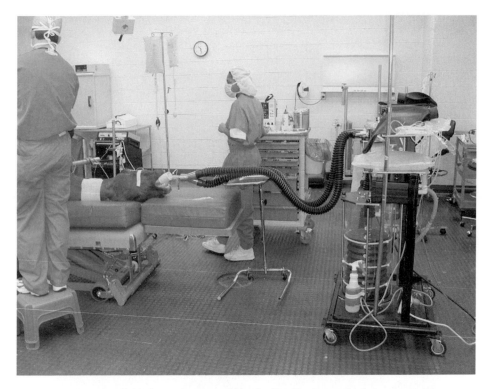

FIG. 10-4   Notice that the polyvinyl chloride (PVC) pipe, which is serving as a mouth speculum, is inserted between the upper and lower incisors, and the endotracheal tube is passed through the lumen.

Intravenous fluid therapy

IV fluid therapy with crystalloids such as lactated Ringer's solution given at a rate of 10 ml/kg/hr is an essential part of quality supportive care. This rate of fluid administration should be increased in dehydrated or hypovolemic patients to offset preexisting fluid losses. In an average size (500-kg) horse, the maintenance fluid rate totals 5 L/hr, and additional volumes may be necessary depending on the patient's condition and surgical losses. In some patients the total fluid requirement may be 30 L or more for the first hour of anesthesia. Because gravity infusion with standard IV administration set and large-bore (12- to 14-gauge) catheters will not permit infusion rates greater than 5 L/hr, fluid pumps or pressure infusors (Fig. 10-7) are often required. The typical fluid pumps used in a small animal intensive care setting will not deliver the necessary volume at the required rate. Roller pumps are commonly used to deliver these larger volumes quickly. If IV fluids are supplied in large (3-L or 5-L) bags, a pressure infusor can be effective in volume delivery. Pressure infusors surround the bag and are inflated with air to "pressurize" the IV fluid bag, thereby increasing the rate of flow. To expedite fluid administration, place a second large-bore IV catheter in the contralateral jugular vein after anesthetic induction.

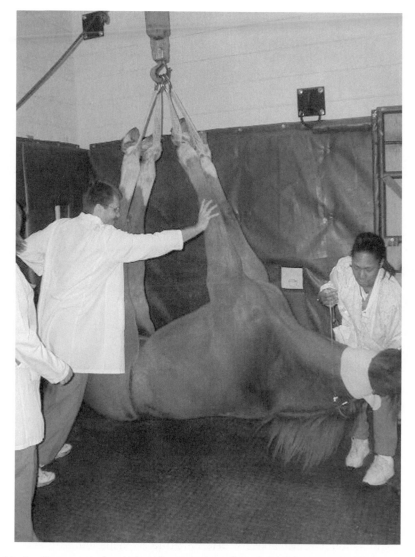

FIG. 10-5   Once anesthesia has been induced and the horse intubated, a hoist is used to lift the horse for positioning on the operating table.

With both IV catheters each attached to a bag of fluids equipped with a pressure infusor, an amount of 20 to 30 L/hr can be readily administered. If medication such as dobutamine is to be infused with the same IV line, another pressure infusor is usually required for the 1-L bag containing dobutamine. Alternately, a small IV catheter can be placed in another small peripheral vein to accommodate gravity infusion of dobutamine.

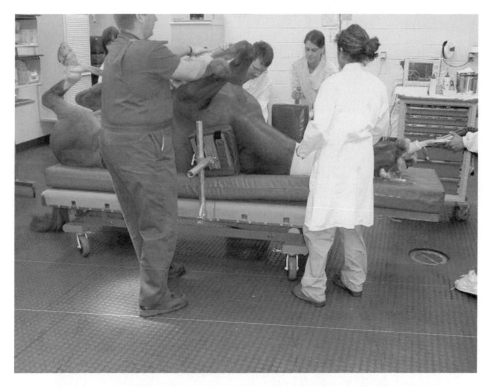

FIG. 10-6   The horse has been positioned in dorsal recumbency on the operating table, and small padded blocks located at the left and right shoulders keep the horse from rolling on its side. Notice the thickness of the padding underneath the horse.

Blood pressure monitoring

In most horses an arterial catheter can be easily placed for blood pressure monitoring. Several sites are available for arterial catheters depending on accessibility and skill. For horses in lateral recumbency, the metatarsal area is easily located and catheterized; it is located on the lateral surface of the metatarsus between the lateral splint bone and third metatarsal bone. In this location, the artery is fairly large, and about 8 cm of the artery length is superficially located in a bony groove bounded by the lateral splint bone and the third metatarsal bone. Other arterial catheter locations (less easily catheterized) include the facial artery and auricular artery. Because of the difficulty in securing the catheter, the carotid artery is rarely used. Once the arterial catheter has been placed, it must be flushed periodically with heparinized saline (5 IU/ml) to maintain patency. An IV extension set and a three-way stopcock allow the catheter to be easily and directly attached to a manometer, or it can be attached to a blood pressure transducer. The transducer converts mechanical energy (from the blood pressure wave) to an electrical signal, which can then be displayed on a monitor (Fig. 10-8).

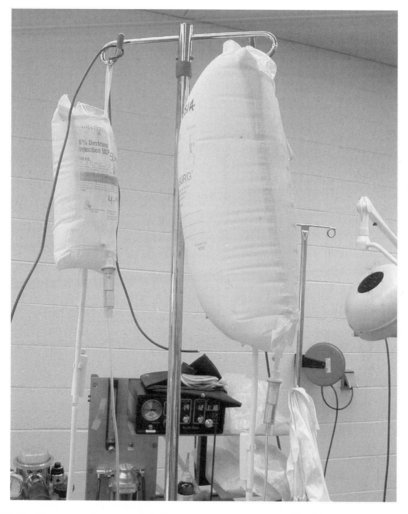

FIG. 10-7 The use of pressure infusors to pressurize IV fluid bags can dramatically increase the rate of administration of IV fluids. The larger bag contains lactated Ringer's solution, whereas the smaller one is a 500-ml bag of 5% dextrose that contains a dilute dobutamine solution.

During anesthesia every effort must be made to maintain blood pressure in the horse at a minimum value of 70 mm Hg mean arterial pressure (MAP). MAP correlates well with perfusion of vital organs, and MAP values less than 70 mm Hg are associated with an increased incidence of postanesthetic myopathy resulting from muscle ischemia. A declining blood pressure is taken as a serious sign indicating deteriorating organ perfusion and must be aggressively treated. Although decreasing the vaporizer dial setting will often improve blood pressure, it usually takes several minutes to appreciate any significant improvement. In the interim, a rapid IV "fluid loading" (10 ml/kg) given over a 10-minute period will usually quickly improve

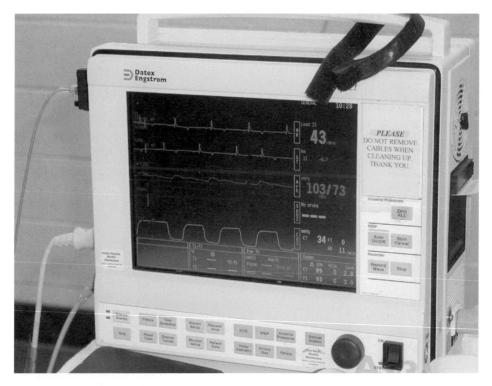

FIG. 10-8 Several monitors are available that can display a blood pressure waveform. This particular monitor also has the capability of ECG, pulse oximetry, capnography, and end-tidal anesthetic agent monitoring.

blood pressure while waiting for the patient to enter a lighter anesthetic plane. In some instances, despite fluid loading and a light plane of anesthesia, blood pressure is unacceptably low. In these situations, a continuous dobutamine infusion may be required. The usual starting dose of dobutamine infusion is 0.5 to 2.0 μg/kg/min (Box 10-2).

Pulse oximetry

Pulse oximetry (SpO_2) has limited utility in adult horses because of the relatively thick tongue, lack of suitable probes, and difficulty in finding other suitable mucous membrane or cutaneous sites. SpO_2 guidelines for the horse during anesthesia are similar to those for small animal patients. With the horse breathing room air, SpO_2 should be at least 90%, and if the horse is breathing an oxygen-enriched mixture delivered by the anesthetic machine, the SpO_2 should be at least 95%.

Capnography

Capnography is becoming more commonly used during anesthesia to evaluate alveolar ventilation. In adult horses, mainstream analyzers will not readily attach to the endotracheal tube, so the typical capnograph used is a side-stream analyzer that

---

BOX 10-2 *How to Calculate and Administer a Dobutamine Drip to a 500-kg Horse**

- Add 50 mg or 4.0 ml of dobutamine (12.5 mg/ml) to 1 L of 5% dextrose solution to yield a 50 µg/ml concentration.
- Give this solution through an adult IV administration set (10 drops per ml) setting the rate at 1 drop per second. This rate provides the adult horse with 6 ml of dobutamine each minute (60 drops per minute, 10 drops per milliliter).
- The horse would receive 300 mg of dobutamine per minute after this regimen (50 µg/ml × 6 ml = 300 µg). The dose administered is 0.6 µg/kg/min, which is near the low end of the range.
- The half-life of dobutamine is 30 to 60 seconds. *Closely* monitor the patient's MAP immediately after beginning the infusion. Slightly decrease the infusion rate as the MAP increases. If MAP remains low after 1 to 2 minutes, the infusion rate may be doubled. *Continue* to monitor MAP.
- If the heart rate increases, arrhythmias occur, or the MAP increases too much, the dobutamine infusion should be slowed or discontinued. Dobutamine, like other sympathomimetic drugs, has an extremely short half-life, and its effects will begin to diminish within 30 to 60 seconds.

*Dosages may vary depending on the source.

---

continuously removes gas from the endotracheal tube (Fig. 10-9) and performs the carbon dioxide (CO_2) analysis at the site of the monitor. Although capnography can be a valuable tool in assessing ventilation, it must be remembered that there may be a significant discrepancy between end-tidal CO_2 levels and those simultaneously determined on arterial blood ($Paco_2$).

Electrocardiography

As in small animal anesthesia, electrocardiographic (ECG) monitoring has limitations. The ECG displays only the electrical activity of the heart and gives no information on the mechanical aspects such as contractile force and blood pressure. Although horses do occasionally have cardiac arrhythmias during anesthesia, the incidence of arrhythmia in the horse is lower than in dogs. Some anesthetic monitors may provide a continuous ECG in addition to other functions, such as pulse oximetry.

Foals

Most foals that weigh less than 100 kg can be easily induced with a nasotracheal tube. Usually a 7-, 8-, or 9-mm diameter tube that is 50 to 60 cm long will be required. The tube often can be placed in the standing foal without sedation in a manner similar to passing a nasogastric tube in adult horses, except that the tube is gently inserted through the larynx and into the trachea. If sedation is necessary, xylazine (0.3 to 0.5 mg/kg IV) is usually adequate. Once the tube is in place, it is attached to the anesthetic machine and induction commenced. During the actual induction, use of a 5- to 7-L/minute oxygen flow and a Bain circuit allows greater mobility, which is useful because some foals tend to move during induction. However, most foals do not resist induction after the tube is positioned. Foals do

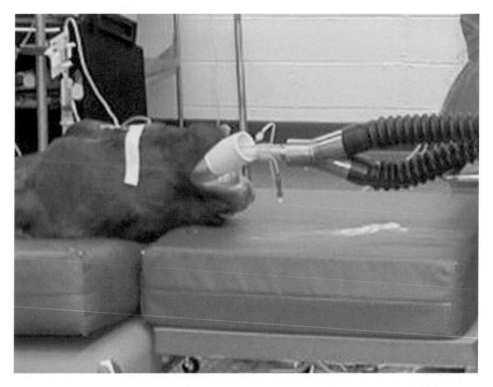

FIG. 10-9 A small-diameter tube can be seen attached to the endotracheal tube between the mouth speculum and the Y connector. This tubing conducts gas from the lumen of the endotracheal tube to the gas analyzer to determine carbon dioxide, oxygen, and inhalant anesthetic concentrations, which in turn will be displayed on the monitor.

not detect the odor of the inhalant anesthetic, because the tube effectively bypasses their olfactory apparatus. Once induction is complete, the tube is replaced with a larger diameter oral endotracheal tube and a standard small animal anesthetic machine with a circle system is used for maintenance.

Injectable anesthetic techniques similar to those used in adult horses have been successfully used in foals. Many foals can be given the standard xylazine (1.1 mg/kg IV) and ketamine (2.2 mg/kg IV) combination. Extremely young foals (younger than 2 months) may not have the same ability to biotransform and excrete drugs as do adult horses. Therefore many anesthetists avoid the use of repetitive injections to maintain anesthesia and prefer inhalant anesthetics for maintenance. From a logistical perspective, inhalant anesthesia is easier in foals because the standard small animal anesthetic machine is adequate for this purpose.

CATTLE

In most operations, cattle remain standing, and anesthesia is actually a combination of sedation, local analgesia, and physical restraint. Numerous restraint devices such as head catches, squeeze chutes, and gating areas are available to facilitate movement of adult cattle from one point to another (Fig. 10-10). Again, from a personnel safety as well as a patient safety perspective, it is important that staff who use restraint/gating devices be thoroughly familiar with their operation.

Cattle do not generally have rough recoveries from general anesthesia such as are seen in the horse. Thus trauma during the recovery period is not common, even in adult cattle. However, because of the rumen volume and the length of time required for ruminal emptying, bloat, regurgitation, and aspiration can a problem during the general anesthetic period. Proper preanesthetic preparation will minimize the risk of bloat and regurgitation but will not totally prevent their occurrence.

Regurgitation may be an active process that occurs during light anesthetic planes as a reflex ejection of a foreign substance (such as the endotracheal tube) from the pharyngeal region. In addition, passive, or silent, regurgitation may occur at surgical levels of anesthesia as a result of the relaxation of the esophageal sphincter. If regurgitation occurs, fluid that collects in the pharyngeal region may be aspirated into the trachea. An endotracheal tube with a properly inflated cuff will tend to minimize the risk of aspiration. For cattle in lateral recumbency, positioning the head and oral cavity lower than the neck region will also tend to decrease the risk of aspiration.

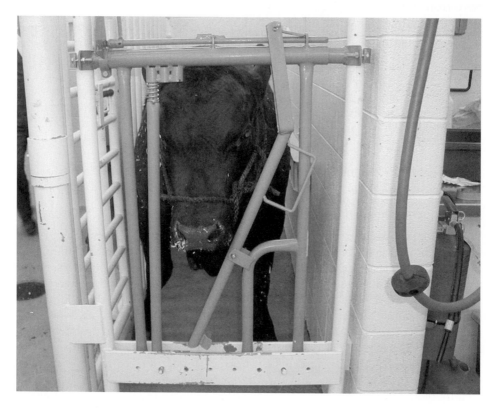

FIG. 10-10   This head catch is used to restrain cattle during insertion of the IV catheter.

Bloat results from continued fermentation within the rumen without the ability to eructate. Generally there is less risk of bloat if cattle are fasted for a period of 48 hours before anesthesia. Although this may not be a feasible time frame for all cattle, feed should be withheld as long as possible before anesthesia in most adult ruminants. Positioning cattle in sternal recumbency also tends to minimize the risk of bloat, but this body position is not suitable for most surgical procedures. Once bloat commences, it is often progressive and results in increased pressure on the diaphragm and reduced alveolar ventilation. It also impairs venous return to the heart via the caudal vena cava. Trocarization can be performed in extreme cases of bloat, but rapid completion of surgery and return to sternal recumbency are effective in less severe cases.

Ruminants also produce copious amounts of saliva (estimated to exceed 50 L per 24 hours in adult cattle). Although it is tempting to use anticholinergics to decrease salivation, studies have indicated that atropine administration simply decreases the viscosity and has minimal if any effect on the total volume produced. Although an atropine dose of 0.06 to 0.10 mg/kg IV has been recommended, the use of anticholinergics in ruminants is controversial. A well-positioned endotracheal tube with a properly inflated cuff is the best preventive measure to avoid aspiration of saliva.

Sedation and Chemical Restraint

Several drugs are available for sedating adult cattle. Xylazine is currently the most commonly used sedative agent. Cattle and most other ruminants are far more sensitive to xylazine than are horses, and the doses used are approximately 10% of the typical horse dosage. The IV dose of xylazine given to cows is approximately 0.10 to 0.15 mg/kg and is lower still (0.075 to 0.10 mg/kg) in bulls. In contrast to xylazine use in the horse, cattle may become recumbent even after only moderate amount of xylazine within these dose ranges. Xylazine sedation can be effectively reversed with tolazoline (0.5 to 1.0 mg/kg IV) or yohimbine (0.1 to 0.2 mg/kg IV).

Acepromazine (0.03 to 0.05 mg/kg IV) will produce slight to moderate sedation in most cattle. Its duration is approximately 90 minutes, or about twice as long as xylazine, but the sedation is not as dramatic as with xylazine.

General Anesthesia

IV anesthetic induction can be performed in much the same manner as in the horse, with drug dosages (except alpha-2 agonists) similar to those used in horses. Because emergence delirium and rough recoveries are seldom a problem in cattle, they are not typically sedated before general anesthesia. Common induction agents include ketamine, telazol, and thiopental either with or without the addition of guaifenesin. When ketamine (2.2 mg/kg IV) is to be used for induction, a low dose of xylazine (0.1 mg/kg IV) given a minute or two earlier is helpful to smooth the induction process. In lieu of xylazine, diazepam (0.11 mg/kg) can be mixed with an equal volume of ketamine immediately before IV injection, or xylazine may be given immediately before the ketamine/diazepam mixture.

With typical field anesthesia drugs, the anesthetic depth of cattle, like that of the horse, is often very light. However, the duration of anesthesia can be extended with a guaifenesin-ketamine-xylazine mixture commonly known as *triple drip*. The formulation of triple drip is different for cattle than for the horse. The final concentration of the component parts of triple drip used for cattle should be guaifenesin (50 mg/ml), ketamine (1 to 2 mg/ml), and xylazine (0.1 mg/ml) (Box 10-3). Triple drip can be used for IV anesthetic induction when infused at 0.5 to 1.0 ml/kg, but at a reduced hourly infusion rate of 2 ml/kg/hr it can be used to effectively extend anesthetic duration.

For longer-term anesthetic maintenance, inhalant anesthetics offer many advantages over injectable combinations and should be seriously considered if anesthetic equipment is available. The same anesthetic machine sizing considerations that apply to the horse apply to adult cattle.

The selection of endotracheal tube sizes is also similar for both cattle and horses. For larger cows and bulls a 30- to 35-mm ID tube will likely be required. For smaller cows, tubes as small as 20-mm ID may be used. Tracheal intubation in adult cattle can be done using a blind technique, as it is in the horse, or by digital palpation of the larynx with one hand while the tube is inserted with the other hand. Regardless of the method of intubation, the tube size should be as large as can gently be inserted into the trachea. After the tube is inserted, the cuff is properly inflated with air. At the conclusion of anesthesia, the animal is positioned in sternal recumbency, the cuff is deflated, and the tube is removed when the swallowing reflex returns (Fig. 10-11).

Monitoring and Supportive Care

Anesthetic depth is assessed in a manner similar to that used in other species. In cattle, the position, patency, and proper cuff inflation of the endotracheal tube are of particular importance because of the possibility of aspiration of regurgitated rumen contents or saliva. Additionally for adult cattle, proper padding and careful positioning will minimize the risk of postanesthetic myopathy. When cattle are placed in lateral recumbency, both the downside front and hindlimb should be pulled forward (craniad) and padding placed between the down and up limbs (Fig. 10-12). In dorsal recumbency, cattle should be squarely positioned on a padded surface so that the body weight is equally distributed over both left and right gluteal regions.

IV fluids given during anesthesia will help maintain intravascular volume and offset the hypotensive effects of the anesthetics. IV fluid rates with crystalloids such as lactated Ringer's solution are 5 to 10 ml/kg/hr for routine maintenance, increas-

---

BOX 10-3 How to Administer Triple Drip to Cattle*

To induce anesthesia, mix the following dosages and administer intravenously at a rate of 0.5 to 1.0 ml/kg:
Guaifenesin, 50 mg/ml
Ketamine, 1.0 to 2.0 mg/ml
Xylazine, 0.1 mg/ml

To extend anesthetic duration, continue administration of triple drip as a constant infusion at the reduced rate of 2.0 ml/kg/hr.

*Dosages may vary depending on the source.

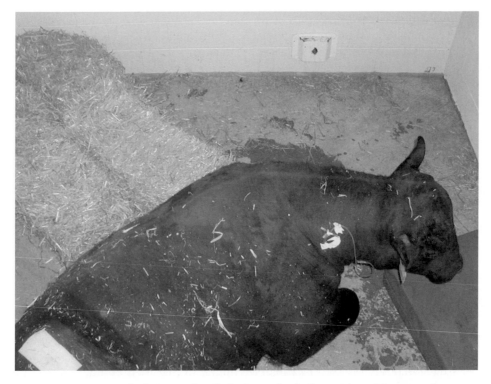

FIG. 10-11 A straw bale is used to help keep the bull positioned in sternal recumbency through the recovery period. Notice that the jugular catheter and IV extension set have been left in place until recovery is complete.

ing to 25 ml/kg/hr for hypotensive patients. Even at moderate infusion rates with larger-bore IV catheters, it can be difficult to administer 5 to 10 L/hr in larger cattle by gravity drip. Pressure infusors or fluid pumps may be required in some situations. Blood pressure can easily be monitored directly from the auricular artery in cattle (Fig. 10-13) using a manometer or transducer, as is done in the horse.

Calves

Young calves can be easily anesthetized with a variety of techniques that are suitable for the dog. Again, the sensitivity of cattle to xylazine and other alpha-2 agonists should be considered and doses reduced appropriately. An IM technique with a combination of xylazine (0.1 mg/kg) and ketamine (5 mg/kg) has proven useful to induce a light plane of anesthesia or as a method to permit oral tracheal intubation. Induction with inhalants can be done either with a mask or with the nasotracheal technique, similar to that in foals. Tracheal intubation can be performed by direct visualization with tube sizes similar in diameter to those used for similar-size dogs. For calves weighing about 150 kg, a typical small animal anesthetic machine with a 5-L reservoir bag works well.

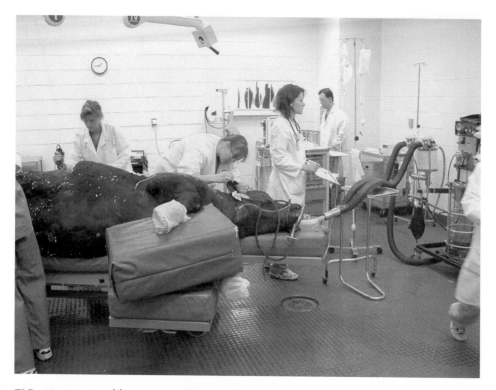

FIG. 10-12 In addition to padding under the bull, pads are used to support the upper limbs during lateral recumbency.

SMALL RUMINANTS

Sheep and goats present similar but not identical challenges to those of adult cattle. Many surgical procedures are performed with the patients under general anesthesia, and many of the same injectable drugs and drug combinations that are used in cattle can be effectively used in sheep and goats. Sheep and goats both exhibit a high sensitivity to xylazine and other alpha-2 agonist drugs, similar to cattle. Given the relatively smaller body size of sheep and goats, the possibility of inadvertent overdose is significant. For this reason, a dilute xylazine solution (20 mg/ml) is recommended for use in small ruminants. Care should also be taken when calculating doses of local anesthetics for smaller ruminants, to avoid systemic toxicity.

Common IV induction techniques include a combination of xylazine (0.05 to 0.10 mg/kg) and ketamine (2.2 mg/kg), or a combination of ketamine (3 mg/kg) and diazepam (0.2 mg/kg) mixed together and given as an IV push. Owing to their relatively small size, both sheep and goats are potential candidates for inhalant anesthetic mask induction as well. Regardless of the general anesthetic used, the issues of bloat and regurgitation need to be addressed by appropriate fasting, body positioning, and tracheal intubation.

The technique for intubation of small ruminants is similar to that performed in the dog. However, visibility tends to be less than in the dog because of their limited ability to completely open the mouth and their saliva production. Once sheep and

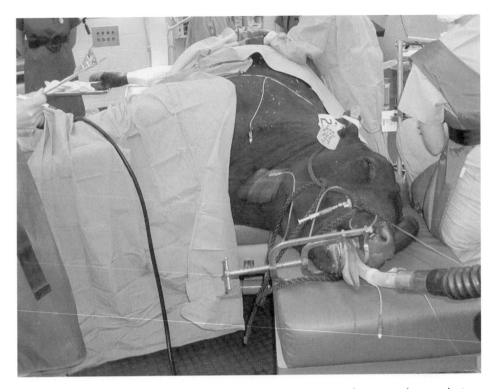

FIG. 10-13   In cattle, the auricular artery is a common site for arterial cannulation and blood pressure determination. A syringe case has been inserted in the ear and taped in place to help immobilize the ear while the arterial catheter is in place. The small tubing leading to the gas analyzer can be clearly seen near the end of the endotracheal tube.

goats are intubated, inhalant anesthetics can be given with a typical small animal anesthetic machine. Depending on the size of the patient, either a 3-L or 5-L reservoir bag can be used.

Swine

Swine can be challenging patients for sedation, chemical restraint, or general anesthesia. Swine have no easily accessible superficial veins, which makes the IV route impossible for all but the most experienced swine practitioners. In addition, the subcutaneous fat layer is so thick that effective IM injections are difficult unless hypodermic needles 1.5 inches or longer are used and properly positioned for injection. Finally, larger swine are extremely difficult to physically restrain (Fig. 10-14).

An 18-gauge 1.5-inch needle is preferred for IM injection, and the most accessible and superficial IM site is located just caudal to the ear and about 2 inches off midline. The most commonly used IM chemical restraint or induction protocols are combinations of a tranquilizer and an opioid (neuroleptanalgesia), often combined with a dissociative anesthetic (ketamine or telazol).

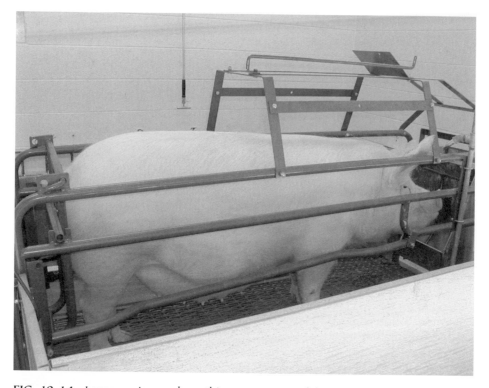

FIG. 10-14   Larger swine such as this sow presented for cesarean section can be difficult to restrain manually. In this case a portable farrowing crate also serves to restrain this sow as preparations are made for anesthetic induction.

Various combinations of tranquilizers and opioids (neuroleptanalgesic combinations) have been used over the last few decades. Of these, the least expensive combination is acepromazine (0.25 to 0.50 mg/kg) and morphine (0.5 to 1.0 mg/kg) given together by IM injection. Many swine can still be aroused from this combination even though they appear sedate. More recently, medetomidine (Domitor), given at a dose of 80 μg/kg IM, and butorphanol (Torbugesic), given at a dose of 0.2 to 0.4 mg/kg, have been shown to provide better chemical restraint. The addition of ketamine or Telazol further improves the quality of chemical restraint.

A combination of telazol-ketamine-xylazine (TKX) can be given by IM injection and provides excellent quality chemical restraint or induction. TKX is formulated by adding 2.5 ml of ketamine (250 mg) and 2.5 ml xylazine (250 mg) as the diluents (in lieu of sterile water or sterile saline) to a bottle of telazol powder. The resultant TKX mixture contains telazol (100 mg/ml), ketamine (50 mg/ml), and xylazine (50 mg/ml). The IM dose for smaller pigs is 1 ml of TKX per 25 kg body weight. The dose of each component is Telazol (4 mg/kg), ketamine (2 mg/kg), and xylazine (2 mg/kg) (Box 10-4). Note that the dose of xylazine used in swine is relatively large compared with the horse (and especially compared with ruminants). In large swine (weighing more than 100 kg), 3 ml TKX may be administered IM and the remaining 2 ml TKX by IV injection in an ear vein after chemical restraint

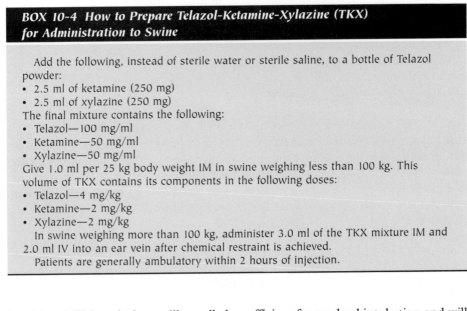

BOX 10-4 How to Prepare Telazol-Ketamine-Xylazine (TKX) for Administration to Swine

Add the following, instead of sterile water or sterile saline, to a bottle of Telazol powder:
- 2.5 ml of ketamine (250 mg)
- 2.5 ml of xylazine (250 mg)

The final mixture contains the following:
- Telazol—100 mg/ml
- Ketamine—50 mg/ml
- Xylazine—50 mg/ml

Give 1.0 ml per 25 kg body weight IM in swine weighing less than 100 kg. This volume of TKX contains its components in the following doses:
- Telazol—4 mg/kg
- Ketamine—2 mg/kg
- Xylazine—2 mg/kg

In swine weighing more than 100 kg, administer 3.0 ml of the TKX mixture IM and 2.0 ml IV into an ear vein after chemical restraint is achieved.

Patients are generally ambulatory within 2 hours of injection.

is achieved. This technique will usually be sufficient for tracheal intubation and will conserve the amount of TKX required. Reversal of xylazine with yohimbine will shorten the duration of anesthesia but worsen the quality of the recovery period. Even without reversal, pigs generally will be ambulatory within 2 hours of injection.

Intubation of swine is notoriously difficult. The presence of a ventral laryngeal diverticulum, limited visibility, inability to open the mouth wide, and relatively narrow dental arcade all contribute to the difficulty. One method of intubation involves using a stylet within the lumen of the endotracheal tube to both stiffen the tube and to permit the end of the tube to be curved to slide through the ventral laryngeal diverticulum. It is helpful to have a 20- to 30-degree ventrad bend to the distal 5 cm of the stylet and another 90-degree ventrad bend at the connector end of the endotracheal tube. The 90-degree bend not only serves as a handle for the stylet but also prevents the stylet from projecting beyond the distal end of the tube. After insertion of the distal end of the tube through the laryngeal opening, the stylet (and tube) are rotated 180 degrees so that the handle is oriented in a dorsad direction. This position facilitates easily sliding the tube with the stylet in place past the ventral laryngeal diverticulum. Regardless of the type of stylet, only the gentlest pressure should be used during tube insertion. The technique of intubation is more one of "rotational fiddling" by twisting the tube and stylet than brute force. Aggressive efforts during intubation will frequently result in laryngeal hemorrhage and edema, leading to possible airway obstruction and death during recovery.

Inhalant anesthetics can be easily administered to swine using a small animal anesthetic machine with a circle system and a reservoir bag of appropriate size for the patient. All currently available inhalants have been successfully used in swine, and recovery from anesthesia is usually rapid and uncomplicated.

Porcine stress syndrome (PSS) or malignant hyperthermia (MH) is associated with anesthesia and has been reported in almost every swine breed, but is most commonly seen in the Pietrain breed. A frequently fatal condition, PSS/MH can be triggered by most inhalant anesthetics, including halothane, isoflurane, and enflurane. Once initiated, this metabolic condition results in an inappropriate heat production by skeletal muscle, hypercapnia, hyperthermia, hyperkalemia, and death. PSS/MH is heritable and is also triggered by stress. Questions should be specifically directed toward any history of unexplained deaths in related swine (for example, death with rapid onset of rigor mortis following shipping, handling, or breeding).

REGIONAL/LOCAL ANESTHETIC TECHNIQUES IN LARGE ANIMALS

Regional anesthesia with local anesthetic drugs is far more commonly done in cattle than in most other large animal species. Although the actual description of specific regional anesthetic techniques is beyond the scope of this chapter, several comments on general principles of regional anesthesia at this point will give the reader an appreciation of how these techniques can be incorporated in anesthetic care and pain management.

Historically, cocaine was the first local anesthetic used. An alkaloid from a species of South American tree leaves, cocaine was first isolated in 1860. Throughout the latter half of the nineteenth century, cocaine was used as a local anesthetic in the eye, for spinal anesthesia in the dog, and for nerve blocks in the horse. The potential for addiction or dependence and the relative toxicity of cocaine promoted searches for a more ideal local anesthetic. An ideal local anesthetic should produce a readily reversible block, have no addiction/dependence potential, have minimal toxic effects, be slowly absorbed systemically from the site of injection, and be rapidly biotransformed and excreted. Lidocaine is currently the most commonly used local anesthetic agent in large animals. For detailed information on the mechanism of action of lidocaine and other local anesthetics, see Chapter 7.

Lidocaine is reported to be toxic at doses as low as 5 mg/kg. Toxicity is most commonly manifested as CNS stimulation, including signs of restlessness and muscle twitching, progressing to seizures. Unconsciousness commonly follows seizures. In addition, on the basis of the mechanism of action of local anesthetics, it is not surprising that both the automaticity and the conduction velocity of cardiac tissue are reduced. This may be manifested as decreased heart rate with a concurrent fall in arterial blood pressure. Hypotension also may be caused by vasodilation, resulting from alteration of the function of the vasomotor center or by direct action on vascular smooth muscle. The incidence of toxic reactions may be reduced by limiting the total dose used and by adding vasoconstrictors (epinephrine, phenylephrine) to the local anesthetic, which will delay absorption from injection site. Skillful deposition of the drug adjacent to the nerve bundle, rather than blind injection into surrounding tissue, will also help limit the total dose.

Use of local anesthetics in large animals may be topical (usually limited to ophthalmic preparations) or injectable. Injections can be made as an infiltration block in which a larger volume of a more dilute solution is injected around the area to be incised or excised. For the paralumbar fossa area of cattle to be blocked with a local infiltration technique, an "inverted L" block can be used. More effective blocks can be achieved by nerve blocks in which the local anesthetic is injected in the immediate area of a nerve that conducts sensory input from a body region more distal to the site of injection. Again, with the paralumbar fossa region as an example, a regional nerve block of several nerves as they exit the spinal cord and cross over the transverse processes of the lumbar vertebrae, can be performed. For a distal extremity operation, such as a claw amputation in cattle, a technique of IV regional anesthesia may be used. When IV regional blocks are done, a tourniquet is applied proximal to the site of venous access and is left in place for the duration of surgery. Optimally the tourniquet is released gradually to avoid sudden high plasma levels of local anesthetic entering the systemic circulation, which may be toxic. Finally, for tail and perineal region analgesia, local anesthetics can be injected in the caudal epidural space (sacrococcygeal or first intercoccygeal space).

Regardless of the local anesthetic technique or drug used, it is extremely important to be aware of the potential for toxicity. Although this is rarely encountered in animals as large as cattle or adult horses, it is possible to reach toxic local anesthetic levels in sheep and goats (especially lambs and kids) because of their small body size. Even in horses and cattle, carelessly performed caudal epidural administration of a seemingly small volume of local anesthetic can produce motor paralysis of the hindlimbs if the drug proceeds craniad to the lumbosacral plexus.

SUMMARY

Anesthesia, whether general or local, can be safely performed in the large animal patient. Safety of personnel must also be ensured. It is important to have a clear understanding of methods of physical restraint and effects of the drugs given, as well as parameters and appropriate monitoring methods to ensure early detection, recognition, and treatment of problems.

KEY POINTS

1. The most effective choice for standing chemical restraint in the horse is a neuroleptanalgesic (NLA), which is a combination of a neuroleptic drug (tranquilizer) and an analgesic (opioid).
2. Xylazine has sedative effects and produces analgesia by activation of alpha-2 receptors in the central nervous system.
3. When a horse is sedated and induced with xylazine and ketamine, xylazine must *always* be administered *before* ketamine.
4. When a basic xylazine/ketamine anesthetic combination is used, it is advisable to use a 5-ml and a 10-ml syringe, respectively, to avoid a potentially fatal consequence of administering ketamine before xylazine.
5. It is imperative that the horse remains recumbent for as short a period as possible to reduce the possibility of postanesthetic myopathies and other injuries.
6. The anesthetic machine used with equine patients has hoses and valve orifices of a larger diameter than those used with small animals. In addition, the reservoir bag is larger (15-30 L), as is the carbon dioxide (CO_2) absorber.
7. The metatarsal artery is the easiest artery for inexperienced personnel to catheterize in a horse.
8. During anesthesia, blood pressure in the horse must be maintained at a minimum of 70 mm Hg mean arterial pressure.
9. In the horse breathing room air, oxygen saturation (SpO_2) should be greater than or equal to 90%. When the horse is breathing oxygen-enriched anesthetic gas, SpO_2 should be equal to or greater than 95%.
10. Nasotracheal tubes can be placed in the standing foal. The tube should be 7, 8, or 9 mm in diameter and approximately 50 to 60 cm long.
11. At the end of anesthesia in large animals, the endotracheal cuff can be deflated and the tube removed when the animal has resumed the swallowing reflex and is in sternal recumbency.
12. Swine veins are extremely difficult to access; therefore, sedation is typically performed via the intramuscular (IM) injection. In addition, swine fat is sufficiently thick such that injections require the use of at least a 1.5-inch hypodermic needle.
13. Two means of decreasing toxic reactions to local anesthetic injections are (1) addition of a vasoconstrictive agent (epinephrine, phenylephedrine) to the local anesthetic and (2) deposition of the drug adjacent to a nerve bundle and not into the surrounding tissue.

REVIEW QUESTIONS

1. The most common site of injection for sedation and standing chemical restraint in the horse is the:
   a. Left jugular vein
   b. Facial vein
   c. Right jugular vein
   d. Lateral saphenous vein
2. Which of the following is an advantage of detomidine (Dormosedan) when compared with xylazine and acepromazine?
   a. Shorter duration of action than xylazine
   b. Slower onset time than acepromazine
   c. Produces sedation and analgesia
   d. Considerably faster onset time than acepromazine

3. A slow oscillatory movement of the eyeball is termed _____:
   a. Nystagmus
   b. Strabismus
   c. Mydriasis
   d. Miosis
4. When xylazine and ketamine are used in combination for equine sedation and induction, it is important to:
   a. Give xylazine before ketamine
   b. Give ketamine only to effect
   c. Understand that a nose-to-knees position may be assumed from the effect of xylazine
   d. All of the above
5. When guaifenesin is added to the basic xylazine/ketamine anesthesia combination for equine anesthesia the agent must be administered in the following order:
   a. Guaifenesin, xylazine, ketamine
   b. Xylazine, guaifenesin, ketamine
   c. Ketamine, xylazine, guaifenesin
   d. Xylazine, ketamine, guaifenesin
6. Adding guaifenesin, diazepam, and butorphanol to a xylazine/ketamine protocol leads to which effects, respectively?
   a. Skeletal muscle relaxation, sedation and skeletal muscle relaxation, analgesia
   b. Analgesia, skeletal muscle relaxation, sedation and skeletal muscle relaxation
   c. Analgesia, skeletal muscle relaxation and sedation, skeletal muscle relaxation
   d. Skeletal muscle relaxation, analgesia, sedation and skeletal muscle relaxation

7. Foals and smaller ponies weighing up to 150 kg require a _____ L reservoir bag, whereas animals weighing more than 150 kg require a

   _____ L reservoir bag.
   a. 10, 5
   b. 5, 10 to 20
   c. 5, 15 to 20
   d. 15 to 20, 5

8. Which of the following inhalant anesthetics provides the best recovery quality for horses?
   a. Sevoflurane
   b. Isoflurane
   c. Halothane
   d. Nitrous oxide
9. What is the maintenance fluid rate of lactated Ringer's solution in a 500-kg horse?
   a. 10 L/hr
   b. 20 L/hr
   c. 8 L/hr
   d. 5 L/hr
10. Where is the metatarsal artery located in the horse?
    a. Medial surface of the metatarsus
    b. Lateral surface of metatarsus
    c. Between medial splint bone and fourth metatarsal
    d. Between lateral splint bone and third metatarsal
11. What drug is commonly administered when the mean arterial pressure (MAP) becomes dangerously low in a horse under anesthesia, after fluid loading is ineffective?
    a. Propranolol
    b. Digoxin
    c. Dobutamine
    d. Glucose
12. An ECG recording provides detailed information concerning contractile force of the heart and blood pressure.
    True   False
13. What size nasotracheal tube is typically placed in a standing foal for anesthetic induction?
    a. 20 to 30 cm long, 3 to 4 mm diameter
    b. 50 to 60 cm long, 7, 8, or 9 mm diameter
    c. 50 to 60 cm long, 2 to 3 mm diameter
    d. 10 to 20 cm long, 7, 8, or 9 mm diameter
14. Which of the following can minimize the risk for aspiration in cattle during anesthesia?
    a. Keep endotracheal tube minimally inflated
    b. Position the head and oral cavity above the body
    c. Position the head and oral cavity below the body
    d. a and c
15. A well-positioned endotracheal tube with proper cuff inflation is the best preventive measure to avoid aspiration of saliva during anesthesia in the large animal.
    True   False

16. Name two reversal agents for xylazine.
   a. Yohimbine and tolazoline
   b. Yohimbine and acepromazine
   c. Tolazoline and naloxone
   d. Yohimbine and naloxone
17. Which artery is commonly catheterized in cattle to directly measure blood pressure?
   a. Facial
   b. Cephalic
   c. Auricular
   d. Medial saphenous

ANSWERS FOR CHAPTER 10

1. c	**2.** d	**3.** a	**4.** d	**5.** b
6. a	**7.** c	**8.** a	**9.** d	**10.** d
11. c	**12.** False	**13.** b	**14.** c	**15.** True
16. a	**17.** c			

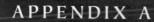
Standard Values and Equivalents

STANDARD VALUES
Metric Weights

$$1 \text{ gram } (1 \text{ g}) = \text{Weight of ml water at } 4° \text{ C}$$
$$1000 \text{ g} = 1 \text{ kilogram (kg)}$$
$$0.1 \text{ g} = 1 \text{ decigram (dg)}$$
$$0.01 \text{ g} = 1 \text{ centigram (cg)}$$
$$0.001 \text{ g} = 1 \text{ milligram (mg)}$$
$$0.001 \text{ mg} = 1 \text{ microgram (μg)}$$

Metric Volumes

$$1 \text{ liter (L)} = 1000 \text{ milliliters (ml) or } 1000 \text{ cubic centimeters (cc)}$$
$$0.001 \text{ L} = 1 \text{ ml}$$
$$1 \text{ deciliter (dl)} = 100 \text{ ml}$$

Solution Equivalents

$$1 \text{ part in } 10 = 10.00\% \ (1 \text{ ml contains } 100 \text{ mg})$$
$$1 \text{ part in } 50 = 2.00\% \ (1 \text{ ml contains } 20 \text{ mg})$$
$$1 \text{ part in } 100 = 1.00\% \ (1 \text{ ml contains } 10 \text{ mg})$$
$$1 \text{ part in } 200 = 0.50\% \ (1 \text{ ml contains } 5 \text{ mg})$$
$$1 \text{ part in } 500 = 0.20\% \ (1 \text{ ml contains } 2 \text{ mg})$$
$$1 \text{ part in } 1000 = 0.10\% \ (1 \text{ ml contains } 1 \text{ mg}) = 1000 \text{ μg per ml}$$
$$1 \text{ part in } 1500 = 0.066\% \ (1 \text{ ml contains } 0.66 \text{ mg})$$
$$1 \text{ part in } 2600 = 0.038\% \ (1 \text{ ml contains } 0.38 \text{ mg})$$
$$1 \text{ part in } 5000 = 0.02\% \ (1 \text{ ml contains } 0.20 \text{ mg})$$
$$1 \text{ part in } 50,000 = 0.002\% \ (1 \text{ ml contains } 0.02 \text{ mg})$$
$$1 \text{ part in } 200,000 = 0.0005\% \ (1 \text{ ml contains } 5 \text{ μg})$$

The number of milligrams in 1 ml of any solution of known percentage strength is obtained by moving the decimal one place to the right. For example, a 1% solution contains 10 mg/ml. By definition, a percent solution contains the specified weight (in grams) of the solute in 100 ml of total solution. For example, a 5% dextrose and water solution contains 5 g of dextrose dissolved in each 100 ml of water.

Approximate Equivalents

Weights

$$1 \text{ kg} = 2.2 \text{ avoirdupois or imperial pounds}$$
$$1 \text{ kg} = 2.6 \text{ apothecary or troy pounds}$$
$$1 \text{ oz} = 30 \text{ g (approx)}$$
$$\text{(Avoirdupois or imperial} = 28.350 \text{ g)}$$
$$\text{(Apothecary or troy} = 31.1045 \text{ g)}$$
$$1 \text{ lb} = 453.6 \text{ g} = 0.4526 \text{ kg} = 16 \text{ oz}$$

Volumes

$$1 \text{ liter} = 10.6 \text{ U.S. quarts} = 33.8 \text{ fluid ounces}$$
$$1 \text{ U.S. pint} = 473.2 \text{ ml}$$
$$1 \text{ quart} = 946.4 \text{ ml}$$

Length

$$1 \text{ meter (m)} = 39.37 \text{ inches (in)}$$
$$1 \text{ in} = \tfrac{1}{12} \text{ ft} = 2.54 \text{ centimeters (cm)}$$

Pressure

$$1 \text{ lb per sq in (psi)} = 0.070 \text{ kg/sq cm}$$
$$= 51.7 \text{ mm of mercury (Hg)}$$
$$= 70.3 \text{ cm of water (H}_2\text{O)}$$
$$1 \text{ mm Hg} = 1.36 \text{ cm H}_2\text{O}$$
$$1 \text{ cm H}_2\text{O} = 0.73 \text{ mm Hg}$$
$$1 \text{ atmosphere} = 760 \text{ mm Hg}$$
$$= 14.7 \text{ lb/in}^2$$
$$= 29.9 \text{ in Hg}$$
$$= 1.03 \text{ kg/cm}^2$$
$$= 33.9 \text{ ft H}_2\text{O}$$
$$= 760 \text{ torr}$$
$$= 1013.25 \text{ millibars}$$
$$= 100 \text{ kilopascals (kPa)}$$

EQUIVALENTS OF CENTIGRADE AND FAHRENHEIT THERMOMETRIC SCALES

Fahrenheit to Centigrade: $°C = (°F - 32) \times \frac{5}{9}$
Centigrade to Fahrenheit: $°F = (°C \times \frac{9}{5}) + 32$

CENTIGRADE DEGREE	FAHRENHEIT DEGREE	CENTIGRADE DEGREE	FAHRENHEIT DEGREE	CENTIGRADE DEGREE	FAHRENHEIT DEGREE
-17	+1.4	5	41.0	27	80.6
-16	3.2	6	42.8	28	82.4
-15	5.0	7	44.6	29	84.2
-14	6.8	8	46.4	30	86.0
-13	8.6	9	48.2	31	87.8
-12	10.4	10	50.0	32	89.6
-11	12.2	11	51.8	33	91.4
-10	14.0	12	53.6	34	93.2
-9	15.8	13	55.4	35	95.0
-8	17.6	14	57.2	36	96.8
-7	19.4	15	59.0	37	98.6
-6	21.2	16	60.8	38	100.4
-5	23.0	17	62.6	39	102.2
-4	24.8	18	64.4	40	104.0
-3	26.6	19	66.2	41	105.8
-2	28.4	20	68.0	42	107.6
-1	30.2	21	69.8	43	109.4
0	32.0	22	71.6	44	111.2
+1	33.8	23	73.4	45	113.0
2	35.6	24	75.2		
3	37.4	25	77.0		
4	39.2	26	78.8	100	212.0

Catheter Comparison Scale (For Comparison of Endotracheal Tube Sizes)

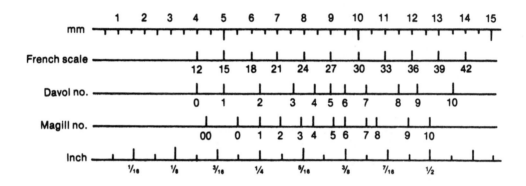

Modified from Lumb WV, Jones EW: Veterinary anesthesia, Philadelphia, 1973, Lea & Febiger.

Equipment for Intravenous (IV) Induction and Inhalation Anesthesia

- Syringes and needles for administering preanesthetic and induction agents
- Alcohol and absorbent cotton
- Plain (nonstretch) gauze for tying endotracheal tube
- Syringe for inflating endotracheal tube cuff
- Laryngoscope
- Mouth gag
- Endotracheal tubes
- Stylet for small endotracheal tubes
- Electric clippers
- Intravenous catheter, administration set, and IV fluid bag
- Lubricating gel for endotracheal tubes (gel containing a local analgesic may be preferred for use in cats)
- Lidocaine spray (for use in cats)
- Ophthalmic ointment or drops (preferably without antibiotic)
- Face mask
- Inhalation anesthesia machine with oxygen and nitrous oxide tanks
- Machine connections, including hoses, Y piece, nonrebreathing circuit
- Reservoir bag
- Cylinder wrench
- Ventilator (if controlled ventilation is required)
- Emergency drugs (contained in crash kit)
- Towels, blankets, or other means of conserving patient's body heat
- Stethoscope, thermometer, penlight, and other monitoring devices
- Scavenging system
- Form for anesthesia record (if required)

Equipment and Drugs for Use in an Emergency Crash Kit

The following list of equipment and supplies may be altered depending on the veterinarian's preference. Some supplies (for example, laryngoscope, Ambu bag, sterile fluids) that are easily accessible within the clinical setting may be omitted from the kit.

EQUIPMENT AND SUPPLIES

- Endotracheal tubes (various sizes)
- Penlight
- Adhesive tape (1-inch)
- Gauze roll (1- or 2-inch)
- Sterile gauze pads
- IV fluid administration set
- Burette for fluid administration
- Intravenous catheters (18-, 20-, and 22-gauge)
- Syringes (1-, 3-, 5-, 20-ml sizes)
- Needles (18-, 20-, and 22-gauge)
- Alcohol swabs
- Sterile surgery instruments, including scalpel handle and blades, hemostats, thumb forceps, scissors, and needle holder
- Sterile suture material (absorbable and nonabsorbable)
- Sterile saline for injection
- Sterile fluids (lactated Ringer's, saline, 5% dextrose)
- Vacutainer needles and tubes (lavender and red top)
- Stethoscope
- Sterile gloves
- Thermometer
- Sterile lubricant and lidocaine gel
- Ambu bag
- Laryngoscope
- Gauze and syringe for inflating endotracheal tube cuff
- Bulb for aspirating fluids
- Tracheostomy tubes
- Oxygen mask

DRUGS

- Epinephrine (1:1000)—may be refrigerated
- Dopamine
- Sodium bicarbonate
- Atropine
- 10% calcium chloride or calcium gluconate
- 2% lidocaine without epinephrine
- Doxapram
- Dexamethasone
- Prednisolone sodium succinate
- Diazepam
- Naloxone
- Yohimbine
- Butorphanol
- Heparin
- Furosemide
- Mannitol 20%
  NOTE: A list of emergency drug dosages should be posted or included in the kit.

Page numbers followed by *f* indicate figures; *t*, tables; *b*, boxes.